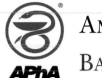

AMERICAN PHARMACEUTICAL ASSOCIATION

BASIC PHARMACY AND PHARMACOLOGY SERIES

BASIC PHARMACOLOGY

PERSPECTIVE PRESS · MORTON PUBLISHING COMPANY

www.morton-pub.com

Morton Publishing

First Edition
Copyright © 2000 by Morton Publishing Company

Printed in the United States of America.

Morton Publishing Company
925 West Kenyon Avenue, Unit 12
Englewood, CO 80110
phone: 1-303-761-4805
fax: 1-303-762-9923

International Standard Book Number
0-89582-506-6

02 03 04 / 9 8 7 6 5 4 3 2

BASIC PHARMACOLOGY
BRIEF TABLE OF CONTENTS

TABLE OF CONTENTS

TABLE OF CONTENTS

TABLE OF CONTENTS

TABLE OF CONTENTS

TABLE OF CONTENTS

TABLE OF CONTENTS

ACKNOWLEDGEMENTS

CONTRIBUTORS

I'd like to thank the following people who have served as the primary co-authors of this book:

Robert P. Shrewsbury, Ph.D., R.Ph., Associate Professor of Pharmaceutics, University of North Carolina-Chapel Hill

> *Bob developed the majority of the material for the Foundations section of this book.*

Melanie Vlosky, R.N., B.S.N., M.Ed.

> *Melanie developed the majority of the material for the Classifications section of this book.*

They have done a great job in drafting material, making suggestions, and providing general assistance. I'd also like to thank the following people who have contributed greatly to this book:

Joseph Medina, R.Ph., Front Range Community College, and Tech Lectures (www.techlectures.com)

> *Joe developed the Drug Charts as well as the end of chapter multiple choice questions.*

Bruce Pleskow, R.Ph.

> *Bruce worked with Melanie in developing the material for the Classifications section of this book.*

EVERYONE ELSE

I'd like to thank Nora E. Meaney-Elman, M.D., for her assistance to Melanie, and Mary F. Powers, Ph.D., R.Ph., in particular for her detailed input. In addition, I'd like to thank some key people who helped develop material that was first used in our text "The Pharmacy Technician" and that we have put to good use here: Samuel Blackman, M.D., Jack Arthur, R.Ph., Ami Teague Deaton and Lori Coleman, Robin Cavallo, and two great artists, Claudette Barjoud and Anna Veltfort.

I'd also like to thank Tammy Newnam for the great art she has developed for this book, Kathy Anderson and Harvey Kane of the American Pharmaceutical Association, and Doug Morton, whose sponsorship makes this book possible. Finally, I'd like to thank my family whose support and patience is essential and deeply appreciated: Joan, Hannah, Joan, Wilma Jean, and Jimmy.

Dennis Hogan, Publisher

PHOTOGRAPHY CREDITS

I'd like to thank the following companies for graciously contributing the photographs of their products that can be found in this book.

Abbott Laboratories
Alcon Laboratories
AstraZeneca LP
Berlex Laboratories
Boehringer Ingelheim, Inc
Dey, L.P.
Eli Lilly & Company
Forest Pharmaceuticals
Genentech Inc.
Glaxo Wellcome Inc.
Hoechst Marion Roussel
Hoffman-LaRoche Inc.
Jones Pharma Incorporated
Merck Archives
Novartis Pharmaceutical Corporation
Novopharm USA INC
Ortho-McNeill Pharmaceutical Company
Par Pharmaceutical, Inc.
Pfizer
Proctor & Gamble
Roberts Pharmaceutical Corporation
Roche
Smith, Kline, Beecham
Tap Pharmaceuticals, Inc.
Whitehall-Robins

HOW TO USE THIS BOOK

This book has been specially designed and developed to make learning easier and more productive. Besides the extensive use of illustrations to both provide information and reinforce text discussion, the book uses a distinctive facing page design that makes it easier to identify important points and make connections between concepts. Illustrations are never a page or two away from the text. Topics are presented *in perspective*. Information is easy to find and understand.

The book is organized into two sections: **Foundations** and **Classifications**. In the Foundations section, we have tried to explain key pharmacological information in a practical and straightforward way. Though it is necessary to use technical terminology, we have tried to avoid being unnecessarily technical, since much about the action and use of drugs can be understood with everyday language. We have also tried to illustrate technical concepts wherever possible, so they may be better understood.

In the Classifications section, we begin each classification with an illustrated anatomy, physiology, and disease state discussion that tries to explain how and why the drug class is used. This is followed by individual discussions of specific drugs that explain common dosages, warnings, and patient information. We have not attempted to cover all common drugs in these discussions. There are simply too many. Instead, we have selected a cross-section that includes many of today's most widely used drugs along with some less common but important ones. These discussions should provide insight into many of the administration and use issues of the drugs in each classification.

For a broader look at a classification, we have added **Drug Charts** at the end of each classification. These are primarily a tool to familiarize yourself with the names of a much larger number of drugs (generic and trade) than we have discussed in the detailed drug descriptions.

Some of the other key features of this book's design are:

→ A **running glossary** represented by the symbol at right is presented throughout the text to emphasize important vocabulary.

→ We have used the **Rx symbol** to indicate points of emphasis and suggestion because these are a recipe for success.

→ End of chapter **Reviews** that provide:

✔ a checklist of the **Key Concepts** in the chapter,

✔ **Match the Terms/Names** sections that test knowledge of terminology or names.

✔ **Multiple Choice** questions in the *choose the best answer* format.

We think you'll find this book a useful guide to understanding the basic principles of pharmacology and the uses and usage issues of many popular drug products. We also hope that you find this to be one of the best texts you will use.

Dennis Hogan, Publisher

AMERICAN PHARMACEUTICAL ASSOCIATION

BASIC PHARMACY AND PHARMACOLOGY SERIES

Dear Student or Instructor,

The American Pharmaceutical Association (APhA), the national professional society of pharmacists in the United States, and Morton Publishing Company, a publisher of educational texts and training materials in healthcare, are pleased to present this outstanding textbook, *Basic Pharmacology*. It is one of a series of distinctive texts and training materials for basic pharmacy and pharmacology training that will be published under this banner: *American Pharmaceutical Association Basic Pharmacy and Pharmacology Series*.

Each book in the series is oriented toward developing an understanding of fundamental concepts. In addition, each text presents applied and practical information on the skills necessary to function effectively in positions such as technicians and medical assistants who work with medications below the prescriber level and whose role in healthcare is increasingly important. Each of the books in the series uses a visual design to enhance understanding and ease of use and is accompanied by various instructional support materials. We think you will find them valuable training tools.

The American Pharmaceutical Association and Morton Publishing thank you for using this book and invite you to look at other titles in this series, which are listed below.

John A. Gans, PharmD
Executive Vice President
American Pharmaceutical Association

Douglas N. Morton
President
Morton Publishing Company

TITLES IN THIS SERIES:

The Pharmacy Technician
Pharmacy Technician Workbook and Certification Review
Basic Pharmacology
Drug Card Workbook

NOTICE

This book is intended as a supporting reference to a training program for individuals who will work or are already working with medications below the prescriber level. Such positions are not authorized to make medication prescription, administration, and use decisions, but nevertheless require a basic knowledge of terminology and pharmacology, the development of which is the purpose of this book. In no way is this book intended as an authoritative reference for prescribing or administering medications. Prescription, administration, and use decisions may only be made by personnel authorized to make them. Legal requirements vary on this by institution and state. Your employer and state can provide you with the most recent regulations, guidelines, and practices that apply to your job, and it is essential that you know and follow them.

To the best of the Publisher's knowledge, the information presented in this book follows general practice as well as federal and state regulations and guidelines. However, please note that you are responsible for following your employer's and your state's regulations, policies, and guidelines.

The Publisher of this book disclaims any responsibility whatsoever for any injuries, damages, or other conditions that result from your practice or use of any information described in this book for any reason whatsoever.

BASIC PHARMACOLOGY

ORIGINS

In earliest times, medicine was based in magic and religion.

Like many ancient peoples, Sumerians living between the Tigris and Euphrates rivers around 4,000 B.C. believed that demons were the cause of illness. They studied the stars and the intestines of animals for clues to the supernatural causes of man's condition and fate. In many cultures, physicians were priests, and sometimes considered gods or demi-gods. The Egyptian Imhotep, for example, born around 3,000 B.C., was a priest and adviser to pharaohs and was the first physician known by name. After his death, he was named a demi-god and eventually a god: the Egyptian God of medicine.

The supernatural approach to treating illness gradually gave way to a more scientific approach, based on observation and experimentation.

Around 400 B.C., the Greek physician Hippocrates developed a more scientific approach which has guided western medicine for much of the time since. He promoted the idea of diagnosing illness based on careful observation of the patient's condition, not supernatural or other external elements. He also wrote the oath which physicians recited for centuries and still honor today: the Hippocratic Oath. From Hippocrates and others following in his footsteps, an approach to medicine in which natural causes were examined scientifically gradually grew to become the dominant approach to treating human illness.

 synthetic man-made; with chemicals, combining simpler chemicals into more complex compounds, to create a new chemical not found in nature.

The God of Medicine

The ancient Greek Aesculapius was said to have been such an extraordinary physician that he could keep his patients from dying and even raise the dead. This skill angered Pluto, the god of the underworld, because it reduced the number of his subjects. At Pluto's request, Zeus killed Aesculapius with a lightning bolt, then named him the God of medicine. Aesculapius's daughter, Panacea, became the Goddess of medicinal herbs.

MEDICAL MYTH

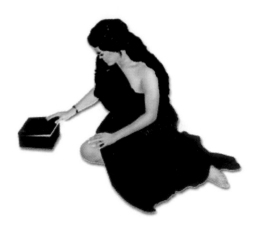

Pandora's Box

As punishment for Prometheus's theft of fire for mankind, the Greek God Zeus created Pandora and had her collect "gifts" for man from the gods. These gifts were really punishments that included disease and pestilence. They were released upon the world when Pandora opened her box.

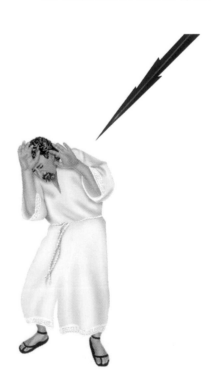

NATURE'S MEDICINE

A Treatment for Malaria

Malaria had long been one of the most deadly diseases in world history, until medicine made from the bark of a Peruvian tree, the Cinchona, was discovered. The medicine was **quinine,** popularly called "Jesuit's powder" for the Spanish priests that sent it to Europe from the New World. Its use along with preventive measures aimed at eradicating the cause of malaria brought the deadly disease under control.

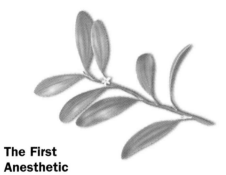

The First Anesthetic

Long before Spanish explorers noticed it, the Indians of the Andes chewed coca leaves for their medicinal effects, which included increased endurance. The active ingredient in the leaves was **cocaine,** which in 1884 was shown to be the first effective local anesthetic by Carl Koller, a Viennese surgeon. This discovery revolutionized surgery and dentistry, since previously anesthesia was administered on a general basis – that is, to the whole body. Eventually, because of its harmful properties when abused, a man-made substitute was developed, called **procain** or **novocain.**

B esides looking to the supernatural, ancient man also looked to the natural world for medical answers.

Early man understood that plants and other natural materials had the power to treat or relieve illness. The ancient Sumerians used about 250 natural medicines derived from plants, many of which are still used today. Around 3000 B.C., the Chinese Emperor Shen Nung is said to have begun eating plants and other natural materials to determine which were poisonous and which were beneficial. One of the first known practitioners of "trial and error" drug testing, he is believed to have established 365 herbs that could be used in health treatments. Over the centuries, this number was gradually expanded by various Chinese physicians into the thousands. Herbal medicine remains a major component of Chinese medicine today.

Through the ages, people have used drugs to treat illnesses and other physical conditions.

Ancient cultures around the world used medicines made from natural sources, many of which contained drugs that we still use today. Over the past two centuries, however, science found ways to create *synthetic* drugs, which often had advantages in cost, effect, and availability. Some of these man-made drugs replaced natural drugs and others were for entirely new uses. Today, while we still rely on many drugs derived from natural sources, we use more than twice as many synthetically produced drugs as naturally produced ones. As a result, the number of illnesses and physical conditions that can be treated with drugs is constantly increasing.

Nature's Aspirin

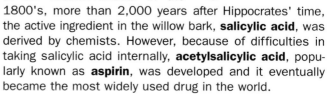

The ancient Greek physicians Hippocrates and Dioscorides both wrote about the pain relieving ability of the bark of a white willow tree that grew in the Mediterranean. In the 1800's, more than 2,000 years after Hippocrates' time, the active ingredient in the willow bark, **salicylic acid**, was derived by chemists. However, because of difficulties in taking salicylic acid internally, **acetylsalicylic acid**, popularly known as **aspirin**, was developed and it eventually became the most widely used drug in the world.

MEDICINE THROUGH THE AGES

— A Timeline —

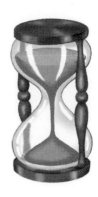

3000 B.C.

The **Egyptian Imhotep,** born around 3,000 B.C., was a priest and adviser to pharaohs and the first physician known by name. After his death, he was named a demi-god and eventually a god: the Egyptian God of medicine.

4000 B.C.

Ancient **Sumerians** studied the stars and animal intestines to divine man's fate and physical condition.

500 B.C.

The **Greek Alcmaeon,** a student of Pythagorus, saw diseases as a result of a loss of the body's natural equilibrium, rather than the work of the gods.

4000 B.C.	3000 B.C.	2000 B.C.	1000 B.C.	500 B.C.	250 B.C.

3000 B.C.

The **Chinese Emperor Shen Nung** is said to have begun tasting plants and other natural materials to determine which were poisonous and which were beneficial. One of the first known practitioners of "trial and error" drug testing, he is credited with establishing hundreds of herbal medicines.

600 B.C.

A cult following **Aesculapius, the Greek God of Medicine,** established centers where medicine was practiced. These early clinics became training grounds for the great Greek physicians of later years.

400 B.C.

A number of medical documents are written by different Greek physicians under the name **Hippocrates.** The works avoid the supernatural and religious and represent an approach to medicine that is grounded in scientific reasoning and close observation of the patient. They contain writings about the conduct of physicians, including the famous Hippocratic oath.

pharmacology the study of drugs – their properties, uses, application, and effects (from the Greek *pharmakon*–drug, and *logos*–word or thought).

materia medica generally pharmacology, but also refers to the drugs in use (from the Latin materia, matter, and medica, medical).

77 B.C.

Dioscorides, a Greek physician working in the Roman Legion, wrote the **De Materia Medica**, five books that described over 600 plants and their healing properties. His work was the main influence for Western pharmaceutics for over sixteen hundred years. One of the remedies he described was made from the bark of a type of willow tree, the active ingredient of which was salicylic acid, the natural drug on which acetylsalicylic acid (aspirin) is based. He also described how to get opium from poppies.

162 A.D.

The Greek physician **Galen** went to Rome and became the greatest name in Western medicine since Hippocrates both through his practice and extensive writings, nearly 100 of which survive. He believed there were four "humours" in man which needed to be in balance for good health, and he advocated "bleeding" to assist that balance. He also believed in the vigorous application of a scientific approach to medicine and his emphasis on education, observation, and logic formed the cornerstone for Western medicine.

100 B.C.

King Mithridates of Pontos practiced an early form of immunization by taking small amounts of poisons so that he could build his tolerance of them. It is said that he was so successful at this that when he eventually decided to kill himself through poisoning, he was unable to, and had to be killed by someone else. The potion Mithridates developed, Mithridaticum, was believed to be good at promoting health and was used for fifteen hundred years.

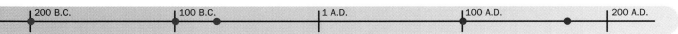

| 200 B.C. | 100 B.C. | 1 A.D. | 100 A.D. | 200 A.D. |

200 B.C.

The first official Chinese "herbal," the **Shen Nung Pen Tsao**, listing 365 herbs for use in health treatments, is believed to have been published. This can be considered an early Chinese forerunner to the FDA approved drug list.

100 A.D.

The **Indian physician Charaka** wrote the **Charaka Samhita**, the first great book of Indian medicine, which among other things described over 500 herbal drugs that had been known and used in India for many centuries.

Note: since the use of drugs goes so far back in history, we use many terms based on Greek or Latin words.

pharmacopeia an authoritative listing of drugs and issues related to their use.

pharmaceutical of or about drugs; also, a drug product.

panacea a cure-all (from the Greek *panakeia,* same meaning).

5

MEDICINE THROUGH THE AGES

— A Timeline —

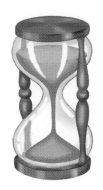

900 A.D.

The **Persian Rhazes** wrote one of the most popular textbooks of medicine in the Middle Ages, the **Book of Medicine Dedicated to Mansur**. A man of science, Rhazes was also an **alchemist** who believed he could turn lesser metal into gold. When he failed to do this, the Caliph ordered him beaten over the head with his own chemistry book until either his head or the book broke. Apparently, it was a tie. Rhazes lost sight in one eye but lived to continue his work.

1500 A.D.

When the Spanish found them, the **Indians of Mexico** had a well established pharmacology that included more than 1,200 drugs and was clearly the result of many hundreds of years of medical practice. One plant, the sarsaparilla, became very popular in Europe for its use on kidney and bladder ailments and can be found to this day in many medicinal teas.

1580 A.D.

In China, **Li Shi Zhen** completed the **Pen Tsao Kang Mu**, a compilation of nearly 2,000 drugs for use in treating illness and other conditions.

1630 A.D.

Jesuits sent **quinine** back to Europe in the early sixteen hundreds. Also called Jesuit's powder, it was the first drug to be used successfully in the treatment of the dreaded disease, malaria.

750 | 1000 | 1250 | 1500 | 1750

1000 A.D.

Perhaps the greatest Islamic physician was **Avicenna**. His writings dominated medical thinking in Europe for centuries. He wrote a five volume encyclopedia, one of which was devoted to natural medications and another to compounding drugs from individual medications.

1500 A.D.

In the early fifteen hundreds, a Swiss alchemist who went by the name of **Paracelsus** rejected the "humoural" philosophy of Galen and all previous medical teaching other than Hippocrates. Though he had many critics, he is generally credited with firmly establishing the use of chemistry to create medicinal drugs. Included in his work is the first published recipe for the addictive drug laudanum, which became a popular though tragically abused drug for the next three hundred years.

1785 A.D.

The **British Physician, William Withering**, publishes his study of the **foxglove** plant and the drug it contained, **digitalis**, which became widely used in treating heart disease. Foxglove had been used since ancient times in various remedies but Withering described a process for creating the drug from the dried leaves of the plant and established a dosage approach.

antitoxin a substance that acts against a toxin in the body; also, a vaccine containing antitoxins, used to fight disease.

antibiotic a substance which harms or kills microorganisms like bacteria and fungi.

1890

Effective **antitoxins** are developed for diptheria and tetanus, giving a major boost to the development of medicines that fight infectious disease.

1803

The German pharmacist **Frederich Serturner** extracts morphine from opium.

1899

Acetylsalicylic acid, popularly known as **aspirin,** is developed because of difficulties in using salicylic acid, a drug contained in certain willow trees that had long been used in the external treatment of various conditions.

1846

In Boston, the first publicized operation using **general anesthesia** is performed. Ether is the anesthetic.

1928

In Britain, **Alexander Fleming** discovers a fungus which produces a chemical that kills bacteria. He names the chemical, **penicillin.** It is the first antibiotic drug.

1943

Russell Marker is able to derive the hormone **progesterone,** the first reliable birth control drug, from a species of Mexican yam.

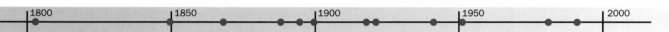

1864

Louis Pasteur's experiments show that microorganisms cause food spoilage, and that heat can be used to kill them and preserve the food. Though others had proposed principles of **"germ theory"** previously, Pasteur's work is instrumental in it becoming widely accepted.

1884

In 1884, **Carl Koller,** a Viennese surgeon, discovers that cocaine, the active ingredient in coca leaves, was useful as a local anesthetic in eye surgery, and cocaine is established as the **first local anesthetic**.

1921

In Toronto, Canada, **Frederick Banting** and **Charles Best** show that an extract of the hormone, **insulin,** will lower blood sugar in dogs and so may be useful in the treatment of the terrible disease diabetes. The biochemist James B. Collip then develops an extract of insulin pure enough to test on humans. The first human trial in January, 1922 proves successful and dramatically changes the prospects for all diabetics.

1951

James Watson and **Francis Crick** identify the structure of **DNA,** the basic component within the cell that contains the organism's genetic code.

1981

First documented cases of **AIDS.**

1988

The **Human Genome Project** is begun with the goal of mapping the entire DNA sequence in the human genome, This information will provide a better understanding of hereditary diseases and allow the development of new treatments for them.

 hormone chemicals produced by the body that regulate body functions and processes.

human genome the complete set of genetic material contained in a human cell.

THE 20TH CENTURY

The average life span in the United States increased by over twenty years in the twentieth century.

At the beginning of the century, the average American lived only into their early fifties. By 1995, the average life expectancy at birth in the United States had risen to 75.8 years. Similar changes were seen throughout the industrialized world and to a lesser extent in developing countries. The growth of hospitals, advances in the treatment of disease, improved medical technology, better understanding of nutrition and health, and the rapid increase in the number of effective drugs and vaccines have all contributed to this profound change in improved life experience.

A major factor in the increased health and life expectancy seen in this century was the dramatic growth in pharmaceutical medicine.

Since the eighteenth century, there was a growing interest and success in developing man-made or synthetic medicines. The development of aspirin in 1899 was followed by more pharmaceutical research and discoveries that spurred the growth of a worldwide industry committed to creating medicines for virtually every illness and condition. The discovery of the antibiotic penicillin was followed shortly by a World War in which its mass production was seen as critical to Allied success. This and other war related drug needs stimulated the pharmaceutical industry to dramatically boost its capacity and production. Ever since, pharmaceutical research and development has grown substantially and continually. Today, the United States is the world's leading producer of medical pharmaceuticals with more than $100 billion in annual worldwide sales.

LIVING LONGER

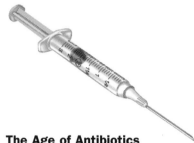

The Age of Antibiotics

In World War I, more soldiers died from infections than the wounds themselves. Although penicillin was discovered as an antibiotic in 1928, it was difficult to produce and for years not much was made of the discovery. With the start of World War II, however, British scientists looked again at penicillin and established that it was effective in fighting infections. Already under attack from Germany and unable to develop mass production methods for penicillin, the British sought help in the United States. In 1942, the Pfizer pharmaceutical company was able to develop a method for mass production of the drug, and by D-Day the Allied army was well stocked with it. Its use saved many thousands of lives during the war and revolutionized the pharmaceutical industry. A period of intense research and discovery in the field of antibiotics began, and many new antibiotics were developed which have dramatically contributed to improved health and increased life expectancy.

Living Longer

Improved pharmaceutical products have had a major effect on the life span of Americans and others in the twentieth century. In the U.S., the life span has increased over 50% in the last century, with much of the increase due to the discovery and use of disease fighting drugs.

source: National Center of Health Statistics

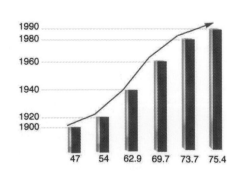

THE DRUG INDUSTRY

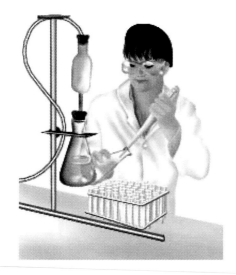

With the increasing availability of powerful drugs, their regulation became more important than ever.

Governments and their leaders have long sought to regulate the use of medicinal drugs because of their effect on the population's health. The explosive growth of pharmaceuticals in the twentieth century made governments throughout the world keenly aware of the importance of setting and maintaining standards for their distribution and use.

In the United States, drug regulation is performed by the Food and Drug Administration.

FDA activity is a major factor in the nation's public health and safety. Before a drug can be marketed, it must be shown through testing that it is safe and effective for its intended use. Once marketed, the FDA monitors drugs to make sure they work as intended, and that there are no serious negative (adverse) effects from their use. If drugs that are marketed are found to have adverse effects, the FDA can recall them (take them off the market).

Patenting Discoveries

As with other scientific and technological areas, patenting new discoveries is an important part of the pharmaceutical development process since it protects against illegal copying of the discovery. The company holding the patent is then able to control the marketing of the product and use this as a way to recover their original investment. Since patenting generally occurs long before a drug is approved, however, a company often has only about ten or so years of patent protection left in which to market their product without competition from direct copies called "generic" versions.

The discovery of new drugs requires a major investment of time, research, and development.

The pharmaceutical industry employs thousands of scientists and devotes about one-sixth of its income to research and development. Bringing a new drug to market is a long and difficult process in which the vast majority of research does not produce a successful drug. Thousands of chemical combinations must be tried in order to find one that might work as hoped. Once a potentially useful drug is created, it must undergo an extensive testing and approval process before it can be made available to the public. In the United States, the length of time from the beginning of development through testing and to ultimate FDA approval is often more than ten years.

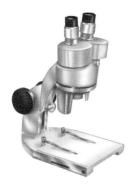

It's in the Genes

One of the most exciting areas of pharmaceutical research is performed by molecular biologists studying human genes. While antibiotics are the answer for many infectious diseases, many other diseases which seemed based on heredity are effectively untreatable. The study of the **human genome** has shown that many diseases are related to genetic defects. This has led to the creation of new drugs that can successfully treat many diseases previously considered untreatable. As a result, the field of biotechnology has become the most dynamic area of pharmaceutical research and development.

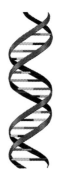

MEDICINE TODAY

A "prescription" drug is one that has been ordered or "prescribed" by a physician or other licensed prescriber to treat a patient. Though physicians occasionally give patients the actual medication, in most cases the individual who dispenses the prescribed medication to the patient is a pharmacist. Pharmacists at more than 50,000 community pharmacies account for approximately half of the distribution of prescription drugs in the United States. The rest reach consumers primarily through hospitals, mass merchandisers, food stores, mail order pharmacies, clinics, and nursing homes– all of which employ pharmacists for the dispensing of medications.

The number of medicines and their use is greater than ever.

The sheer number of available drugs, their different names and costs, multiple prescriptions from different physicians for the same patient, and the involvement of third-party insurers are among the many factors which make the use of prescription drugs a complex area for everyone involved, and especially for patients.

In this increasing complex environment, powerful computerized tools are essential.

Computers put patient profiles, drug product information, inventory, pricing, and other important data within easy access. They identify potentially dangerous interactions, generate instructions for patients, resolve billing details with insurers, and coordinate many aspects of a patient's pharmaceutical care. As a result, more prescriptions are dispensed than ever before. In addition, more information about drug products is provided and used.

---

 formulary a list of drugs that are approved for use, from which individual drugs may be selected.

third party insurance a party other than the dispenser or the patient that pays for all or part of the cost of a prescription.

COMPUTERIZATION

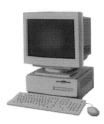

Though the environment for dispensing and using drug products is highly complex, computerized systems are used to ensure safety and efficiency. Systems vary in features depending upon whether they are for suppliers, insurers, dispensers, etc., but they generally communicate with each other, allowing the coordination of tremendous amounts of information on patients and drug products. Examples of the information they contain:

Patient

Complete patient profiles, including their prescribers, insurer, medical and medication history. Drug interactions are routinely identified for patients taking multiple medications.

Prescriber

Prescriber profiles, including state identification numbers, and affiliations with facilities and insurers.

Drug Product

Identified by various means: brand name, generic name, product code, category, suppliers, etc.

Education/Counseling

Patient information about usage, possible interactions, allergies, etc.

Insurance

Policy information, including deductibles, co-pay amounts, generic substitution information, etc.

ECONOMIC TRENDS

In thirty years, the cost of health care in the United States rose over 2,500 percent! As a result, there have been increasing efforts by government, industry, and consumers to find ways to control the costs of care. Though drugs represent only a small fraction of overall health care expenses, they have also been included in these efforts.

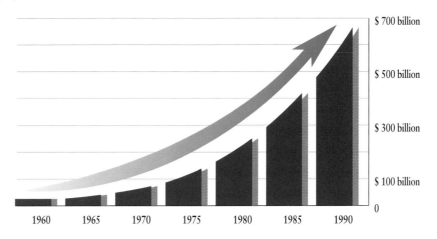

	$ 700 billion
	$ 500 billion
	$ 300 billion
	$ 100 billion
	0

1960   1965   1970   1975   1980   1985   1990

➡ A result of the **managed care** movement is that the majority of prescriptions are now paid by private third parties such as HMO's and other insurance companies, instead of directly by consumers.

➡ Along with this is a trend toward the use of closed **formularies**, lists of drugs which are approved for use. These lists rely substantially on substituting generic drugs in place of more expensive brands that may be prescribed by the physician. By 1996, the use of generics had doubled in ten years to 40% of dispensed prescriptions.*

➡ Another cost cutting trend is the increasing use of "therapeutic substitution" in which a chemically different drug that performs a similar function is substituted, usually because it is less expensive.

*source for text: Pharmaceutical Research and Manufacturers of America;
source for illustration: U.S. Statistical Abstract*

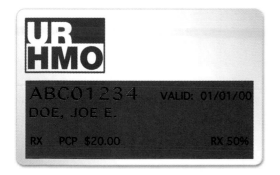

Third Party Payment

Third party payment programs are simply another party besides the patient or the dispenser that pays for some or all of the cost of medication – essentially, an insurer. Although many individuals are uninsured, most people have some form of private or public health insurance. In the U.S., these include public programs such as Medicaid and Medicare as well as private programs such as HMOs and basic health insurance. Many but not all such programs include prescription drug coverage. When they do, the patient usually has a prescription drug benefit card such as the one shown at left that identifies the prescription plan and the patient.

REVIEW

KEY CONCEPTS

✔ People have used drugs derived from plants to treat illnesses and other physical conditions for thousands of years.

✔ The ancient Greeks used the bark of a white willow tree to relieve pain. The bark contained salicylic acid, the natural forerunner of the active ingredient in aspirin.

✔ Cocaine was the first effective local anesthetic.

✔ The foxglove plant contains the drug digitalis, which has been widely used in treating heart disease.

✔ Louis Pasteur's experiments show that microorganisms cause food spoilage, and that heat can be used to kill them and preserve the food.

✔ Frederick Banting and Charles Best showed that an extract of the hormone, insulin, lowered blood sugar in dogs and might be useful in the treatment of diabetes.

✔ Alexander Fleming discovered the antibiotic chemical, penicillin.

✔ The Human Genome Project is an attempt to map the entire DNA sequence in the human genome. This information will provide a better understanding of hereditary diseases and how to treat them.

✔ The average life span in the United States increased by over twenty years in the Twentieth Century.

✔ In World War I, more soldiers died from infections than the wounds themselves.

✔ Increasing costs of health care have brought increased efforts to control the cost of prescription drugs, on aspect of which is the use of closed "formularies" that rely substantially on substituting generic drugs in place of more expensive brands.

✔ Computerized management systems put customer profiles, product, inventory, pricing, and other essential information within easy access. One result has been that more prescriptions and information is dispensed than ever before.

SELF TEST

MATCH THE TERMS.   *answers can be checked in the glossary*

antibiotic	combining simpler chemicals into more complex ones, creating a new chemical not found in nature.
antitoxin	an authoritative listing of drugs and issues related to their use.
hormone	of or about drugs; also, a drug product.
human genome	a cure-all.
materia medica	the study of drugs—their properties, uses, application, and effects.
panacea	generally pharmacology, but also refers to the drugs in use.
pharmaceutical	a substance that acts against a toxin in the body
pharmacology	a substance which harms or kills microorganisms like bacteria and fungi.
pharmacopeia	chemicals produced by the body that regulate body functions and processes.
synthetic	the complete set of genetic material contained in a human cell.

CHOOSE THE BEST ANSWER.   *answers are in the back of the book*

1. Derived from the bark of the Peruvian tree, "Jesuit's Powder," used along with preventive measures, helps keep this disease under control.
   a. smallpox
   b. malaria
   c. polio
   d. tuberculosis

2. The first local anesthetic used in surgery was
   a. salicylic acid.
   b. acetylsalicylic acid.
   c. aspirin.
   d. none of the above.

3. Life expectancy in the United States in the 20th century increased by:
   a. approximately 50%.
   b. approximately 100%.
   c. approximately 125%.
   d. approximately 150%.

4. The FDA is required to
   a. ensure that a drug is safe and effective for its intended use.
   b. to monitor a drug after it is marketed to ensure it works as intended.
   c. to monitor a drug for any adverse effects.
   d. all of the above.

DRUG REGULATION

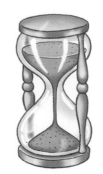

— A TIMELINE —

There are many laws in the United States concerning the safety and effectiveness of food, drugs, medical devices and cosmetics. Regardless of whether a product is produced in the United States or is imported, it must meet the requirements of these laws. The leading enforcement agency at the federal level for these regulations is the Food and Drug Administration. On these pages are brief descriptions of U.S. federal laws and their significance.

Food and Drug Act of 1906

Prohibited interstate commerce in adulterated or misbranded food, drinks, and drugs. Government pre-approval of drugs is required.

1927 Food, Drug and Insecticide Administration

The law enforcement agency is formed that would be renamed in 1930 as the Food and Drug Administration.

1950 Alberty Food Products v. U.S.

The United States Court of Appeals rules that the purpose for which a drug is to be used must be included on the label.

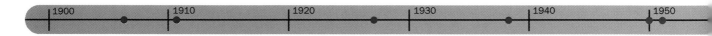

1911 Sherley Amendment

This law was enacted in response to the Supreme Court's interpretation that the 1906 Food and Drugs Act only applied to misleading information about the ingredients of a drug, as opposed to its effects. It prohibits false and misleading claims about the **therapeutic** effects of a drug.

1938 Food, Drug and Cosmetic (FDC) Act

In response to the fatal poisoning of 107 people, primarily children, by an untested sulfanilamide concoction, this comprehensive law requires new drugs be shown to be safe before marketing.

1951 Durham-Humphrey Amendment

This law defines what drugs require a prescription by a licensed practitioner and requires them to include this **legend** on the label: "Caution: Federal Law prohibits dispensing without a prescription."

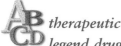 *therapeutic* serving to cure or heal.

legend drug any drug which requires a prescription and either of these "legends" on the label: "Caution: Federal law prohibits dispensing without a prescription," or "Rx only."

1962 Kefauver-Harris Amendments

Requires drug manufacturers to provide proof of both safety and effectiveness before marketing the drug.

1966 Fair Packaging and Labeling Act

This requires all consumer products in interstate commerce to be honestly and informatively labeled.

1970 Controlled Substances Act (CSA)

The CSA classifies drugs that may be easily abused and restricts their distribution. It is enforced by the Drug Enforcement Administration (DEA) within the Justice Department.

1983 Orphan Drug Act

Provides incentives to promote research, approval and marketing of drugs needed for the treatment of rare diseases.

1987 Prescription Drug Marketing Act

Restricts distribution of prescription drugs to legitimate commercial channels and requires drug wholesalers to be licensed by the states.

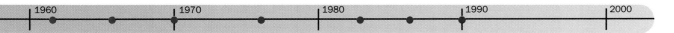

1960   1970   1980   1990   2000

1970 Poison Prevention Packaging Act

Requires child-proof packaging on all controlled and most prescription drugs dispensed by pharmacies. Non-child-proof containers may only be used if the prescriber or patient request one.

1976 Medical Device Amendment

Requires pre-market approval for safety and effectiveness of life-sustaining and life-supporting medical devices.

1990 Omnibus Budget Reconciliation Act (OBRA)

Among other things, this act required pharmacists to offer counseling to Medicaid patients regarding medications.

1997 FDA Modernization Act

Changed the legend requirement to "**Rx only**," with a phase in period until February, 2003.

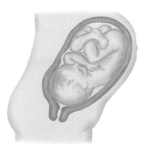

The Thalidomide Lesson

In 1962, a new sleeping pill containing the drug, thalidomide, was found to cause severe birth defects when used by pregnant women. This included lost limbs and other major deformities that affected thousands of children in Europe, where the drug had been widely used. In the United States, the drug was not yet approved for marketing and was only being used in tests, so it affected a small number of children. However, the nature of the defects and the number of children affected created a public demand in the U.S. for tighter drug regulation that resulted in the Kefauver-Harris Amendments. From then on, drugs would have to be shown to be both safe and effective before they could be marketed in the United States.

NEW DRUG APPROVAL

All new drugs, whether made domestically or imported, require FDA approval before they can be marketed in the United States.

A new drug is any drug proposed for marketing after 1938 that was not already recognized as safe and effective. This represents the vast majority of drugs on the market.

Before it will be approved, a new drug must be shown to be both safe and effective and that its benefits substantially outweigh its risks.

It is the responsibility of the drug manufacturer (not the FDA) to provide proof of this to the FDA's **Center for Drug Evaluation and Research (CDER)**. The proof is based on extensive testing which begins in the laboratory, where chemical analysis is performed, and moves on to animal testing and then clinical trials with people. The FDA estimates that the testing process currently takes 8.5 years.

Clinical trials **involve testing the drug on people.**

Clinical tests begin with small numbers of participants over a short period of time and eventually expand into large groups of participants over long periods. Trial participants must give their informed consent. Among other things, it means the person must be told of the risks of the treatment along with other treatment options in language they can understand. Participants are also free to leave the trial at any time they wish.

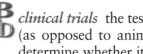

clinical trials the testing of a new drug on people (as opposed to animal or laboratory testing) to determine whether it merits FDA approval.

placebo an inactive substance given in place of a medication.

pediatric having to do with the treatment of children.

Testing Children

Children are not included in trials until a drug has been fully tested on adults. Drugs which have not been tested on children generally state on the label that their safety and effectiveness has not been established for children. Some drugs, however, may carry label information for pediatric use that is based on studies of adults and other pediatric treatment information.

TESTING

Animal Testing

Once laboratory testing of a proposed new drug is finished, the drug is tested on animals before it will be tested on humans. Drug companies try to use as few animals and to treat them as humanely as possible. Since different species often react differently, more than one species is usually tested. Drug absorption into the bloodstream is monitored carefully. Only a fraction of a percent of drugs tested on animals are ever tested on humans.

Placebos

Placebos are inactive substances, not real medications, that are administered to give the patient the impression he or she is receiving a potentially effective medication. This provides a valuable comparison against patients who receive a test drug. Patients in trials must freely agree to the possibility that they may be given a placebo. They must also be informed of an effective treatment if one is available.

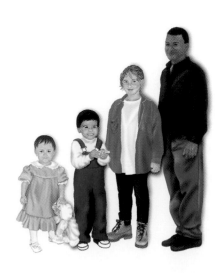

Testing Phases in Humans

There are **three phases** of testing a new drug in humans. Testing begins with a small number of participants for a short time and this gradually increases to a large number of participants over long periods of time. The goals of each phase also change from indicating a minimal level of safety to ultimately verifying the safety, effectiveness and dosage for widespread use. Only about 25% of drugs tested in phase 1 successfully complete phase 3.

phase 1

➡ **20-100 patients**
➡ **time: several months**
➡ **purpose: mainly safety**

phase 2

➡ **up to several hundred patients**
➡ **time: several months to two years**
➡ **purpose: short-term safety but mainly effectiveness**

phase 3

➡ **several hundred to several thousand patients**
➡ **time: one to four years**
➡ **purpose: safety, dosage, and effectiveness**

source: Food and Drug Administration

During the trial phase, a proposed new drug is called an *investigational new drug* (IND).

It is available for use only within the trial groups unless granted a special "treatment" status which is sometimes given to provide relief to critically ill patients outside of clinical trials. An example of this is AZT, which was used on thousands of AIDS patients who were not part of a clinical trial prior to the drug receiving FDA approval. It is worth noting, however, that such drugs are extremely expensive and are excluded from coverage by most insurers and HMOs.

Tests are "controlled" by comparing the effect of a proposed drug on one group of patients with the effect of a different treatment on other patients.

Patients have the same condition and similar characteristics and are placed in control groups at random to make sure the groups have essentially the same characteristics. The different treatment may be no drug at all, a placebo, a drug known to be effective, or a different dose of the same drug.

The patients in a trial are always "blind" to the treatment.

They are not told which control group they are in. In a "double-blind" test, neither the patients nor the physicians know what the medication is. So patients or their physicians may not be influenced into imagining effects one way or the other. Medical results alone determine the drug's effectiveness and its safety.

Medical Products Other Than Drugs

Medical devices and biological products such as insulin and vaccines must also meet FDA testing and approval requirements. The **Center for Devices and Radiological Health (CDRH)** is responsible for devices. The **Center for Biologics Evaluation and Research (CBER)** is responsible for biological products made from living organisms.

MARKETED DRUGS

A patent for a new drug gives its manufacturer an exclusive right to market the drug for a specific period of time under a *brand name*. During this time, the manufacturer attempts to recover the costs of the drug's research and development. A drug patent is in effect for 17 years from the date of the drug's discovery. Since the testing and approval process takes years to complete, for many years drugs reached the market with only half their patent time left. To compensate for this, the Hatch-Waxman Act of 1984 provided for up to five year extensions of patent protection to the patent holders to make up for time lost while products went through the FDA approval process.

Once a patent for a brand drug expires, other manufacturers may copy the drug and release it under its pharmaceutical or "generic" name.

Manufacturers of generic drugs do not need to perform the safety and effectiveness testing required of new drugs. However, they need to demonstrate that the drug is **pharmaceutically equivalent** to the patented brand drug – that it has same active ingredients, same dosage form, same route of administration, and same strength, and that it is **therapeutically equivalent** – that the body's use of the drug is the same. This is measured by the rate and extent to which the active ingredients are absorbed into the bloodstream.

Over-the-counter (OTC) drugs are drug products that do not require a prescription.

They can be used upon the judgment of the consumer. There are over 100,000 OTC drugs in 80 therapeutic categories marketed. The FDA publishes acceptable ingredients for OTC drugs in "Drug Monographs." The manufacturer of an OTC drug must follow monograph requirements to be able to market their drug without undergoing the FDA new drug approval process. Though some OTC drugs were available before FDA approval was required, the FDA has been reviewing them under the "OTC Drug Review Program," and all new OTC drugs require FDA approval.

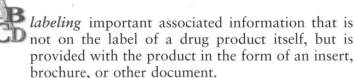

labeling important associated information that is not on the label of a drug product itself, but is provided with the product in the form of an insert, brochure, or other document.

LABELS AND LABELING

While all drugs are required to have clear and accurate information for all labels, inserts, packaging, and so on, there are different information requirements for various categories of drugs. Information requirements for OTC drugs are designed to enable consumers to use them without medical advice. Manufacturers of prescription drugs do not have to include directions for use on their labels since such directions must be supplied by the prescriber and dispenser. In many cases, important associated information may not fit on the label itself, and it will be provided in the form of an insert, brochure, or other document that is referred to as **labeling.**

Look Alike, Sound Alike

Federal laws require that a drug and/or its container not be imitative of another drug so that the consumer will be misled. Nevertheless, there are many drugs with similar sounding names in similar looking packages. It is therefore essential to pay close attention to the details of drug names and packaging. Using the wrong drug can have very serious consequences.

OTC LABELS

Over-the-counter medications do not require a prescription but sometimes prescriptions are written for them for insurance or other reasons. **OTC medications are not without risks,** and in many cases patients should seek the advice of a physician or pharmacist before using them.

The following information should be contained on the labels of over-the counter-medications.

- ➡ product name
- ➡ name and address of manufacturer or distributor
- ➡ list of all active and other ingredients
- ➡ amount of contents
- ➡ adequate warnings
- ➡ adequate directions for use

Many over-the-counter products have labels that are difficult to read, understand, or both. At right is a label format proposed by the FDA to make it easier to read and understand the information currently contained on over-the-counter medication labels. Note that this format is not a requirement.

a proposed FDA label format
for OTC medications

Active Ingredient (In Each Tablet)   **Purpose**

Chlorpheniramine Maleate 4 mg..Antihistamine

Uses: for the temporary relief of these symptoms of hay fever
- ▶ sneezing
- ▶ runny nose
- ▶ itchy,watery eyes

Warnings

Ask a Doctor Before Use
If You Have:

- ▶ glaucoma
- ▶ a breathing problem such as emphysema or chronic bronchitis
- ▶ difficulty in urination due to enlargement of the prostate gland

If You Are:

- ▶ taking sedatives or tranquilizers

When Using This Product:

- ▶ marked drowsiness may occur
- ▶ alcohol, sedatives, and tranquilizers may increase the drowsiness effect
- ▶ avoid alcoholic beverages
- ▶ use caution when driving a motor vehicle or operating machinery
- ▶ excitability may occur, especially in children

If pregnant or breast-feeding, ask a health professional before use.
Keep out of reach of children. In case of overdose, get medical help right away.

Directions:

Adults and children over 12 years:	Take 1 tablet every 4 to 6 hours as needed. Do not take more than 6 tablets in 24 hours.
Children 6 to under 12 years:	Take 1/2 tablet every 4 to 6 hours as needed. Do not take more than 3 tablets in 24 hours.
Children under 6 years:	Ask a doctor.

SAMPLE LABELS

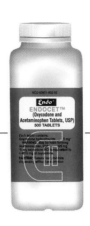

MANUFACTURER STOCK LABEL

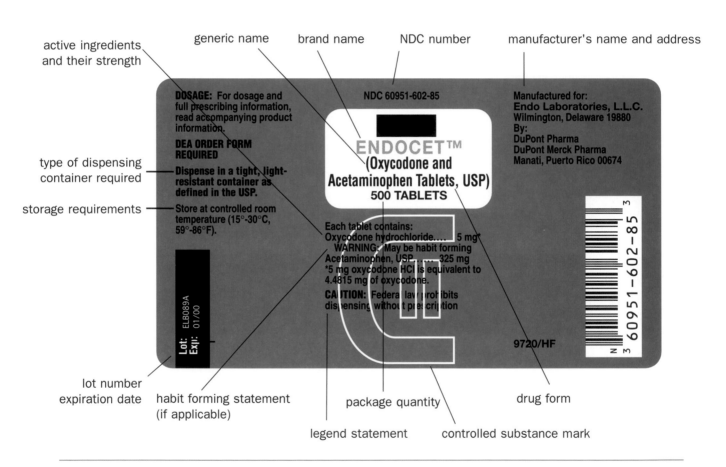

active ingredients and their strength

generic name

brand name

NDC number

manufacturer's name and address

DOSAGE: For dosage and full prescribing information, read accompanying product information.

DEA ORDER FORM REQUIRED

type of dispensing container required — **Dispense in a tight, light-resistant container as defined in the USP.**

storage requirements — **Store at controlled room temperature (15°-30°C, 59°-86°F).**

NDC 60951-602-85

ENDOCET™ (Oxycodone and Acetaminophen Tablets, USP) 500 TABLETS

Each tablet contains:
Oxycodone hydrochloride.... 5 mg*
   WARNING: May be habit forming
Acetaminophen, USP... 325 mg
*5 mg oxycodone HCl is equivalent to 4.4815 mg of oxycodone.

CAUTION: Federal law prohibits dispensing without prescription

Manufactured for:
Endo Laboratories, L.L.C.
Wilmington, Delaware 19880
By:
**DuPont Pharma
DuPont Merck Pharma
Manati, Puerto Rico 00674**

9720/HF

Lot: ELB089A
Exp: 01/00

3 60951-602-85

lot number
expiration date

habit forming statement (if applicable)

package quantity

legend statement

controlled substance mark

drug form

Labeling

In addition to a container label, manufacturer prescription drugs must also be accompanied by labeling which includes information on the following: clinical pharmacology, indications and usage, contraindications, warnings, precautions, adverse reactions, drug abuse and dependence, dosage, and packaging. This information is designed to inform both the prescriber and the dispenser regarding the drug.

ABCD **NDC (National Drug Code) number** the number assigned by the manufacturer. The first five digits indicate the manufacturer. The next four indicate the medication, its strength, and dosage form. The last two indicate the package size.

controlled substance mark the mark (CII-CV) which indicates the control category of a drug with a potential for abuse.

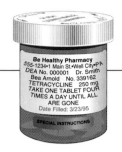

DISPENSED PRESCRIPTION DRUG LABEL

Minimum requirements on prescription labels for most drugs generally are as follows:

✔ name and address of dispenser

✔ prescription serial number.

✔ date of prescription or filling

✔ name of prescriber

And any of the following that are stated in the prescription:

✔ name of patient

✔ directions for use

✔ cautionary statements

Certain drugs have greater requirements, and many states impose greater requirements.

Typical elements on a prescription label:

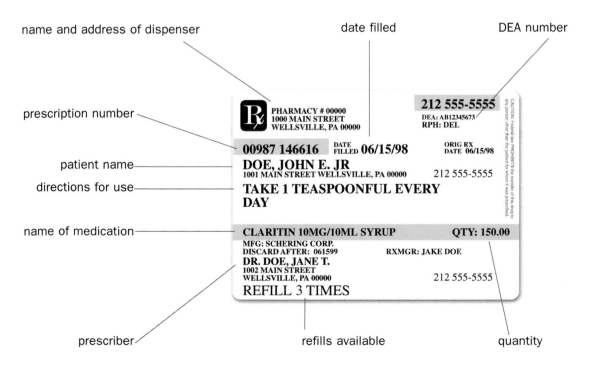

name and address of dispenser

date filled

DEA number

prescription number

patient name

directions for use

name of medication

prescriber

refills available

quantity

CONTROLLED SUBSTANCES

The government tightly controls the use of drugs that can be easily abused.

The 1970 Controlled Substances Act (CSA) identified five groups or schedules of such drugs as **controlled substances** and put strict guidelines on their distribution. It required manufacturers, distributors, or dispensers of controlled substances to register with the Drug Enforcement Administration (DEA) of the Justice Department. This created a "closed system" in which only registered parties can distribute these drugs.

The five control schedules are as follows*:

Schedule I:

➡ Each drug has a high potential for abuse and no accepted medical use in the United States. It may not be prescribed. Heroin, various opium derivatives, and hallucinogenic substances are included on this schedule.

Schedule II:

➡ Each drug has a high potential for abuse and may lead to physical or psychological dependence, but also has a currently accepted medical use in the United States. Amphetamines, opium, cocaine, methadone, and various opiates are included on this schedule.

Schedule III:

➡ Each drug's potential for abuse is less than those in Schedules I and II and there is a currently accepted medical use in the U.S., but abuse may lead to moderate or low physical dependence or high psychological dependence. Anabolic steroids and various compounds containing limited quantities of narcotic substances such as codeine are included on this schedule.

Schedule IV:

➡ Each drug has a low potential for abuse relative to Schedule III drugs and there is a current accepted medical use in the U.S., but abuse may lead to limited physical dependence or psychological dependence. Phenobarbital, the sedative chloral hydrate, and the anesthetic methohexital are included in this group.

Schedule V:

➡ Each drug has a low potential for abuse relative to Schedule IV drugs and there is a current accepted medical use in the U.S., but abuse may lead to limited physical dependence or psychological dependence. Compounds containing limited amounts of a narcotic such as codeine are included in this group.

*21 USC Sec. 812 as of 1/96. Note: these schedules are revised periodically. It is important to refer to the most current schedule.

REGULATIONS

Labels

Manufacturers must clearly label controlled drugs with their control classification.

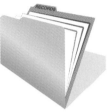

Record keeping

Distributors are required to maintain accurate records of all controlled substance activity. This includes accurate records of inventory as well as drugs dispensed. Schedule-II prescription records must be kept separate from non-controlled drug records, though they may be kept with other controlled drug records.

Security for Controlled Drugs

Schedule II drugs must be stored in a locked tamperproof narcotics cabinet that is usually secured to the floor or wall. Schedule III, IV, and V drugs may be kept openly on storage shelves in retail and hospital settings.

Joint responsibility

By law, both the prescriber and the dispenser of the prescription have joint responsibility for the legitimate medical purpose of the prescription. This is intended to ensure that controlled substances not be prescribed for inappropriate reasons.

DEA Number

All prescribers of controlled substances must be authorized by the DEA. They are assigned a DEA number that must be used on all controlled drug prescriptions.

SAMPLE LABELS AND ORDER FORM

Manufacturer containers and labels for C-II, C-III, and C-IV controlled drug products. Note that the control substance marks are prominent.

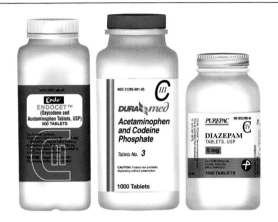

A sample C-I and C-II order form. It must be signed by a registered person, in triplicate. Note that C-III, C-IV, and C-V don't require federal order forms. Because of the lower potential for abuse they are controlled by the record keeping requirements for all controlled substances.

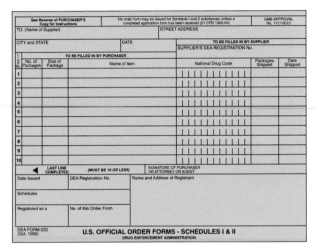

CONTROLLED SUBSTANCE PRESCRIPTIONS

Controlled-Substance Prescriptions

Controlled-substance prescriptions have greater requirements at both federal and state levels than other prescriptions, particularly Schedule II drugs. On controlled substance prescriptions, the DEA number must appear on the form and the patient's full street address must be entered.

On Schedule II prescriptions, the form must be signed by the prescriber (no phoned or faxed prescriptions allowed). In many states, there are specific time limits that require Schedule II prescriptions be promptly filled. Quantities are limited and no refills are allowed. When the prescription is filled, the pharmacist draws a line across it indicating it has been filled.

Federal requirements for Schedules III-V are less stringent than for Schedule II. Refills and faxed prescriptions are allowed, for example. However, state and other regulations may be stricter than federal requirements, so it is necessary to know the requirements for your specific job setting.

DEA Numbers

DEA numbers are required by federal law but administered by the states. They have two letters followed by seven single-digit numbers, e.g., AB1234563. **The following should always be true of a DEA number on a prescription form:** if the sum of the first, third and fifth digits is added to twice the sum of the second, fourth, and sixth digits, the total should be a number whose last digit is the same as the last digit of the DEA number.

PUBLIC SAFETY

Though the FDA approval process is quite thorough, it is impossible to fully prove that a drug is safe for use.

No matter how many people participate in the clinical trials, the number is always just a fraction of the number that will use a drug once it is approved. So there is always the risk that the drug may produce adverse side effects when used on a larger population. To monitor this, the FDA maintains a reporting program called **MedWatch** that encourages health care professionals to report adverse effects that occur from the use of an approved drug or other medical product. MedWatch does not monitor vaccines. That is performed by the Vaccine Adverse Event Reporting System.

The FDA has several options if it determines that a marketed drug presents a risk of illness, injury, or gross consumer deception.

It may seek an **injunction** that prevents the manufacturer from distributing the drug; it may seize the drug; or it may issue a **recall.** Of these, recalls are considered the most effective, largely because they involve the cooperation of the manufacturer, which after all is the only party that knows where the drugs have been distributed. As a result, recalls are the FDA's preferred means of removing dangerous drugs from the market.

adverse effect an unintended side affect of a medication that is negative or in some way injurious to a patient's health.

injunction a court order preventing a specific action, such as the distribution of a potentially dangerous drug.

recall the action taken to remove a drug from the market and have it returned to the manufacturer.

A Manufacturer Recall

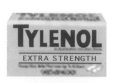

When someone tampered with a small number of Tylenol capsule packages and fatally poisoned seven people, Johnson & Johnson immediately recalled the capsules from the market. This swift and responsible action resulted in a highly favorable public response and increased popularity for Tylenol – and Johnson & Johnson.

RECALLS

Recalls are, with a few exceptions, voluntary on the part of the manufacturer. However, once the FDA requests a manufacturer recall a product, the pressure to do so is substantial. The negative publicity from not recalling would significantly damage a company's reputation, and the FDA would probably take the manufacturer to court, where criminal penalties could be imposed. The FDA can also require recalls in certain instances with infant formulas, biological products, and devices that pose a serious health hazard. Manufacturers may of course recall drugs on their own and do so from time to time for any number of reasons.

Recall Classifications

There are three classes of recalls:

Class I

Where there is a strong likelihood that the product will cause serious adverse effects or death.

Class II

Where a product may cause temporary but reversible adverse effects, or in which there is little likelihood of serious adverse effects.

Class III

Where a product is not likely to cause adverse effects.

How an FDA requested recall works:

Reports of adverse effects

The FDA receives enough reports of adverse effects or misbranding that it decides the product is a threat to the public health. It contacts the manufacturer and recommends a recall.

Manufacturer agrees to recall

If the manufacturer agrees to a recall, they must establish a recall strategy with the FDA that addresses the depth of the recall, the extent of public warnings, and a means for checking the effectiveness of the recall. The depth of the recall is identified by wholesale, retail, or consumer levels. The effectiveness may require anything from no follow-up to a complete follow-up check of everyone who should have been notified of the recall. Checks can be made by personal visit, phone calls, or letters.

Customers contacted

Once the strategy is finalized, the manufacturer contacts its customers by telegram, mailgram, or first-class letters with the following information:

✔ the product name, size, lot number, code or serial number, and any other important identifying information.

✔ reason for the recall and the hazard involved.

✔ instructions on what to do with the product, beginning with ceasing distribution.

Recalls listed publicly

Recalls are listed in the weekly FDA Enforcement Report.

LEGAL ENVIRONMENT

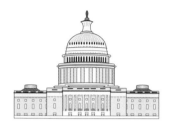 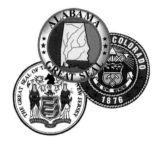

FEDERAL LAW

Federal laws provide a foundation for the state laws that govern the dispensing of prescription drugs in every state. In addition to the specific drug laws enforced by the FDA and DEA, there are federal laws regulating the treatment of patients (especially in nursing homes) that apply to various aspects of drug dispensing and use. These laws also guarantee certain patient rights which must be observed by all. These rights include: privacy and confidentiality, right to file complaints, information necessary for informed consent, and the right to refuse treatment. It is necessary for all health care workers to know the specific patient rights that apply to their workplace.

STATE LAW

In each state, there is a **state board of pharmacy** responsible for licensing all prescribers and dispensers. State boards also administer state regulations for the practice of pharmacy in the state. In many cases, state regulations are stricter than federal, and the stricter state regulation must be followed. By definition, this means that the lesser federal requirements are also being met. Therefore, following both state and federal regulations is mandatory.

Each state has specific regulations which may or may not be different from other states. For example, a few states allow pharmacists to prescribe under limited conditions. Many allow nurse practitioners and physician assistants to prescribe. When states allow non-physicians to prescribe, they limit their **scope of authority.** That is, a non-physician prescriber may only prescribe for certain conditions and must follow a strict set of rules (called a **protocol**) that determines the prescription. Non-physician prescribers include dentists, veterinarians, pharmacists, nurse practitioners, and physician assistants, among others. Since states differ on many aspects of pharmacy practice, including who may and may not prescribe, it is necessary to know your own state's regulations.

States regulate the work of non-prescribers such as medical assistants and technicians in part by holding the prescriber, supervisor, or employer involved responsible for their performance. They are generally required to provide a description to the employee of all the regulations (federal, state, and local) that apply to their job, to monitor performance, and to assure **compliance** with the appropriate regulations.

compliance doing what is required.
negligence failing to do something that should or must be done.

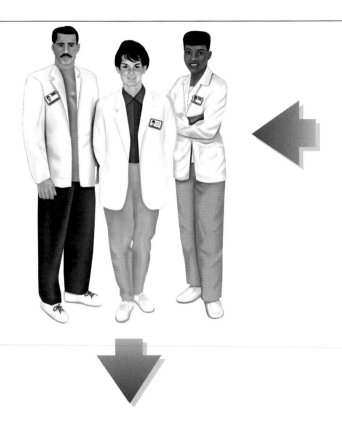

OTHER STANDARDS

Besides the FDA, DEA, and the State Board of Pharmacy, there are various professional bodies and associations which set and maintain pharmacy standards. These include:

➡ **United States Pharmacopeia:** The USP is a voluntary not-for-profit organization that sets standards for the manufacture and distribution of drugs and related products in the United States. These standards are directly referred to by federal and state laws and are published in the "United States Pharmacopeia and the National Formulary."

➡ **Joint Commission on Accreditation of Health Care Organizations:** JCAHO is an independent non-profit organization that establishes standards and monitors compliance for nearly twenty thousand health care programs in the United States. JCAHO-accredited programs include hospitals, health care networks, HMOs, and nursing homes, among others.

➡ **American Society of Health-System Pharmacists:** The ASHP is a 30,000 member association for pharmacists practicing in hospitals, HMOs, long-term care facilities, home care agencies, and other health care systems. It is an accrediting organization for pharmacy residency and pharmacy technician training programs.

➡ **The American Society for Consultant Pharmacists:** The ASCP sets standards for practice for pharmacists who provide medication distribution and consultant services to nursing homes.

LIABILITY

Legal liability means you can be prosecuted for misconduct. This is true even if you are directed to do it by a supervisor, physician, patient, or customer. Misconduct doesn't necessarily mean you intended to do something, or even that you actively did it. You can be guilty of misconduct by simply failing to do something you should have done. This is called **negligence**, and is the most common form of misconduct. Here are some ways you can be negligent:

➡ failing to maintain patient confidentiality.
➡ failing to recognize expired drugs.
➡ calculation errors.
➡ dispensing the wrong medication.
➡ incorrect handling of controlled substance.
➡ inaccurate record keeping.

 Basic criminal and civil laws also apply to health care professionals, which means that crimes like theft, discrimination, sexual harassment, fraud, etc. are punishable just as they would be outside of your job.

REVIEW

KEY CONCEPTS

- ✔ In the United States, the leading enforcement agency at the federal level for regulations concerning drug products is the Food and Drug Administration.
- ✔ The distribution of drugs that may be easily abused is controlled by the Drug Enforcement Administration (DEA) within the Justice Department.
- ✔ Before it is approved for marketing, a new drug must be shown to be both safe and effective and that its benefits substantially outweigh its risks.
- ✔ Federal law defines what drugs require a prescription by a licensed practitioner.
- ✔ Manufacturers' containers for prescription drugs must have this legend on the label: "Caution: Federal Law prohibits dispensing without a prescription." By 2003, it must be changed to "Rx only."
- ✔ Pharmacists must offer counseling to patients regarding medications.
- ✔ Federal law requires child-proof packaging on all controlled and most prescription drugs dispensed by pharmacies.
- ✔ Placebos are inactive substances, not real medications, that are used to test the effectiveness of drugs.
- ✔ Once a patent for a brand drug expires, other manufacturers may copy the drug and release it under its pharmaceutical or "generic" name.
- ✔ All drugs are required to have clear and accurate information for all labels, inserts, packaging, and so on, but there are different information requirements for various categories of drugs.
- ✔ The minimum requirements on prescription labels for most drugs are as follows: name and address of dispenser, prescription serial number, date of prescription or filling, name of prescriber, name of patient, directions for use, and cautionary statements.
- ✔ Controlled drugs have greater requirements for labeling.
- ✔ Manufacturers must clearly label controlled drugs with their control classification.
- ✔ All prescribers of controlled substances are assigned a DEA number which must be used on all controlled drug prescriptions.
- ✔ There is always the risk that an approved drug may produce adverse side effects when used on a larger population.
- ✔ Recalls are, with a few exceptions, voluntary on the part of the manufacturer.
- ✔ Federal laws provide a foundation for the state laws which govern pharmacy practice in every state.
- ✔ State boards of pharmacy are responsible for licensing all prescribers and dispensers and administering regulations for the practice of pharmacy in the state.
- ✔ Legal liability means you can be prosecuted for misconduct.

SELF TEST

MATCH THE TERMS.

answers can be checked in the glossary

Terms: adverse effect, controlled substance mark, injunction, labeling, legend drug, liability, NDC (National Drug Code), negligence, pediatric, placebo, recall, therapeutic

Definitions:
- a court order preventing a specific action, such as the distribution of a potentially dangerous drug.
- an inactive substance given in place of a medication.
- an unintended side affect of a medication that is negative or in some way injurious to a patient's health.
- any drug which requires a prescription and this "legend" on the label: Rx only.
- failing to do something you should have done
- having to do with the treatment of children.
- important associated information that is not on the label of a drug product itself.
- means you can be prosecuted for misconduct.
- serving to cure or heal.
- the action taken to remove a drug from the market and have it returned to the manufacturer.
- the mark (CII-CV) which indicates the control category of a drug with a potential for abuse.
- the number on a manufacturer's label indicating the manufacturer and product information.

CHOOSE THE BEST ANSWER. *answers are in the back of the book*

1. Pharmacies located in health care institutions (hospitals, etc.) are required to follow regulations of this organization.
   a. ASHP
   b. USP
   c. ASCP
   d. JCAHO

2. The practice of pharmacy is influenced by federal and state laws. Which major federal law deals with the issue of safety caps?
   a. Federal Food, Drug and Cosmetic Act (FDC)
   b. The Controlled Substance Act (CSA)
   c. The Poison Prevention Packaging Act
   d. The Hazardous Substance Labeling Act

3. Of the following Schedule of drugs, which one deals with drugs that have no accepted medical use in the United States?
   a. Schedule I
   b. Schedule II
   c. Schedule III
   d. Schedule IV

4. Recalls, action taken to remove a drug from the market, are based on different classes. Which class of Recall indicates there is a strong likelihood that the product will cause serious adverse effects or death.
   a. Class I
   b. Class II
   c. Class III
   d. Class IV

HOW DRUGS WORK

Drugs produce their individual effects on the body as either desired effects or undesired effects.

Once they are in the blood, drugs are circulated throughout the body. The properties of both the drug and the body influence where the drug will go, and what concentration it will have at each place. The place where a drug causes an effect to occur is called the **site of action**. Some of the effects caused by the drug are desired effects, and some are undesired. *The objective of drug therapy is to deliver the right drug in the right concentration to the right site of action at the right time to produce the desired effect.*

When a drug produces an effect, it is interacting on a molecular level with cell material or structure.

The cell material directly involved in the action of the drug is called its **receptor.** The receptor is often described as a lock into which the drug molecule fits as a key, and only those drugs able to bind chemically to the receptors in a particular site of action can produce effects in that site. This is why specific cells only respond to certain drugs, even though their receptors are exposed to any drug molecules that are present in the body. This is also why drugs are **selective** in their action. That is, they only act on specific targeted receptors and the tissues they affect.

Receptors are located on the surfaces of cell membranes and inside cells.

There are many different types of receptors, having many different roles in the body's processes. Most receptors can be found throughout the body, though some occur in only a few places. Receptor activation is responsible for most of the pharmacological responses in the body.

---

biopharmaceutics the study of the factors associated with drug products and physiological processes, and the resulting systemic concentrations of the drugs.

site of action the location where an administered drug produces an effect.

receptor the cellular material at the site of action that interacts with the drug.

selective (action) the characteristic of a drug that makes its action specific to certain receptors and the tissues they affect.

DRUG ACTION AT THE SITE OF ACTION

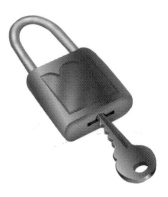

Like a lock and key, only certain drugs are able to interact with certain receptors.

Primary Types of Action

When drugs interact with the site of action, they can:

➡ act through physical action, as with the protective effects of ointments upon topical application;

➡ react chemically, as with antacids that reduce excess gastric acid;

➡ modify the metabolic activity of pathogens, as with antibiotics;

➡ change the characteristics of plasma to draw water out of tissues and into the blood.

➡ incorporate into cellular material to interfere with normal cell function.

➡ join with other chemicals to form a complex that is more easily excreted.

➡ modify the biochemical or metabolic process of the body's cells or enzyme systems.

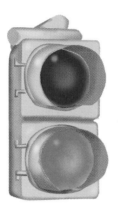

antagonists
block action

agonists activate
receipts

Other Drug Actions

➥ Some drugs work by changing the ability of ions to move into or out of cells. For example, sodium or calcium ion channels can open and allow movement of the ions into nerve cells, stimulating them. With potassium channels, the opposite can happen. The channels can open and allow the movement of potassium ions out of nerve cells, blocking their function.

➥ Some drugs modify the creation, release, or control of nerve cell hormones that regulate different physiological processes.

When drug molecules bind with a receptor, they can cause a reaction that stimulates or inhibits cell functions.

The pharmacological effects of this are called **agonism** or **antagonism**. **Agonists** are drugs that activate receptors and produce a response that may either accelerate or slow normal cell processes, depending on the type of receptor involved. For example, epinephrine-like drugs act on the heart to increase the heart rate, and acetylcholine-like drugs act on the heart to slow the heart rate. Both are agonists. **Antagonists** are drugs that bind to receptors but do not activate them. They block the receptors' action by preventing other drugs or substances from interacting with them.

The number of receptors available to interact with a drug will directly influence the effect.

A minimum number of receptors have to be occupied by drug molecules to produce the desired effect. If there are too few drug molecules to occupy the necessary number of receptors, there will be little or no effect. In this case, increasing the dosage will increase the effect. On the other hand, once all receptors are occupied, increasing the dosage will not increase the effect.

Receptors can be changed by drug use.

For example, long term stimulation of cells with an agonist can reduce the number or sensitivity of the receptors, and the effect of the drug is reduced. Extended use of an antagonist can increase the number or sensitivity of receptors, and if the antagonist is stopped abruptly, the cells can have an extreme reaction to an agonist. To avoid such withdrawal symptoms, some drugs must be gradually discontinued.

 agonist drugs that activate receptors to accelerate or slow normal cell function.

antagonist drugs that bind with receptors but do not activate them. They block receptor action by preventing other drugs or substances from activating them.

CONCENTRATION & EFFECT

It is difficult to measure the amount of a drug at the site of action and therefore to predict an effect based upon it.

One problem is that many factors influence a drug's movement from the site of administration to the site of action (metabolism, excretion, membrane permeability, etc.). It can also be physically impossible to measure the site of action either because of its unknown location or small size.

One way to monitor the amount of a drug in the body and its effect at the site of action is to use a *dose-response curve.*

A specific dose of a drug is given to one subject and the effect or response is measured. When a series of such doses is given to a number of people, the results show that some people respond to low doses but others require larger doses for a response to be produced. This is due to **human variability**: different people have different characteristics that affect how a drug product behaves in them. Some differences are due to the product itself, but most come from how the drug is transported from the site of administration to the site of action, and how it interacts with the receptor.

Another way to monitor a drug's concentration in the body and its related effect is to determine its concentration in the body's fluids.

Of the body's fluids, blood is generally used because of its rapid and intensive interaction between the site of administration and the site of action. As a result, knowing a drug's concentration in the blood can be directly related to its effect and this is the most common way to analyze the potential effect of a drug.

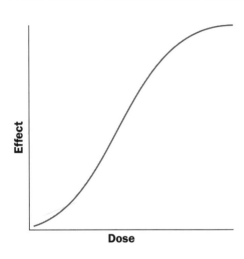

A typical dose-response curve shows that responses increase as the doses are increased.

Blood Concentration-Time Profiles

Blood concentration-time profiles have these applications:

➡ Manufacturers use their data to evaluate their drug products

➡ Pharmacy professionals use them to visualize the consequences of incorrectly compounding a formulation or of using the wrong route of administration.

➡ Researchers and clinicians use them to measure human variability in drug formulation performance (e.g., influence of age, gender, nationality, or disease).

➡ Physicians and pharmacists use them to monitor the drug therapy of patients.

dose response curve a graph of the responses in different patients to a series of doses .

blood concentration-time profile a graph of the blood concentration of a drug over time.

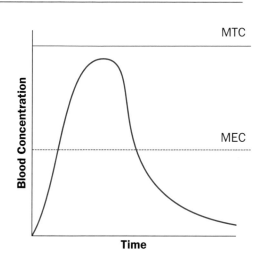

An advantage of using blood concentrations as a measure of "drug amount in the body" is that blood can be repeatedly sampled. When sampling covers several hours or more, a **blood concentration-time profile** can be developed. Plasma or serum concentrations can also be used, and the same profiles will also result.

For most drugs, changes in the blood concentration-time profile reflect changes in concentration at the site of action and therefore changes in effect.

There are exceptions to this. The concentration of some drugs in the site of action produces an action hours or days later. Other drugs show no relationship between blood concentrations and concentrations in the site of action. Still others don't depend on blood concentrations at all to produce an effect.

A Sample Profile

The illustration above shows a typical blood concentration–time curve for a drug given orally. The blood concentration begins at zero at the time the drug is administered (before it has been absorbed into the blood). With time, the drug leaves the formulation and enters the blood, causing concentrations to rise. To produce an effect, they must achieve a **minimum effective concentration (MEC).** This is when there is enough drug at the site of action to produce a response. The time this occurs is called the **onset of action.** With most drugs, when blood concentrations increase, so does the intensity of the effect, since *blood concentrations reflect the site of action concentrations that produce the response.*

Some drugs have an upper blood concentration limit beyond which there are undesired or toxic effects. This limit is called the **minimum toxic concentration (MTC).** The range between the minimum effective concentration and the minimum toxic concentration is called the **therapeutic window.** *When concentrations are in this range, most patients receive the maximum benefit from their drug therapy with a minimum of risk.*

The last part of the curve shows the blood concentrations declining as absorption is complete. The time between the onset of action and the time when the minimum effective concentration is reached by the declining blood concentrations is called the **duration of action.** The duration of action is the time the drug should produce the desired effect.

 minimum effective concentration (MEC) the blood concentration needed of a drug to produce a response.

onset of action the time MEC is reached and the response occurs.

therapeutic window a drug's blood concentration range between its minimum effective concentration and minimum toxic concentration.

ADME PROCESSES & DIFFUSION

Blood concentrations are the result of four simultaneously acting processes: absorption, distribution, metabolism, and excretion.

These four processes are referred to as the **ADME** processes, but may also be called **disposition**. Metabolism and excretion combined are often referred to as **elimination**.

The transfer of drug into the blood from an administered drug product is called absorption.

When a drug product is first administered, absorption is the primary process. Distribution, metabolism, and excretion will also occur, but the amount of drug available for them is much less than the amount of drug available for absorption. So these processes have little effect. As more of the drug is absorbed into the blood, it is available to undergo the other processes and their roles increase.

A drug's distribution will be affected by physiological functions and its own properties.

Though blood may deliver the drug to body tissue, if the drug cannot penetrate the tissue's membranes, it will not interact with the receptors inside. The opposite situation can also occur. A drug may be able to enter a tissue, but if there is not enough blood flow to the tissue, little of the drug will enter. Distribution is also influenced by drug binding to proteins in the blood or in tissues.

The ADME processes are all illustrated by blood concentration–time curves.

Concentrations rise during absorption, but as absorption nears completion, metabolism and elimination become the primary processes, and they cause the blood concentration to decline.

In the first part of a blood concentration–time curve, absorption is the primary process and concentrations rise. As absorption nears completion, metabolism and excretion become the primary processes, with distribution occurring throughout.

 Even though the ADME processes occur simultaneously, they are studied separately to understand the critical factors responsible for each process.

disposition a term sometimes used to refer to all of the ADME processes together.

passive diffusion the movement of drugs from an area of higher concentration to lower concentration.

active transport the movement of drug molecules across membranes by active means, rather than passive diffusion.

hydrophobic water repelling; cannot associate with water.

hydrophilic capable of associating with or absorbing water.

lipoidal fat like substance.

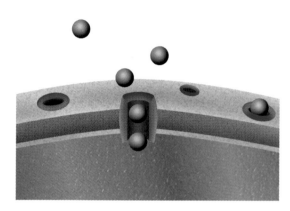

A diagram showing drug molecules penetrating a cell membrane. These molecules generally move from areas of higher concentration to areas of lower concentration in a process called passive diffusion.

Ionization and Unionization

Most drugs are weak organic acids and bases that will come apart (**dissociate**) and attach to other chemicals (**associate**) in solutions. When acids dissociate, they become **ionized**. That is, they carry an electric charge. When bases dissociate, they become **unionized** (have no charge).

Unionized drugs penetrate biological membranes more easily than ionized drugs for these reasons:

➡ unionized drugs are more soluble in fats (**lipids**).

➡ charges on biological membranes bind or repel ionized drug.

➡ ionized drugs associate with water molecules, creating larger particles with reduced penetrating capability.

Besides the four ADME processes, a critical factor of drug concentration and effect is how drugs move through biological membranes. Before an effective concentration of a drug can reach its site of action, it must overcome many barriers, most of which are biological membranes.

Biological membranes are complex structures composed of lipids (fats) and proteins.

They are generally classified in three types: those made up of *several layers of cells*, such as the skin; those made up of *a single layer of cells*, as in the intestinal lining; and those of *less than one cell* in thickness, as in the membrane of a single cell.

Most drugs penetrate biological membranes by *passive diffusion*.

Drugs in the body's fluids will generally move from an area of higher concentration to an area of lower concentration until the concentrations in each area are balanced, or in a state of equilibrium. This process is called passive diffusion. It is the most common way a drug penetrates biological membranes and is a primary factor in the distribution process. This movement from higher to lower concentration causes most orally administered drugs to move from the intestine to the blood and from the blood to the site of action.

Drug concentration is not the only factor influencing diffusion.

Membranes are **lipoidal** (fat-like), and drugs that are more lipid (fat) soluble will penetrate them better than those that are not. These drugs are called **hydrophobic**. They hate or repel water and are attracted to fats. **Hydrophilic** drugs (drugs attracted to water) can also penetrate membranes, however. It is thought that they move through water-filled passages called **aqueous pores** which allow water (and any drug contained in it) into cells.

In addition to passive diffusion, some drugs may be carried across membranes by *specialized transport mechanisms*.

This type of **active transport** (as opposed to passive) is thought to explain how certain substances that do not penetrate membranes by passive diffusion nevertheless succeed in entering a cell.

ABSORPTION

Once a drug is released from its dosage formulation, the process that transfers it into the blood is called *absorption*.

Absorption occurs to some extent with any route of administration. For example, even a drug in an intravenous suspension or emulsion must first be released from the dosage form to be absorbed into the blood. However, since most drugs are given orally, this page and the next several will look at the ADME processes from the perspective of oral administration.

One of the primary factors affecting oral drug absorption is the *gastric emptying time*.

This is the time a drug will stay in the stomach before it is emptied into the small intestine. Since stomach acid can degrade many drugs and since most absorption occurs in the intestine, gastric emptying time can significantly affect a drug's action. If a drug remains in the stomach too long, it can be degraded or destroyed, and its effect decreased. Gastric emptying time can be affected by a various conditions, including the amount and type of food in the stomach, the presence of other drugs, the person's body position, and their emotional condition. Some factors increase the gastric emptying time, but most slow it.

Once a drug leaves the stomach, its rate of movement through the intestines directly affects its absorption.

Slower than normal intestinal movement can lead to increased drug absorption because the drug is in contact with the intestinal membrane longer. Faster than normal intestinal movement can produce the opposite result since the drug moves through the intestinal tract too rapidly to be fully absorbed.

Bile salts and enzymes from the intestinal tract also affect absorption.

Bile salts improve the absorption of hydrophobic and certain other drugs. Enzymes added to the intestinal tract's contents from pancreatic secretions destroy certain drugs and consequently decrease their absorption. Enzymes in the intestinal wall also destroy drugs as they pass from the gut into the blood, decreasing their absorption.

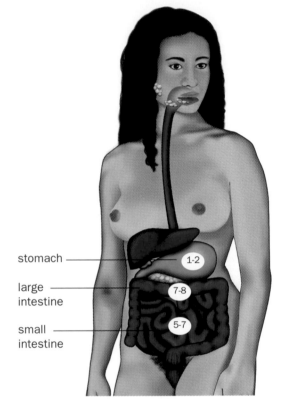

stomach
large intestine
small intestine

gastrointestinal organs and their pH

Most drugs are given orally and absorbed into the blood from the small intestine. The small intestine's large surface area makes absorption easier. However, there are many conditions in the stomach that can affect absorption positively or negatively before the drug even reaches the small intestine. Once in the intestines, there are many additional factors that can affect a drug's absorption.

 gastric emptying time the time a drug will stay in the stomach before it is emptied into the small intestine.

DISTRIBUTION

Distribution involves the movement of a drug within the body once the drug has reached the blood.

Blood carries the drug throughout the body and to its sites of action, as well as to the organs responsible for the metabolism and excretion of the drug.

The blood flow rates to certain organs have a significant effect on distribution.

Drugs are rapidly distributed to organs having high blood flow rates such as the heart, liver, and kidneys. Distribution to areas such as muscle, fat, and skin is usually slower because they have lower blood flow rates.

The permeability of tissue membranes to a drug is also important.

Most tissue membranes are easily penetrated by most drugs. Small drug molecules (those having a low molecular weight) and drugs that are hydrophobic will generally diffuse through tissue membranes with ease. Some tissue membranes have specialized transport mechanisms that assist penetration. A few tissue membranes are highly selective in allowing drug penetration. The **blood-brain barrier,** for example, limits drug access to the brain and the cerebral spinal fluid.

Protein binding **can also affect distribution.**

Many drugs will "bind" to proteins in blood plasma, forming a complex. The large size of such complexes prevents the bound drug from entering its sites of action, metabolism, and excretion—making it inactive. Only free or "unbound" drug can move through tissue membranes. Another drug with a stronger binding characteristic can displace a less well bound drug, making it pharmacologically active again and increasing its effect.

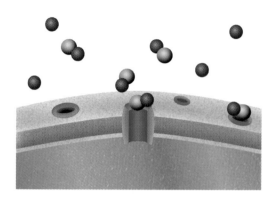

Protein Binding

Many drugs bind to proteins in blood plasma to form a complex that is too large to penetrate cell openings. So the drug remains inactive.

Protein binding can be considered a type of drug storage within the body. Some drugs bind extensively to proteins in fat and muscle, and are gradually released as the blood concentration of the drug falls. These drugs remain in the body a long time, and therefore have a long duration of action.

Selective Action

Though drugs are widely distributed throughout the body once they reach the bloodstream, they can have action that is selective to certain tissues or organs. This is due both to the specific nature of receptor action as well as to various factors that can affect the distribution of the drug. This is why drugs can be targeted to specific therapeutic effects.

Since most receptors can be found in multiple areas throughout the body, most drugs have multiple effects. This is why a drug may be used for different therapies. It is also one reason they have side effects. For example, terbutaline is used for bronchodilation. It will also delay labor in pregnant women.

blood–brain barrier a barrier membrane between the blood and the brain that blocks certain harmful substances from entering the brain.

complex when molecules of different chemicals attach to each other, as in protein binding.

protein binding the attachment of a drug molecule to a plasma or tissue protein, effectively making the drug inactive, but also keeping it within the body.

METABOLISM

Drug metabolism refers to the body's process of transforming drugs.

The transformed drug is called a **metabolite.** Most metabolites are inactive and are excreted. However, the metabolites of some drugs are active, and they will produce effects on the individual until they are further metabolized or excreted.

The primary site of drug metabolism in the body is the liver.

Enzymes are complex proteins that cause chemical reactions in other substances. The enzymes produced by the liver interact with drugs and transform them into metabolites.

In response to the chronic administration of certain drugs, the liver will increase its enzyme production.

This is called **enzyme induction,** and it results in greater metabolism of a drug. As a result, larger doses of the drug must be administered to produce the same therapeutic effects. Some drugs decrease or delay enzyme activity, a process called **enzyme inhibition.** In this case, smaller doses of the drug will be needed to avoid toxicity from drug accumulation.

The liver may secrete drugs or their metabolites into bile that is stored in the gall bladder.

The gall bladder empties the bile (and any drugs or metabolites in it) into the intestine in response to food entering the intestinal tract. This is called **enterohepatic cycling.** Any drugs or metabolites contained in the bile may be reabsorbed or simply eliminated with the feces.

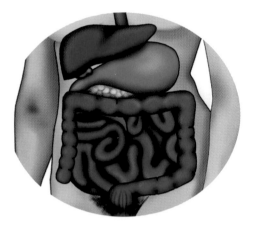

First Pass Metabolism

With oral administration, once a drug is absorbed from the enteral tract, it is immediately delivered to the liver. It will then be transferred into the general systemic circulation.

Before it reaches the circulatory system, however, the drug can be substantially degraded or destroyed by the liver's enzymes. This is called "first-pass metabolism" and is an important factor with orally administered drugs. Because of it, certain drugs must be administered by other routes. Any route other than oral either partially or completely bypasses first-pass metabolism.

---

metabolite the substance resulting from the body's transformation of an administered drug.

enzyme a complex protein that causes chemical reactions in other substances

enzyme induction the increase in enzyme activity that results in greater metabolism of drugs.

enzyme inhibition the decrease in enzyme activity that results in reduced metabolism of drugs.

first pass metabolism the substantial degradation of a drug caused by enzyme metabolism in the liver before the drug reaches the systemic circulation.

enterohepatic cycling the transfer of drugs and their metabolites from the liver to the bile in the gall bladder and then into the intestine.

EXCRETION

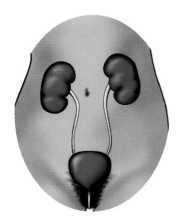

Factors Affecting Urinary Excretion

➡ If the kidney's process of filtration becomes impaired, excretion will be reduced and drugs will accumulate in the blood. In such cases, the dosage of drugs must be decreased or the dosage interval lengthened.

➡ Some drugs affect the excretion of others. In such cases, the affected drug will accumulate in the blood, and the dosage of the affected drug must be decreased or the dosage interval lengthened.

➡ The pH of the urine can affect the reabsorption of some drugs. A high pH can increase excretion of weak acids such as salicylates and phenobarbital. The opposite effect can occur with a low (acidic) pH.

Most drugs and their metabolites are excreted by the kidneys through the urine.

Some orally administered drugs are not easily absorbed from the gastrointestinal tract and as a result are significantly excreted in the feces. Excretion can also occur through the bile and certain drugs are removed from the lungs through the expired breath.

The kidneys filter the blood and remove waste (including drugs and metabolites) from it.

As blood flows through a kidney, some of the plasma water is filtered from it into the kidney **nephron** (the functional unit of the kidney) in a process called **glomerular filtration**. As the water moves through the nephron, waste substances are secreted into the fluid, with urine as the end result. Some drugs can be filtered and reabsorbed back into the blood during this process, and some drugs are not filtered at all but are secreted into the urine by specialized processes.

The rate of urinary excretion is much faster than that of fecal excretion.

Drugs that will be excreted through the feces generally take a day to be excreted, whereas drugs may be excreted through the urine within hours of administration.

nephron the functional unit of the kidneys.
glomerular filtration the blood filtering process of the kidneys.

BIOEQUIVALENCE

The amount of a drug that is available to the site of action and the rate at which it is available is called the *bioavailability* of the drug. By FDA definition, it is measured by determining *the relative amount of an administered dose of a drug that reaches the general systemic circulation and the rate at which this occurs.* As a result, it can be measured by a blood concentration-time curve.

Comparing the bioavailability of one dosage form to another determines their *bioequivalency*.

The FDA requires drug manufacturers to perform bioequivalency studies on their products before they are approved for marketing. In such studies, the bioavailability of the active ingredients in a test formulation is compared to that in a standard formulation. Bioequivalency studies are also used to compare bioavailability between different dosage forms (tablets, capsules, etc), different manufacturers, and different production lots.

A B C D *bioavailability* the relative amount of an administered dose that reaches the general circulation and the rate at which this occurs.

bioequivalence the comparison of bioavailability between two dosage forms.

BIOEQUIVALENCE

Bioequivalent Drug Products

Bioequivalent drug products are pharmaceutical equivalents or alternatives which have *essentially* the same rate and extent of absorption when administered at the same dose of the active ingredient under similar conditions.

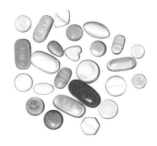

Differences Between Equivalents

Exact bioequivalency between drug products (where blood concentration–time curves for each product are identical) doesn't occur, and is not expected. There are simply too many variables that can contribute to differences between products. In tablets, for example, there can be different amounts or types of fillers, binders, lubricants, and other components. The particle size of the drug itself may be slightly different. The manufacturing process may also produce different results in size, hardness, or other characteristics (especially for different manufacturers, but also for the same manufacturer at different times or different plants). Changes in these or various other factors can affect the bioavailability of a drug. Though there can be differences in the bioavailability of a drug between bioequivalent products because of this, the differences must be slight and not significant.

The following terms are used by the FDA to define the type of equivalency between drug products:

Pharmaceutical Equivalents

Pharmaceutical equivalents are drug products that contain identical amounts of the same active ingredients in the same dosage form, and that meet the same applicable standards of identity, strength, quality, and purity, including potency and, where applicable, content uniformity, disintegration times, and/or dissolution rates. They do not have to contain the same inactive ingredients, or have the same shape, release mechanisms, packaging, or expiration time. Since pharmaceutical equivalents may have different inactive ingredients, different pharmaceutically equivalent products may not be equally suitable for a patient. Some patients may be unusually sensitive to an inactive ingredient in one product that another product does not contain.

➡ same active ingredients
➡ same amounts
➡ same dosage form
➡ inactive ingredients can be different

Pharmaceutical Alternatives

Pharmaceutical alternatives are drug products that contain the identical active ingredients, but not necessarily in the same amount or dosage form. Each such drug product must individually meet the applicable standards of its dosage form. They do not have to contain the same inactive ingredients, or have the same shape, release mechanisms, packaging, or expiration time.

➡ same active ingredients
➡ amounts can be different
➡ dosage form can be different

Therapeutic Equivalents

Therapeutic equivalents are pharmaceutical equivalents which produce the same therapeutic effect in patients.

Note: a related term is **therapeutic alternative**. This refers to drugs that have different active ingredients but produce similar therapeutic effect.

➡ pharmaceutical equivalents that produce the same effects in patients.

 pharmaceutical equivalent drug products that contain identical amounts of the same active ingredients in the same dosage form.

pharmaceutical alternative drug products that contain the same active ingredients, but not necessarily in the same amount or dosage form.

therapeutic equivalent pharmaceutical equivalents that produce the same effects in patients.

REVIEW

KEY CONCEPTS

- ✔ The objective of drug therapy is to deliver the right drug, in the right concentration, to the right site of action at the right time to produce the desired effect.

- ✔ Only those drugs able to bind chemically to the receptors in a particular site of action can produce effects in that site. This is why specific cells only respond to certain drugs.

- ✔ Receptor activation is responsible for most of the pharmacological responses in the body.

- ✔ Agonists are drugs that activate receptors and produce a response that may either accelerate or slow normal cell processes. Antagonists are drugs that bind to receptors but do not activate them. They prevent other drugs or substances from interacting with receptors.

- ✔ The primary way to monitor a drug's concentration in the body and its related effect is to determine its blood concentrations.

- ✔ To produce an effect, a drug must achieve a minimum effective concentration (MEC). This is when there is enough drug at the site of action to produce a response.

- ✔ The range between the minimum effective concentration and the minimum toxic concentration is called the therapeutic window. When concentrations are in this range, most patients receive the maximum benefit from their drug therapy with a minimum of risk.

- ✔ Blood concentrations are the result of four simultaneously acting processes: absorption, distribution, metabolism, and excretion.

- ✔ The transfer of drug into the blood from an administered drug product is called absorption.

- ✔ Besides the four ADME processes, a critical factor of drug concentration and effect is how drugs move through biological membranes. Most drugs penetrate biological membranes by passive diffusion.

- ✔ Most drugs are given orally and absorbed into the blood from the small intestine. One of the primary factors affecting oral drug absorption is the gastric emptying time.

- ✔ Many drugs bind to proteins in blood plasma to form a complex that is too large to penetrate cell openings. So the drug remains inactive.

- ✔ The primary site of drug metabolism in the body is the liver. Enzymes produced by the liver interact with drugs and transform them into metabolites.

- ✔ The kidneys filter the blood and remove waste (including drugs and metabolites) from it.

- ✔ The amount of a drug that is available to the site of action and the rate at which it is available is called the bioavailability of the drug.

- ✔ Bioequivalent drug products are pharmaceutical equivalents or alternatives which have essentially the same rate and extent of absorption when administered at the same dose of the active ingredient under similar conditions.

- ✔ Pharmaceutical equivalents are drug products that contain identical amounts of the same active ingredients in the same dosage form, but may contain different inactive ingredients.

- ✔ Pharmaceutical alternatives are drug products that contain the identical active ingredients, but not necessarily in the same amount or dosage form.

SELF TEST

answers can be checked in the glossary

agonist

antagonist

bioavailability

bioequivalence

enzyme induction

first pass metabolism

passive diffusion

protein binding

receptor

selective (action)

site of action

the location where an administered drug produces an effect.

the cellular material which interacts with the drug.

the characteristic of a drug that makes its action specific to certain receptors.

drugs that activate receptors to accelerate or slow normal cell function.

drugs that bind with receptors but do not activate them.

the movement of drugs from an area of higher concentration to lower concentration.

the attachment of a drug molecule to a protein, effectively making the drug inactive.

the increase in enzyme activity that results in greater metabolism of drugs.

the substantial degradation of a drug caused by enzyme metabolism in the liver.

the relative amount of an administered dose that reaches the general circulation and the rate at which this occurs.

the comparison of bioavailability between two dosage forms.

CHOOSE THE BEST ANSWER. *answers are in the back of the book*

1. Most drugs and their metabolites are excreted by the
   a. liver
   b. kidneys
   c. gall bladder
   d. gastrointestinal tract

2. The percentage or fraction of the administered dose of a drug that actually reaches systemic circulation and the rate at which this occurs is the drug's
   a. bioequivalence
   b. bioavailability
   c. biotransformation
   d. gastric emptying time

3. In metabolism, the breakdown of drugs into metabolites is caused by
   a. passive diffusion
   b. glomerular filtration
   c. enterohepatic cycling
   d. enzymes

4. In the blood concentration-time curve, the range between the Minimum Toxic Concentration (MTC) and the Minimum Effective Concentration (MEC) is called
   a. the onset of action
   b. the concentration at site of action
   c. the duration of action
   d. the therapeutic window

HUMAN VARIABILITY

Human variability in biopharmaceutics and disposition is a significant factor in the outcome of drug activity and effect. Differences in age, weight, genetics, and gender are among the significant factors that influence the differences in response to medication among people.

Age

Human life is a continuous process but it is usually characterized as having stages. The distinctions between the stages are relative and vary among individuals, but they are based on relevant physiological characteristics. The stages are generally considered as:

➡ **Neonate**, up to one month after birth

➡ **Infant**, between the ages of one month and two years

➡ **Child**, between two years and twelve years of age

➡ **Adolescent**, between the ages of 13 and 19 years

➡ **Adult**, between 20 and 70 years

➡ **Elder**, older than 70 years of age

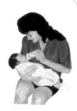

Drug distribution, metabolism, and excretion are quite different in the **neonate** and **infant** than in adults because their organ systems are not fully developed. They are not able to eliminate drugs as efficiently as adults. Older infants reach approximately adult levels of protein binding and kidney function, but liver function and the blood-brain barrier are still immature.

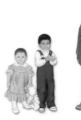

Children metabolize certain drugs more rapidly than adults. Their rate of metabolism increases between 1 year and 12 years of age depending on the child and the drug. Afterwards, metabolism rates decline with age to normal adult levels. Some of the drugs eliminated faster in children include clindamycin, valproic acid, ethosuximide, and theophylline.

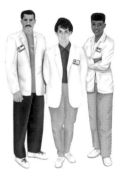

Adults

Adults experience a decrease in many physiological functions from 30 to 70 years of age, but these decreases and their affects on drug activity are gradual.

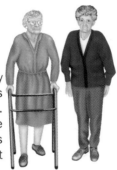

The Elderly

The elderly typically consume more drugs than other age groups. They also experience physiological changes that significantly affect drug action.

➡ Changes in gastric pH, gastric emptying time, intestinal movement, and gastrointestinal blood flow all tend to *slow the rate of absorption*.

➡ Changes in the cardiovascular system (including lower cardiac output) tend to *slow distribution* of drug molecules to their sites of action, metabolism, and excretion.

➡ Though there is probably a decrease in the liver's production of metabolizing enzymes, the metabolism of drugs does not appear to slow.

➡ A decline in kidney function (including glomerular filtration and drug secretion) occurs that tends to *slow urinary excretion of drugs*.

Gender

Gender is generally not considered a major influence on drug action. Most research has involved men, with the findings applied to women. One particular reason has been to avoid exposing a fetus or potential fetus to unknown risks.

However, some gender based differences in drug response appear to be related to hormonal fluctuations in women during the menstrual cycle. For women with clinical depression, for example, higher dosage levels of antidepressant medication may be necessary when menstrual symptoms are worst.

Distribution may also be somewhat different between men and women simply as a result of differences in body composition (males have more muscle, women more fat).

Pregnancy

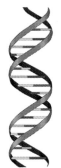

A number of physiological changes (including delayed gastric emptying and decreased movement in the gastrointestinal tract) occur in women in the latter stages of pregnancy.

These changes tend to *reduce the rate of absorption.* Drug binding may be reduced. *Urinary excretion increases,* and the rate of excretion for a number of drugs is much greater in pregnant women than in non-pregnant women.

Genetics

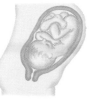

Genes determine the types and amounts of proteins produced in the body, with each person being somewhat different. Since drugs interact with proteins in plasma, tissues, receptor sites, and elsewhere, genetic differences can result in differences in drug action.

Genetics can also cause variations in metabolism in which people with certain genetic characteristics will not metabolize a drug that most people metabolize, or will metabolize it at an abnormal rate. In such cases, the individual may experience no therapeutic effect at all, or perhaps even an adverse or toxic effect instead.

Body Weight

Weight adjustments are generally not made for dosage regimens because the other variability factors tend to be more significant. However, weight adjustments may be needed for individuals whose weight is more than 50% higher than the average adult weight. Weight adjustments are also made for children, or unusually small, emaciated, or obese adult patients.

Psychological

Though the specific reasons are unknown, it is clear that psychological factors can influence individual responses to drug administration. For example, in clinical trials in which placebos are used, patients receiving them often report both therapeutic and adverse effects. This may account for some variability in patient responses to an administered (non-placebo) drug. At a fundamental level, it is a factor in patient willingness to follow prescribed dosage regimens.

ADVERSE EFFECTS

Drugs generally produce a mixture of *therapeutic* (desired) and *adverse effects* (undesired effects). An adverse effect can be any symptom or disease process and involve any organ. They may be common or rare, localized or widespread, mild or severe depending on the drug and the patient. Some adverse effects occur with usual doses of drugs (often called **side effects**). Others are more likely to occur only at higher than normal dosages.

Central Nervous System Effects

CNS effects may result from CNS stimulation (e.g., agitation, confusion, delirium, disorientation, hallucinations) or CNS depression (dizziness, drowsiness, sedation, coma, impaired respiration and circulation).

Hepatotoxicity

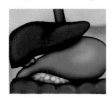

"Hepato" means "of the liver." Hepatotoxity includes hepatitis, hepatic necrosis, and biliary tract inflammation or obstruction. It is relatively rare but potentially life-threatening. Commonly used hepatotoxic drugs include acetaminophen, halothane, isoniazid, chlcrpromazine, methotrexate, nitrofurantoin, phenytoin, and aspirin.

ABCD *adverse effect* an undesired effect of drug therapy.

anaphylactic shock a potentially fatal hypersensitivity reaction producing severe respiratory distress and cardiovascular collapse.

hepato a prefix meaning "of the liver."

hypersensitivity an abnormal sensitivity generally resulting in an allergic reaction.

COMMON ADVERSE EFFECTS

Hypersensitivity or Allergy

Almost any drug, in almost any dose, can produce an allergic or hypersensitive reaction in a patient. It generally happens because a patient develops antibodies to a drug he or she has taken. Once this occurs, the drug will interact with the antibodies, releasing histamines and other substances that produce reactions that can range from mild rashes to potentially fatal **anaphylactic shock.**

Allergic reactions can occur within minutes or weeks of drug administration. Anaphylactic shock occurs within minutes. It is a hypersensitivity reaction that can lead to cardiovascular collapse and death if untreated. Its symptoms include severe respiratory distress and convulsions. Immediate emergency treatment with epinephrine, antihistamines, or bronchodilator drugs is required.

Gastrointestinal Effects

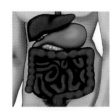

Anorexia, nausea, vomiting, constipation, and diarrhea are among the most common adverse reactions to drugs. More serious effects include ulcerations and colitis (irritable bowel disease).

Nephrotoxicity

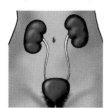

Kidney failure can occur with gentamicin and other aminoglycosides, and with ibuprofen and other nonsteroidal anti-inflammatory drugs.

Drug Dependence

Chronic usage of narcotic analgesics, sedative-hypnotic agents, antianxiety agents, and amphetamines often results in physiological or psychological dependence. Physiological dependence is accompanied by unpleasant physical withdrawal symptoms when the dose is discontinued or reduced. Psychological dependence involves an emotional or mental fixation on drug usage.

Idiosyncrasy

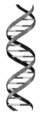

Idiosyncrasy is the unexpected reaction to a drug the first time it is given to a patient. Such reactions are generally thought to be caused by genetic characteristics that alter the patient's drug metabolizing enzymes.

Teratogenicity

This is the ability of a substance to cause abnormal fetal development when given to pregnant women. Drug groups considered teratogenic include analgesics, diuretics, antihistamines, antibiotics, and antiemetics.
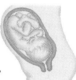

Hematological Effects

Blood coagulation, bleeding, and bone marrow disorders are potentially life threatening and can be caused by various drugs. Anticoagulants can cause excessive bleeding. Antineoplastic drugs may cause bone marrow depression.

Carcinogenicity

This is the ability of a substance to cause cancer. Several drugs are carcinogens, including some hormones and anticancer drugs.

 carcinogenicity the ability of a substance to cause cancer.

idiosyncrasy an unexpected reaction the first time a drug is taken, generally due to genetic causes.

nephrotoxicity the ability of a substance to harm the kidneys.

DRUG-DRUG INTERACTIONS

The administration of more than one drug at a time to a patient can cause *drug-drug interactions.* The probability of a drug-drug interaction increases with the number of drugs a patient takes. Such interactions can affect the disposition of one or more drugs and *result in either increases or decreases in therapeutic effects or adverse effects.* Some drug-drug interactions may not alter drug disposition but will still change the therapeutic effect.

Drug-drug interactions that *increase* the therapeutic or adverse effects of drugs:

➡ **Additive effects** occur when two drugs with similar pharmacological actions are taken.

   Example: alcohol + sedative drug = increased sedation

➡ **Synergism** or **potentiation** occurs when two drugs with different sites or mechanisms of action produce greater effects when taken together than either does when taken alone.

   Example: acetaminophen + codeine = increased analgesia

➡ **Interference** by one drug with the elimination of a second drug may intensify the effects of the second drug.

   Example: cimetidine inhibits drug metabolizing enzymes in the liver and therefore interferes with the metabolism of many drugs. When these drugs are given at the same time as cimetidine, their blood concentration increases and they are more likely to cause adverse reactions or toxic effects.

➡ **Displacement** of one drug from protein binding sites by a second drug increases the effects of the displaced drug. This occurs because the blood concentration of the now free displaced drug is increased.

   Example: aspirin + warfarin = increased anticoagulant effect

Time Course of Drug Interactions

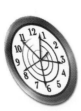

The time it takes for drug-drug interactions to occur can vary substantially. Some interactions occur almost immediately while others may take weeks. Knowing the time course of an interaction allows quick identification and treatment of potential interactions. It also allows clinicians to evaluate the relative importance of an interaction from two drugs compared to their therapeutic effects. For example, if an interaction requires one to two weeks to occur, short term administration over a few days may not cause a significant adverse effect.

An understanding of the ways drug-drug interactions occur is important. Examples of some common types are on these pages.

Drug-drug interactions that *decrease* the therapeutic effects of drugs:

➡ An **antidote** to a particular drug is given to **block or reduce its toxic effects.**

Example: naloxone + morphine = relief of morphine induced respiratory depression. Naloxone molecules displace morphine molecules from their receptor sites on nerve cells, preventing the morphine molecules from causing further effect.

➡ **Decreased intestinal absorption** of oral drugs occurs when drugs combine to produce nonabsorbable compounds.

Example: aluminum or magnesium hydroxide + oral tetracycline = binding of tetracycline to aluminum or magnesium. This causes decreased absorption and a decreased antibiotic effect of the tetracycline dose.

➡ When drugs activate metabolizing enzymes in the liver, it **increases the metabolism** of other drugs affected by the same enzymes. Enzyme inducing drugs include some anticonvulsants, barbiturates, and antihistamines.

Example: phenobarbital + warfarin = decreased effects of warfarin

➡ Some drugs **increase excretion** by raising urinary pH and lessening renal reabsorption.

Example: sodium bicarbonate + phenobarbital = increased excretion of phenobarbital. The sodium bicarbonate raises urine pH and ionizes the phenobarbital, increasing its excretion.

additive effects the increase in effect when two drugs with similar pharmacological actions are taken.

antidote a drug that antagonizes or blocks the toxic effect of another drug.

displacement when one drug displaces another from a protein binding site, increasing the concentration of the displaced drug in the blood.

interference when one drug interferes with the elimination of another, increasing its concentration in the blood as a result.

synergism (potentiation) when two drugs with different sites or mechanisms of action produce greater effects when taken together than when taken alone.

DRUG-DRUG INTERACTIONS (cont'd)

ABSORPTION

There are several means by which one drug may affect the gastrointestinal absorption of another:

➡ **drug binding** in the gastrointestinal tract

➡ **alterations in gastrointestinal movement**

➡ **alterations in gastrointestinal pH**

Drug Binding

Some drugs can form nonabsorbable complexes by binding to other drugs, resulting in decreased absorption. For example, iron salts can affect the absorption of several tetracyclines, methlydopa, and levodopa this way.

Gastric Emptying

Certain drugs will affect gastric emptying and therefore the absorption of other drugs. For example, use of propantheline will delay acetaminophen absorption. On the other hand, use of metoclopramide will increase acetaminophen absorption, since metoclopramide increases the rate of gastric emptying. Another problem with reducing gastric emptying time is that drugs that are degraded by gastric acid have a longer time to degrade, resulting in a decreased amount of drug available for absorption from the intestine.

Gastric pH

Drugs that alter the gastrointestinal pH can have a complex effect on other administered drugs. Some of the factors affected by pH are:

➡ the amount of unionized drug available for absorption

➡ the rate of dissolution

➡ gastric emptying

➡ degradation

DISTRIBUTION

Displacement

One drug can displace another from a plasma protein binding site and so increase the amount of the free drug available for distribution. This will increase its pharmacological effect and its elimination, since more of the drug is available for metabolism and excretion.

The biggest consequence of displacement interactions is the *change in pharmacological effect.* If drugs are highly protein bound, displacement tends to have a greater effect than with drugs that are not highly bound. For example, warfarin is 98% plasma protein bound, with only 2% of it free or unbound. If a drug interaction displaces only 2% of the bound warfarin, then 96% will be bound, but 4% will now be free. That is a 100% increase in the free concentration of warfarin, and it might double its pharmacological effect. By comparison, for a drug that is only 50% bound, displacing 2% will cause only a minor increase in the free concentration.

Such displacement interactions generally occur within the first week or two of administration. When they do occur, many turn out to be self-correcting after a few days, at which point the concentration of displaced drug often returns to pre-interaction levels, even if the patient continues to take both drugs.

METABOLISM

Enzyme Induction

Some drugs are capable of increasing the metabolizing enzymes in the liver. This process is called enzyme induction. It increases the metabolism of drugs and usually results in a *reduction in pharmacological effect.* Examples of enzyme inducers include phenobarbital, carbamazepine, phenytoin, and rifampin. Cigarette smoking and chronic alcohol use may also induce metabolism.

The time course of drug interactions from enzyme induction is slower than for many other types of interactions. Though enzyme induction may be dose related, it can also be caused by age, genetics, or liver disease. As a result, it is a difficult type of interaction to predict.

Enzyme Inhibition

The other alteration in metabolism is called enzyme inhibition, which usually occurs when two drugs compete for binding sites on the liver's metabolizing enzymes. This generally *increases the plasma concentration (and consequently the pharmacological effect) of at least one of the drugs.* Enzyme inhibition is one of the most common drug interactions. In fact, if a drug is known to be metabolized by the liver, manufacturers often study its potential for enzyme inhibition early in the drug development process.

Unlike enzyme induction, which has a much slower time course, enzyme inhibition has a rapid onset, generally within 24 hours, and tends to disappear quickly once the inhibitor is discontinued. Enzyme inhibition is also easier to predict since it appears to be dose related. It is also true that drugs that share a similar chemical structure often share the potential for enzyme inhibition.

EXCRETION

Filtration

Drug interactions that actually change the filtration rate itself are rare. Changes in the filtration rate are more likely to occur in response to specific drugs, such as those that change the systemic blood pressure, for example. Whatever the cause, changes in the filtration rate will also change the rate of drug excretion.

Kidney Secretion

There are different transport systems in the kidneys for basic drugs and acidic drugs. Basic drugs do not seem to compete for the acidic drug transport system, or visa versa. However, two basic drugs or two acidic drugs may compete for the same transport system and this can cause one or both of the drugs to accumulate in the blood. For example, probenecid competes with penicillin and reduces penicillin's secretion. Probenecid also inhibits the secretion of cephalosporins. An example of such a competition involving basic drugs involves quinidine and digoxin. Quinidine reduces digoxin excretion by 30% to 50%.

Urinary Reabsorption

Urinary reabsorption, a passive transport process, is influenced by the pH of the urine and the extent of ionization of the drug. In acidic urine, acidic drugs tend to be reabsorbed while basic drugs are not. As a result, they are excreted in the urine. In alkaline urine, acidic drugs will not be reabsorbed but will instead be excreted in the urine, while basic drugs will be reabsorbed. An example of these interactions is quinidine, which is a base. The excretion of quinidine is reduced nearly 90% when the urine pH is increased from less than 6.0 to over 7.5.

DRUG-DIET INTERACTIONS

Dietary intakes and patterns vary widely among individuals and can contribute to variability in the disposition of drugs. Differences may be attributed to various factors, including food preferences and availability, diets designed for weight gain or loss, and variations for seasonal, religious, and therapeutic reasons.

ABSORPTION

The physical presence of food in the gastrointestinal tract can alter absorption in a number of ways:

➡ interacting chemically (e.g., certain medications and tetracycline)

➡ improving the water-solubility of some drugs by increasing bile secretion

➡ affecting the performance of the dosage form (e.g., altering the release characteristics of polymer-coated tablets)

➡ altering gastric emptying

➡ altering intestinal movement

➡ altering liver blood flow.

As a result, some drugs have increased bioavailability and some have decreased bioavailability in the presence of food. For example, the bioavailability of propranolol is enhanced by the presence of food.

The bioavailability of a drug is generally decreased when the presence of food slows absorption. For example, when tablets or capsules are taken with food, they dissolve more slowly, slowing absorption as a result.

Food may also combine with a drug to form an insoluble drug-food complex. This is how tetracycline interacts with dairy products, such as milk and cheese. It combines with the calcium in milk products to form an insoluble, non-absorbable compound that is excreted in the feces.

DISTRIBUTION

The presence of food can also influence drug distribution. For example, high-fat meals can increase fatty acid levels in the blood. The fatty acids bind to the same plasma protein binding sites as many drugs. This displaces previously bound drug and increases the free concentration of that drug, leading to an increased effect.

There are also differences in the plasma protein binding of certain drugs between well-nourished and undernourished people.

ADMINISTRATION TIMES

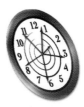

Interactions that alter drug absorption can be minimized by separating the administration of drugs and food intake about 2 hours.

 drug-diet interactions when elements of ingested nutrients interact with a drug and this affects the disposition of the drug.

METABOLISM

Most foods are complex mixtures of carbohydrate, fat, and protein. Research studies designed to determine the influence of diet on drug metabolism have diets in which one of these nutrients is increased, another decreased, and the third nutrient and total caloric intake are kept constant. In general, high-protein (low-carbohydrate) diets are associated with accelerated metabolism while high-carbohydrate (low-protein) diets appear to decrease metabolism. The substitution of fat calories for carbohydrate seems not to affect drug metabolism rates.

In general, mildly or moderately undernourished adults have normal or enhanced metabolism of drugs and severely malnourished adults have decreased drug metabolism. As with any diet, however, there are many variables in malnourishment that can produce an affect on metabolism.

EXCRETION

Reducing dietary protein appears to decrease filtration, increase reabsorption, and increase secretion in the kidney. The total effect of restricted protein intake will depend on the urinary excretion characteristics of the specific drug.

SPECIFIC FOODS

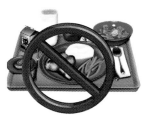 Some foods contain substances that react with certain drugs. For example, eating foods containing tyramine while using monoamine oxidase inhibitors (MAOI) may produce severe hypertension or intracranial hemorrhage. MAOIs include isocarboxazid, phenelzine, and procarbazine. Foods containing tyramine include beer, red wine, aged cheeses, yeast products, chicken livers, and pickled herring.

Certain cruciferous vegetables (i.e., brussels sprouts, cabbage) stimulate the metabolism of a few drugs. Other foods that might also have the similar effect are alfalfa, turnips, broccoli, cauliflower, or spinach. Some of the same foods are also involved with an interaction with oral anticoagulants such as warfarin. Spinach and other greens contain vitamin K, and vitamin K inhibits the action of oral anticoagulants. A patient ingesting foods containing vitamin K while taking an anticoagulant would not receive a therapeutic effect from the drug.

DISEASE STATES

The disposition and effect of some drugs can be influenced by the presence of diseases other than the one for which a drug is used. Hepatic, cardiovascular, renal, and endocrine disease all increase the variability in drug response.

HEPATIC

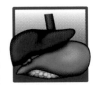

There are a variety of liver diseases that affect hepatic function differently. Some, but not necessarily all, require that special care should be taken when administering drugs to patients with hepatic diseases.

Cirrhosis tends to decrease the hepatic metabolism of drugs. On the other hand, **acute viral hepatitis** decreases metabolism in about half of drugs, but has no affect on the metabolism of the other half. **Obstructive jaundice** appears to diminish drug elimination.

The effect of hepatic disease on drug absorption is not well understood. However, to the extent that liver activity is decreased, it appears that the first-pass effect is also reduced. This results in increased bioavailability for drugs that are usually severely degraded by first-pass metabolism. Another factor that increases bioavailability is that patients with cirrhosis can develop a condition in which a significant amount of the blood coming from the intestine bypasses liver cells and enters the circulatory system directly. When this happens, the bioavailability of drugs that would otherwise be degraded by first-pass metabolism rises substantially.

CIRCULATORY

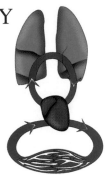

Circulatory disorders are generally characterized by diminished blood flow to one or more organs of the body. Since blood flow influences drug absorption, distribution, and elimination, this may also affect the action of drugs.

Decreased blood flow from cardiovascular disorders can delay or cause erratic drug absorption. As a result, intravenous administration may be needed to obtain a desired effect.

Decreased blood flow can also affect the metabolizing action of the liver. For example, when blood flow to the liver is decreased, the metabolism of lidocaine also decreases.

hepatic disease liver disease.

cirrhosis a chronic and potentially fatal liver disease causing loss of function and resistance to blood flow through the liver.

acute viral hepatitis a virus caused systemic infection that causes inflammation of the liver.

obstructive jaundice an obstruction of the bile excretion process.

RENAL

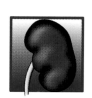

In patients with renal disease, the urinary excretion of drugs decreases in proportion to the decrease in kidney function.

Such decreases can be measured by monitoring the amount of creatinine excreted in the urine. Creatinine is produced by muscle activity in the body and is excreted at a standard rate by healthy kidneys. In diseased kidneys, the rate of creatinine clearance decreases as an indication that kidney function (including glomerular filtration) decreases. In such cases, drug excretion is reduced and to avoid excessive accumulation of the drug in the blood, the dosage must be reduced.

THYROID

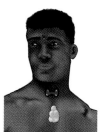

Changes in thyroid function can affect many of the aspects of absorption, excretion, and metabolism.

In **hypothyroidism** (a condition in which the thyroid is underactive), the bioavailability of a few drugs (i.e., riboflavin, digoxin) is increased. In **hyperthyroidism** (an overactive thyroid condition) their bioavailability is decreased because of changes in gastrointestinal movement.

Some other changes affected by thyroid conditions are:

➥ Renal blood flow is decreased in hypothyroidism and increased in hyperthyroidism.

➥ The activity of metabolizing enzymes in the liver is reduced in hypothyroidism and increased in hyperthyroidism.

➥ The metabolism of theophylline, propranolol, propylthiouracil, and methimazole is increased by hyperthyroidism.

hypothyroidism a condition in which thyroid hormone secretions are below normal, often referred to as an underactive thyroid.

hyperthyroidism a condition in which thyroid hormone secretions are above normal, often referred to as an overactive thyroid.

REVIEW

KEY CONCEPTS

✔ Differences in age, weight, genetics, and gender are among the significant factors that influence the differences in medication responses among people.

✔ Drug distribution, metabolism, and excretion are quite different in the neonate and infant than in adults because their organ systems are not fully developed.

✔ Children metabolize certain drugs more rapidly than adults.

✔ The elderly typically consume more drugs than other age groups. They also experience physiological changes that significantly affect drug action.

✔ A number of physiological changes that occur in women in the latter stages of pregnancy tend to reduce the rate of absorption.

✔ Genetic differences can cause differences in the types and amounts of proteins produced in the body, which can result in differences in drug action.

✔ Almost any drug, in almost any dose, can produce an allergic or hypersensitive reaction in a patient. Anaphylactic shock is a potentially fatal hypersensitivity reaction.

✔ Anorexia, nausea, vomiting, constipation, and diarrhea are among the most common adverse reactions to drugs.

✔ Teratogenicity is the ability of a substance to cause abnormal fetal development when given to pregnant women.

✔ Drug-drug interactions can result in either increases or decreases in therapeutic effects or adverse effects.

✔ Additive effects occur when two drugs with similar pharmacological actions are taken.

✔ Synergism or potentiation occurs when two drugs with different sites or mechanisms of action produce greater effects when taken together than either does when taken alone.

✔ Interference by one drug with the elimination of a second drug may intensify the effects of the second drug.

✔ Displacement of one drug from protein binding sites by a second drug increases the effects of the displaced drug.

✔ Decreased intestinal absorption of oral drugs occurs when drugs combine to produce nonabsorbable compounds.

✔ When drugs activate metabolizing enzymes in the liver, it increases the metabolism of other drugs affected by the same enzymes.

✔ Some drugs increase excretion by raising urinary pH and lessening renal reabsorption.

✔ The physical presence of food in the gastrointestinal tract can alter absorption.

✔ Some foods contain substances that react with certain drugs, e.g., foods containing tyramine can react with monoamine oxidase inhibitors (MAOIs).

✔ The disposition and effect of some drugs can be influenced by the presence of diseases other than the one for which a drug is used. For example, decreased blood flow from cardiovascular disorders can delay or cause erratic drug absorption.

SELF TEST

MATCH THE TERMS.   *answers can be checked in the glossary*

additive effects

anaphylactic shock

antidote

carcinogenicity

cirrhosis

hepato

hypersensitivity

idiosyncrasy

nephrotoxicity

synergism

teratogenicity

a prefix meaning "of the liver."

the ability of a substance to cause abnormal fetal development when given to pregnant women.

an abnormal sensitivity generally resulting in an allergic reaction.

a potentially fatal hypersensitivity reaction producing severe respiratory distress and cardiovascular collapse.

an unexpected reaction the first time a drug is taken, generally due to genetic causes.

the ability of a substance to harm the kidneys.

the ability of a substance to cause cancer.

the increase in effect when two drugs with similar pharmacological actions are taken.

when two drugs with different sites or mechanisms of action produce greater effects when taken together than taken alone.

a drug that antagonizes the toxic effect of another drug.

a chronic and potentially fatal liver disease causing loss of function and resistance to blood flow through the liver.

CHOOSE THE BEST ANSWER.   *answers are in the back of the book*

1. What organ is associated with the adverse effect of nephrotoxicity?
   a. liver
   b. kidney
   c. gall bladder
   d. gastrointestinal tract

2. When two drugs with different sites or mechanisms of action produce greater effects when taken together then when either does when taken alone is called:
   a. an additive effect
   b. a synergestic effect
   c. an interference effect
   d. a displacement effect

3. Enzyme induction and inhibition would be part of which process?
   a. absorption
   b. distribution
   c. metabolism
   d. excretion

4. An unexpected adverse effect to a drug the first time it is given to a patient is considered what type of reaction?
   a. hypersensitivity
   b. anaphylaxis
   c. idiosyncrasy
   d. autoimmune

TERMINOLOGY

Root	Prefix
Suffix	C.V.

Medical dictionaries contain thousands of words that are used in medicine and pharmacy.

Many of the words don't look like words commonly used in literature or speech, and at first glance they can be quite intimidating. However, the secret to learning medical science terminology is to learn that there is a system or order to it.

Medical science terminology is made up of a small number of root words.

Most of these root words originate from either Greek or Latin words. Words developed from the Greek language are most often used to refer to diagnosis and surgery. Words from the Latin language generally refer to the anatomy of the body.

Numerous suffixes and prefixes are attached to the root word.

The suffixes and prefixes give specific meaning to the use of the root word. The suffix is a modifier attached to the end of the root word, and the prefix is attached to the front of the root word. So each medical science term will have at least one root word and then a suffix or prefix to complete the meaning. It is not required that every root word have both a suffix and a prefix. Each root could have just one. In general, prefixes are used less frequently than suffixes.

Combining vowels are used to connect the prefix, root, or suffix parts of the term.

In some cases the combining vowel can be used to combine two root words. And there are some cases where the combining vowels are not used at all. Sometimes a combining vowel is added to make the word easier to pronounce. The most common combining vowel is the letter "o".

ROOT WORDS

The root word is the foundation of medical science terminology. Root words can immediately identify what part of the body a term relates to. For example, consider this list of common root words and the parts of the body to which they refer:

Root	Part of Body
card	heart
cyst	bladder
gastr	stomach
hemat	blood
hepat	liver
my	muscle
pector	chest
neur	nerve
pneum	lung
ocul	eye
derma	skin
ven	vein
mast	breast
oste	bone
nephr	kidney
ot	ear

If a phrase contains the word "cardiac," it is referring to the heart, since "card" is the root word of the word cardiac. The word "ocular" would refer to the eye since "ocul" is the root word of the word ocular.

nomenclature a system of names specific to a particular field.

root word the base component of a term which gives it a meaning that may be modified by other components.

prefix a modifying component of a term located before the other components of the term.

suffix a modifying component of a term located after the other components of the term.

 Learning the most popular roots, suffixes and prefixes will help you to understand a large amount of pharmaceutical terminology.

Medical Term

Medical and pharmaceutical nomenclature is a system made up of these four elements.

- ➡ **root words** ➡ **prefixes**
- ➡ **suffixes** ➡ **combining vowels**

PREFIXES

A prefix is added to the beginning of a root word to clarify its meaning. For example, *"derma"* is the root word for skin, or things related to the skin, and *"xero"* is a prefix used to describe things that are dry. So:

xero + derma = xeroderma

➡ *meaning:* a "dry skin" condition.

Consider another example. The root word for vision is *"opia,"* and the prefix for double is *"dipl."* So:

dipl + opia = diplopia

➡ *meaning:* double vision.

For a final example, consider the prefix *"sub"* and the root *"lingu."* "Sub" means under or beneath, and "lingu" is the root word for tongue. So:

sub + lingu = sublingu

➡ would mean "under the tongue."

However, there are few English words ending in "u," and so this combination is further modified with the typical suffix *"al"* which means "pertaining to," as in:

sub + lingu + al = sublingual

➡ *meaning:* pertaining to under the tongue.

SUFFIXES

The suffix is added to the end of a root word to clarify the meaning. Sometimes the connection is made without the aid of a connecting vowel.

Root	Suffix
gastr (stomach)	**itis** (inflammation)

➡ **gastritis**: inflammation of the stomach

Root	Suffix
neur (nerve)	**algia** (pain)

➡ **neuralgia**: a pain in the nerve

Sometimes a **combining vowel** (CV) is used to complete the connection of the different word parts.

1st Root	2ndRoot	Suffix	CV
pneum (lung)	**thorax** (chest)		o

➡ **pneumothorax**: area of the chest containing the lungs

1st Root	2ndRoot	Suffix	CV
card (heart)	**my** (muscle)	**pathy** (disease)	i, o

➡ **cardiomyopathy**: disease in the heart muscle tissue

COMBINING THE ELEMENTS

The last combination possibility is to have a prefix and a suffix attached to a root word.

Prefix	Root	Suffix
hypo (low)	**glyc** (sugar)	**emia** (blood)

➡ **hypoglycemia**: low blood sugar

Prefix	Root	Suffix
hyper (high)	**thyroid** (thyroid)	**ism** (state of)

➡ **hyperthyroidism**: too much thyroid activity

And then there is always the possibility that a combining vowel (CV) will be used within a word.

Prefix	Root	Suffix	CV
peri (around)	**dont** (teeth)	**ic** (pertaining to)	o

➡ **periodontic**: around the teeth

ORGAN SYSTEM TERMINOLOGY

A good way to learn medical science terminology is to learn it based on the different organ systems in the body.

There are names for structures and parts of organ systems that form the root words used in medical science terminology. These names have to be learned. Then they can be applied to understand or to construct words.

The cardiovascular system distributes blood throughout the body using blood vessels called arteries, capillaries, and veins. Blood transports nutrients to the body's cells and carries waste products away from them. Blood is made up of red blood cells, white blood cells, platelets, and plasma. **Erythrocytes** (red blood cells) transport oxygen from the lungs to the body and carbon dioxide from the cells to the lungs. **Leukocytes** (white blood cells) fight bacterial infections by producing antibodies.

Blood is pumped through the cardiovascular system by the heart. Valves within the heart maintain the flow of blood in only one direction. Conductive tissue that is unique to the heart muscle is responsible for the heartbeat.

When blood is forced out of the heart, the increased pressure on the system is called the **systolic** phase. When blood pressure is monitored, this pressure is reported (in mm Hg) as the first number of a two number sequence. The **diastolic** phase, or relaxation phase, is the second number reported in blood pressure monitoring. Blood pressures are reported as systole/diastole, i.e., 120/80. A sphygmomanometer is used to measure blood pressure.

CARDIOVASCULAR SYSTEM

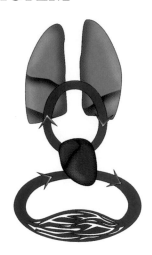

Cardiovascular Root Words

angi	vessel
aort	aorta
card	heart
oxy	oxygen
pector	chest
phleb	vein
stenosis	narrowing
thromb	clot
vas(cu)	blood vessel
ven	vein

Prefix	Root Word	Suffix	CV	Term	Meaning
hyper (high)		tension (pressure)		**hypertension**	high blood pressure.
	thromb (clot)	sis (abnormal condition)	o	**thrombosis**	condition of having blood clots in the vascular system.
	phleb (vein)	itis (inflammation)		**phlebitis**	inflammation of a vein.
	arter (artery)	sclerosis (hardening)	i, o	**arteriosclerosis**	hardening of the arteries.
	card (heart) my (muscle)	pathy (disease)	i, o	**cardiomyopathy**	disease of the heart muscle.
	my (muscle) card (heart)	ial (condition of)	o	**myocardial**	concerning heart muscle.
tachy (fast)	card (heart)	ia (condition of)		**tachycardia**	abnormally rapid heart action.

ENDOCRINE SYSTEM

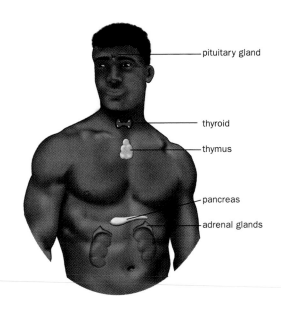

pituitary gland

thyroid

thymus

pancreas

adrenal glands

Endocrine Root Words

lipid	fat
nephr	kidney
thym	thymus
adrena	adrenal
gluc	sugar
pancreat	pancreas
somat	body

The endocrine system consists of the glands that secrete **hormones**, chemicals that assist in regulating body functions.

Several organs act as endocrine glands as well as members of other organ systems. For example, the liver, stomach, pancreas, and kidneys are members of endocrine system as well as other organ systems. Organs that belong primarily to the endocrine system include the **pituitary gland**, the **adrenal glands**, the **thyroid gland**, and the **gonads** (ovaries and testes).

The pituitary gland produces multiple hormones and is located at the base of the brain. It controls the body's growth and releases hormones into the bloodstream that control much of the activity of the other glands. The thyroid gland is located just below the larynx and releases hormones important for regulating body metabolism. There are also four smaller **parathyroid** glands located on the thyroid gland. The **thymus** gland is located beneath the sternum. The **pancreas** is best known for its production of insulin and glucagon. The small adrenal glands are located on top of the kidneys. They produce such hormones as aldosterone, cortisol (hydrocortisone), androgens, and estrogens. The medulla region of the adrenal glands produce adrenaline (epinephrine) and noradrenaline (norepinephrine).

Prefix	Root Word	Suffix	CV	Term	Meaning
end (within)		crine (secrete)	o	**endocrine**	pertaining to the glands that secrete onto the bloodstream.
hyper (high)	lipid (fat)	emia (blood)		**hyperlipidemia**	increase of lipids in the blood.
hypo (low)	thyroid (thyroid gland)	ism (condition)		**hypothyroidism**	a deficiency of thyroid secretion.
	somat (body)	ic (pertaining to)		**somatic**	pertaining to the body.

 The majority of the terms in the combining tables on body system terminology are for disorders or conditions.

ORGAN SYSTEM TERMINOLOGY

GASTROINTESTINAL TRACT

The gastrointestinal (GI) tract is located in the abdomen, and is surrounded by the peritoneal lining. The GI tract contains the organs that are involved in the digestion of foods and the absorption of nutrients. These organs include the stomach, small and large intestine, gallbladder, liver, and pancreas.

The GI tract is sometimes inappropriately referred to as the **alimentary canal.** The alimentary canal refers to the system that goes from the mouth to the anus. The alimentary canal contains organs such as lips, tongue, teeth, salivary glands, pharynx, esophagus, rectum, and anus, in addition to the GI tract.

Several organs contribute to the digestion of foods by secreting enzymes into the small intestine when food is present. Ducts carry bile from the liver (hepatic duct) and the gallbladder (cystic duct) to the duodenum. The pancreas is located behind the stomach and also contributes enzymes to the digestive process.

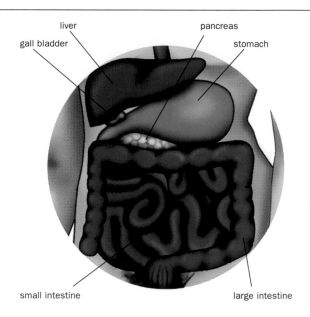

liver   pancreas

gall bladder   stomach

small intestine   large intestine

Gastrointestinal Root Words

chol	bile
col	colon
duoden	duodenum
enter	intestine
esophag	esophagus
gastr	stomach
hepat	liver
lapar	abdomen
pancreat	pancreas

Prefix	Root Word	Suffix	CV	Term	Meaning
an (no)	orexia (appetite)			**anorexia**	loss of appetite.
a (no)	phagia (swallow)			**aphagia**	inability to swallow.
	appendic (appendix)	itis (inflammation)		**appendicitis**	inflammation of the appendix.
	col (colon)	itis (inflammation)		**colitis**	inflamed or irritable colon.
dia (across, through)	rrhea (discharge)			**diarrhea**	liquid or unformed bowel movements.
	duoden (duodenum)	al (pertaining to)		**duodenal**	pertaining to the duodenum.
	hemat (blood)	emesis (vomit)		**hematemesis**	vomiting of blood.
	hepat (liver)	itis (inflammation)		**hepatitis**	inflammation of the liver from various causes.
	hepat (liver)	oma (tumor)		**hepatoma**	liver tumor.
	gastr (stomach)	itis (inflammation)		**gastritis**	inflammation of the stomach.
	gastr (stomach) } enter (abdomen) }	itis (inflammation)	o	**gastroenteritis**	inflammation of the stomach and the intestinal tract.

INTEGUMENTARY SYSTEM

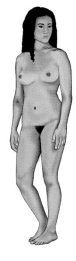
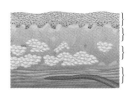

} epidermis
} dermis
} subcutaneous
} muscle

The covering of the body is referred to as the integumentary system. It is the body's first line of defense, acting as a barrier against disease and other hazards. It also helps control body temperature by releasing heat through sweat or by restricting blood vessels to act as insulation. It includes the skin, hair, and nails.

The skin is composed of the **epidermis** and **dermis.** The epidermis has no blood or nerves and is constantly discarding dead cells. The dermis, which is made of living cells, contains capillaries, nerves, and lymphatics. The dermis also contains the subcutaneous glands, sweat glands, and hair.

Hair is made of keratinized cells. Finger nails and toenails are also composed of keratin. The mammary glands, or breasts, are also considered part of the integumentary system.

The subcutaneous layer of tissue is beneath the dermis but is closely interconnected to it. It separates the skin from the other organs (the muscular system, for example, as in the illustration).

Integumentary Root Words

necr	death (cells, body)
derma	skin
cutane	skin
mast	breast
onych	nail

Prefix	Root Word	Suffix	CV	Term	Meaning
	derma (skin)	itis (inflammation)		**dermatitis**	skin inflammation.
erythro (red)	derma (skin)			**erythroderma**	abnormal redness of skin.
	lact (milk)	tation (act of secreting)		**lactation**	secretion of milk.
	mast (breast)	ectomy (removal)		**mastectomy**	surgical removal of breast.
	onych (nail)	mycosis (fungal infection)	o	**onychomycosis**	fungal infection of nails.
pach (thick)	derma (skin)		y	**pachyderma**	abnormal thickness of skin.
sub (under)	cutane (skin)	ous (pertaining to)		**subcutaneous**	beneath the skin.
trans (through)	derma (skin)	al (pertaining to)		**transdermal**	through the skin.

ORGAN SYSTEM TERMINOLOGY

LYMPHATIC SYSTEM

The lymphatic system is responsible for collecting plasma water that leaves the blood vessels, filtering it for impurities through its lymph nodes, and returning the lymph fluid back to the general circulation. The lymphatic system is the center of the body's immune system.

The largest organ in the system is the spleen. It is responsible for removing old red blood cells from the circulation. It is also a storage organ for **lymphocytes,** a type of white blood cell that attacks bacteria and disease cells. Lymphocytes release antibodies that destroy disease cells and provide immunity against them.

The thymus, tonsils, spleen, and adenoids are lymphoid organs outside the network of the lymphatic system.

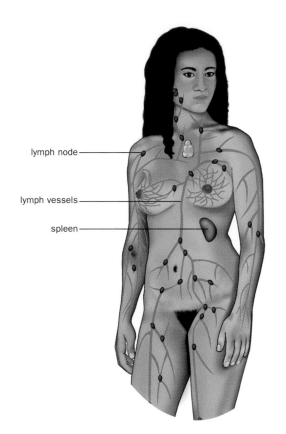

lymph node

lymph vessels

spleen

Lymphatic Root Words

aden	gland
cyt	cell
hemo, hemat	blood
lymph	lymph
splen	spleen

Prefix	Root Word	Suffix	CV	Term	Meaning
	aden (gland)	pathy (disease)	o	**adenopathy**	lymph node disease.
	hemat (blood)	oma (tumor)		**hematoma**	a collection of blood, often clotted.
	hemo (blood)	philia (attraction)		**hemophilia**	a disease in which the blood does not clot normally.
	lymph (lymph tissue)	oma (tumor)		**lymphoma**	lymphatic system tumor.
leuk (white)		emia (blood condition)		**leukemia**	a disease of blood forming tissues.
	thym (thymus)	oma (tumor)		**thymoma**	tumor of the thymus.

lymphocytes a white blood cell that helps the body defend itself against bacteria and diseased cells.

MUSCULAR SYSTEM

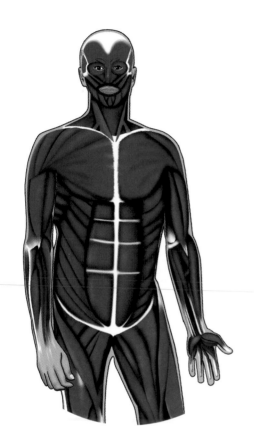

The word muscle comes from the Latin *mus* (mouse) and *cle* (little) because muscle movements resemble a mouse moving under a cover.

The body contains more than 600 muscles which give shape and movement to it. The skeletal muscles are attached to the bones by tendons. The muscles themselves are striated, i.e., made up of fibers.

The action of most muscles is called voluntary, because it is controlled consciously. Involuntary muscles operate automatically and are found in the heart, the stomach, or in walls of blood vessels.

Some muscles produce an outward or **flexor** movement and these are called agonist muscles. Antagonist muscles are the ones that contract or bring the limb back to the original position.

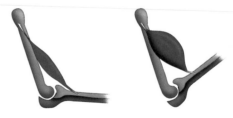

expansion and contraction of muscles

Root Words

my	muscle
fibr	fiber
tendin	tendon

Prefix	Root Word	Suffix	CV	Term	Meaning
	fibr (fiber) } my (muscle)	algia (pain)	o	**fibromyalgia**	chronic pain in the muscles.
	my (muscle)	plasty (repair)	o	**myoplasty**	plastic surgery of muscle tissue.
	tendin (tendon)	itis (inflammation)		**tendinitis**	inflammation of a tendon.

 flexor movement an expansion or outward movement by muscles.

ORGAN SYSTEM TERMINOLOGY

NERVOUS SYSTEM

The most complex of the body organ systems is the nervous system, the body's system of communication. The **neuron** (nerve cell) is the basic functional unit in this system. There are over 100 billion neurons in the brain alone. Neurons also transmit information from the brain to the entire body.

The primary parts of this system are the brain and the spinal cord, called the **central nervous system (CNS)**. The **peripheral nervous system** is composed of nerves that branch out from the spinal cord.

There are subdivisions of the peripheral nervous system called the **autonomic nervous system** and the **somatic nervous system**. The autonomic nervous system controls the automatic functions of the body, e.g., breathing, digestion, etc.

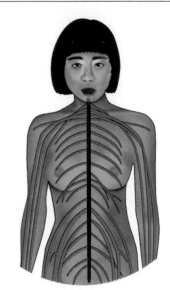

central and peripheral nervous systems

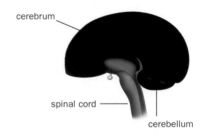

brain and spinal cord

Nervous System Root Words

cerebr	cerebrum
encephal	brain
mening	meninges
myel	spinal cord
neur	nerve

Prefix	Root Word	Suffix	CV	Term	Meaning
	encephal (brain)	itis (inflammation)		**encephalitis**	inflammation of the brain.
	neur (nerve)	algia (pain)		**neuralgia**	severe pain in a nerve.
	neur (nerve)	oma (tumor)		**neuroma**	tumor of nerve cells.

SKELETAL SYSTEM

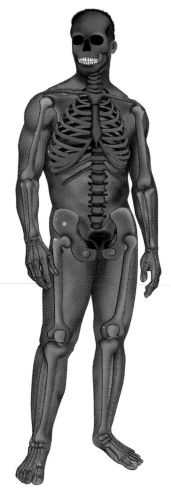

axial (red) and appendicular (blue) skeleton

The skeletal system protects soft organs and provides structure and support for the body's organ systems. Made up largely of hard **osseus** tissue, it is a living system that undergoes dynamic changes throughout life.

The system's 206 bones are called **axial** (skull and spinal column) or **appendicular** (arms, legs, and connecting bones). They are held together at joints by connective tissue called ligaments and cartilage. Joints range from rigid to those allowing full motion (e.g., the ball and socket joints of the hips and shoulders).

Skeletal System Root Words

arthr	joint
calcane	heel bone
carp	wrist
crani	cranium
dactyl	finger or toe
femor	thigh bone
fibul	small, outer lower leg bone
humer	humerus
myel	bone marrow, spinal cord
oste	bone
patell	kneecap
ped, pod	foot
pelv	pelvis
phalang	bones of fingers and toes
rachi	spinal cord, vertebrae
spondy	backbone, vertebrae
stern	sternum, breastbone
tibi	large lower leg bone
vertebr	backbone, vertebrae

Prefix	Root Word	Suffix	CV	Term	Meaning
	arthr (joint)	algia (pain)		**arthralgia**	joint pain.
	arthr (joint)	itis (inflammation)		**arthritis**	inflammation of a joint.
	carp (wrist)	al (pertaining to)		**carpal**	pertaining to the carpus in the wrist.
	crani (cranium)	malacia (softening)	o	**craniomalacia**	softening of the skull.
	oste (bone) arthr (joint)	itis (inflammation)	o	**osteoarthritis**	chronic disease of bones and joints.
	oste (bone) carcin (cancer)	oma (tumor)	o	**osteocarcinoma**	cancerous bone tumor.
	rachi (vertebrae)	itis (inflammation)		**rachitis**	inflammation of the spine.

ORGAN SYSTEM TERMINOLOGY

FEMALE REPRODUCTIVE SYSTEM

The female reproductive system produces hormones (**estrogen, progesterone**), controls menstruation, and provides for childbearing. The system contains the vagina, uterus, fallopian tubes, ovaries, and the external genitalia.

There are also two gland organs associated with the system: Bartholin's glands and mammary glands (located in breast tissue). The mammary glands produce and secrete milk at childbirth.

The vagina is a muscular tube that leads from an external opening to the cervix and uterus. The uterus is a hollow, pear-shaped organ that is the normal location for pregnancy. The fallopian tubes transport eggs from the ovary to the uterus. The ovaries are located on each side of the uterus. In sexually mature females, the uterus is prepared for the possibility of fertilization and pregnancy each month.

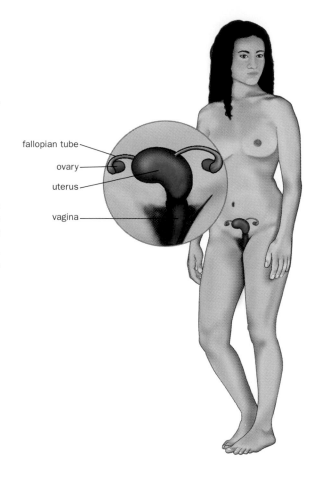

fallopian tube
ovary
uterus
vagina

Root Words

gynec	woman
hyster	uterus
lact	milk
mamm	breast
mast	breast
metr	uterus
ovari	ovary
salping	fallopian tube
toc	birth
uter	uterine

Prefix	Root Word	Suffix	CV	Term	Meaning
a (no)	men (menstrual)	orrhea (discharge)		**amenorrhea**	absence of menstruation.
dys (difficult)	men (menstrual)	orrhea (discharge)		**dysmenorrhea**	menstrual pain.
dys (difficult)	toc (birth)	ia (condition of)		**dystocia**	difficult labor.
end (within)	metri (uterus)	sis (abnormal)	o	**endometriosis**	abnormal growth of uteral tissue within the pelvis.
	gynec (woman)	logy (study of)	o	**gynecology**	the study of the female reproductive organs.
	mast (breast)	itis (inflammation)		**mastitis**	inflammation of the breast.
	salping (fallopian)	cyesis (pregnancy)	o	**salpingocyesis**	fetal development in the fallopian tube.
	vagin (vagina)	itis (inflammation)		**vaginitis**	inflammation of the vagina.

MALE REPRODUCTIVE SYSTEM

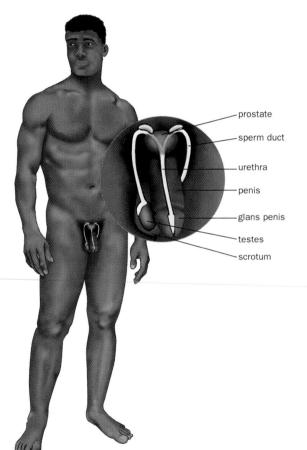

prostate
sperm duct
urethra
penis
glans penis
testes
scrotum

The male reproductive system produces sperm and secretes the hormone **testosterone**. The primary male sex organs are the testicles. They are the oval shaped organs enclosed in the scrotum.

The seminal glands, located at the base of the bladder, produce part of the seminal fluid. They have ducts that lead into sperm ducts called the vas deferens which carry the sperm from the testes. The prostate gland is located at the upper end of the urethra. The penis (glans penis) is the external organ for urination and sexual intercourse. The tip of the penis is covered by the prepuce (foreskin). The urethra, by which urine and semen leave the body, is inside the penis.

Root Words

andr	male
balan	glans penis
orchid, test	testis, testicle
prostat	prostate gland
sperm	sperm
vas	vessel, duct
vesicul	seminal vescles

Prefix	Root Word	Suffix	CV	Term	Meaning
a (no)	sperm (sperm)	ia (condition of)		**aspermia**	inability to produce semen.
	balan (glans penis)	itis (inflammation)		**balanitis**	inflammation of the glans penis.
crypt (hidden)	orchid (testis)	ism (state of)		**cryptorchidism**	failure of testes to drop into the scrotum.
	prostat (prostate)	itis		**prostatitis**	inflammation of prostate.
	prostat (prostate)	lith (stone)	o	**prostatolith**	a prostate stone.
	semin (testis)	oma (tumor)		**seminoma**	tumor of the testes.

ORGAN SYSTEM TERMINOLOGY

RESPIRATORY SYSTEM

The respiratory system brings oxygen into the body through inhalation and expels carbon dioxide gas through exhalation. It produces sound for speaking and helps cool the body.

The lungs have specialized tissues called **alveoli** that exchange the gases between the blood and the air. Respiratory muscles (especially the diaphragm) expand the lungs automatically, causing air to be inhaled into the upper respiratory tract. As air enters through the nose, it is warmed, moistened, and filtered. The pharynx directs food into the esophagus and air into the trachea. The larynx contains the vocal cords. The trachea, or windpipe, connects to the two **bronchi** (bronchial tubes) that enter the lungs.

Inside the lungs, the broncial tubes branch out and lead to the alveolar sacs that are the site of gas exchange within the lungs. The pleural cavity surrounds the lungs and provides lubrication for respiration.

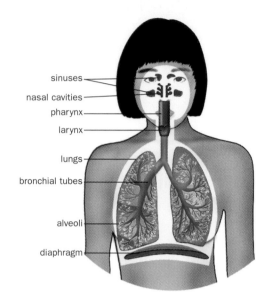

Root Words

aer	air
aero	gas
pneum	lung, air
pulmon	lung
pector	chest
nasal	nose
sinus	sinus
laryng	larynx
bronch	bronchus
ox	oxygen
capnia	carbon dioxide

Prefix	Root Word	Suffix	CV	Term	Meaning
a (no)	pnea (to breathe)			**apnea**	temporary failure to breathe.
	bronch (bronchus)	itis (inflammation)		**bronchitis**	inflammation of bronchial membranes.
cyan (blue)		sis (condition of)	o	**cyanosis**	blue discoloration of skin.
dys (difficult)	pnea (to breathe)			**dyspnea**	labored breathing.
hyper (high)	capnia (CO_2)			**hypercapnia**	excessive carbon dioxide in the blood.
hypo (low)	ox (oxygen)	ia (condition of)		**hypoxia**	abnormally low blood oxygen level.
	laryng (larynx)	itis (inflammation)		**laryngitis**	inflammation of the larynx.
para (around)	nasal (nose)			**paranasal**	near or along the nasal cavities.
	pector (chest)	algia (pain)		**pectoralgia**	chest pain.
	pneum (lung)	nia (condition of)	o	**pneumonia**	inflammation of the lungs.
	pulmon (lung)	ary (pertaining to)		**pulmonary**	pertaining to the lungs.
	sinus (sinus)	itis (inflammation)		**sinusitis**	inflammation of the sinuses.

URINARY SYSTEM

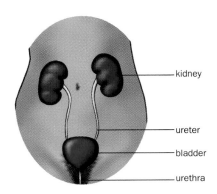

kidney

ureter

bladder

urethra

The urinary system is responsible for removing wastes from the body. The urinary system includes the kidneys, ureters, urinary bladder, and urethra.

The primary organ of the urinary system is the kidney, which filters the blood for unwanted material and makes urine. The **nephron** is the functional unit of the kidney. Plasma water from the blood passes through the nephron and through processes of reabsorption, filtration, and secretion is converted into urine.

Urine is excreted from the kidney through the ureters to the bladder. It is excreted from the bladder through the urethra.

Root Words

cyst	bladder
vesic	bladder
ren	kidney
nephr	kidney
uria	urine, urination

Prefix	Root Word	Suffix	CV	Term	Meaning
an (no)	uria (urine)			**anuria**	inability to produce urine.
	cyst (bladder)	itis (inflammation)		**cystitis**	inflammation of the bladder.
	cyst (bladder)	lith (stone)	o	**cystolith**	a bladder stone.
	nephr (kidney)	itis (inflammation)		**nephritis**	inflammation of the kidney.
poly (much)	uria (urine)			**polyuria**	excessive urination.
	ure (urine)	emia (blood condition)		**uremia**	toxic blood condition caused by kidney insufficiency or failure.

ORGAN SYSTEM TERMINOLOGY

SENSES: HEARING

The sense of hearing, as well as the maintenance of body equilibrium, is performed by the ear. The external ear consists of a funnel shaped structure which captures sound waves and channels them through an opening to the **tympanic membrane** (eardrum). The opening also contains glands that make earwax that protects the external ear.

The **middle ear** consists of three bony structures (malleus, incus, and stapes) that transmit sound from a vibrating tympanic membrane to the cochlea. The eustachian tube connects the middle ear to the nose and throat, serving to equalize the air pressure on both sides of the tympanic membrane.

The inner ear is called the **labyrinth** for obvious reasons. It consists of three areas: vestibule, cochlea, and semicircular canals. The cochlea contains the organ of hearing. When sound waves are transmitted to it, it converts them into nerve impulses that are sent to the brain for interpretation. The semicircular canals are responsible for body equilibrium.

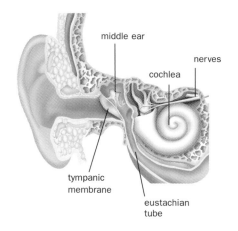

Root Words

ot	ear
cusis	hearing condition
acous	hearing
audi	hearing
salping	eustachian tube
tympan	eardrum
myring	eardrum
cerumin	wax-like, waxy

Prefix	Root Word	Suffix	CV	Term	Meaning
	labyrinth (inner ear)	itis (inflammation)		**labyrinthitis**	inflammation of the inner ear.
	ot (ear)	algia (pain, ache)		**otalgia**	pain in the ear.
	ot (ear)	mycosis (fungal infection)	o	**otomycosis**	fungal ear infection.
	ot (ear)	orrhea (drainage)		**otorrhea**	ear infection with discharge.
para (partial)	cusis (hearing condition)			**paracusis**	hearing disorder.
	tympan (eardrum)	itis (inflammation)		**tympanitis**	inflammation of the middle ear.

SENSES: SIGHT

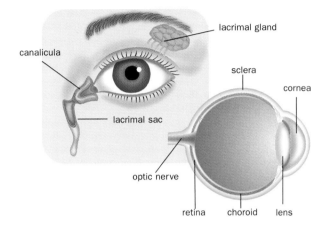

lacrimal gland

canalicula

sclera

cornea

lacrimal sac

optic nerve

retina   choroid   lens

The eyes are the organs that provide sight. The eyelids protect the eye and assist in its lubrication. The **conjunctiva** is the blood-rich membrane between the eye and the eyelid. There are several glands that secrete fluids to protect and lubricate the eye: the **lacrimal glands** above each eye secrete tears and the meibomian glands produce sebum. Excess fluid drains into the canalicula (tear ducts).

The eye has three layers. The outer layer is composed of the sclera and the **cornea.** The sclera is the white part of the eye. The cornea is transparent so the iris (the color of the eye) and the pupil (the opening of the eye) are visible. The middle layer is called the choroid and contains blood vessels that nourish the entire eye. In the third layer, the lens focuses light rays on the **retina.** The vitreous humor (one of two fluids in the eye) lies between the retina and the lens. Rods and cones within the retina are responsible for visual reception. The **optic nerve** within the retina transmits the nerve impulses to the brain.

Root Words

blephar	eyelid
cor	pupil
dacry, lacrim	tear, tear duct
corne, kerat	cornea
retin	retina
irid, iri	iris
bi, bin	two
opia	vision

Prefix	Root Word	Suffix	CV	Term	Meaning
ambly (dull)	opia (vision)			**amblyopia**	reduction in vision.
	blephar (eyelid)	itis (inflammation)		**blepharitis**	inflammation of eyelids.
	blephar (eyelid)	optosis (dropping)		**blepharoptosis**	drooping of upper eyelid.
	conjunctiv (conjunctiva)	itis (inflammation)		**conjunctivitis**	inflammation of the conjunctiva.
end (within)	opthalm (eye)	itis (inflammation)		**endopthalmitis**	inflammation of the inside of the eye.
	irid (iris)	plegia (paralysis)	o	**iridoplegia**	paralysis of the iris.
	ocul (eye)	mycosis (fungus infection)	o	**oculomycosis**	fungal disease of the eye.
	retin (retina)	itis (inflammation)		**retinitis**	inflammation of the retina.

PRESCRIPTION ABBREVIATIONS

Abbreviations for many medical terms are regularly used in prescriptions.

Many of these abbreviations are from Latin words, though a number are from English. They are commonly used on prescriptions and medical orders to communicate essential information on formulations, preparation, dosage regimens, and administration.

MOST COMMON ABBREVIATIONS

Note that while it is not necessary to know the latin term from which an abbreviation comes, it has been included for reference.

	Abbreviation	Meaning	Latin term
ROUTE	a.d.	right ear	auris dexter
	a.s.	left ear	auris sinister
	a.u.	each ear	auris utro
	i.m., IM	intramuscular	
	inj.	injection	injectio
	i.v., IV	intravenous	
	i.v.p., IVP	intravenous push	
	IVPB	intravenous piggyback	
	o.d.	right eye	oculus dexter
	o.s.	left eye	oculus sinister
	o.u.	each eye	oculus utro
	p.o.	by mouth	per os
	SQ, SC, subc	subcutaneously	
	top.	topically, locally	
FORM	aq	water	aqua
	aqua. dist.	distilled water	
	caps	capsules	capsula
	DW	distilled water	
	elix.	elixir	
	liq.	liquid	liquor
	NS	normal saline	
	supp.	suppository	suppositorum
	syr.	syrup	syrupus
	tab.	tablet	tabella
	ung.	ointment	ungentum
TIME	a.c.	before food, before meals	ante cibum
	a.m.	morning	ante meridien
	a.t.c.	around the clock	
	b.i.d.,bid	twice a day	bis in die
	h	hour, at the hour of	hora
	h.s.	at bedtime	hora somni
	p.c.	after food, after meals	post cibum
	p.r.n., prn	as needed	pro re nata
	q.i.d., qid	four times a day	quater in die
	q	each, every	quaque
	q.d.	every day	quaque die
	q.h.	every hour	quaque hora
	stat.	immediately	statim
	t.i.d., tid	three times a day	ter in die

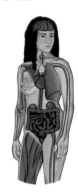

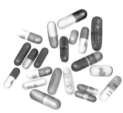

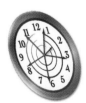

Note that some prescribers will leave out periods in written abbreviations, and that some may use capital letters, while other may not.

	Abbreviation	Meaning	Latin term
MEASUREMENT	ī	one, ī	
	a.a. or aa	of each	ana
	ad	to, up to	ad
	aq. ad	add water up to	
	dil.	dilute	dilutus
	div.	divide	
	f, fl.	fluid	
	g., G., gm.	gram	
	gtt.	drop	guttae
	L	liter	
	mcg.	microgram	
	mEq.	milliequivalent	
	mg.	milligram	
	ml.	milliliter	
	q.s.	a sufficient quantity	quantum sufficiat
	q.s. ad	add sufficient quantity to make	quantum sufficiat ad
	ss	one-half	
	tbsp.	tablespoon	
	tsp.	teaspoon	
OTHER	c	with	cum
	d.t.d.	give of such doses	dentur tales doses
	disp.	dispense	
	f, ft.	make, let it be made	fac, fiat, fiant
	l	left	laevus
	s	without	sine
	ut dict., u.d.	as directed	ut dictum

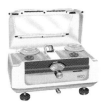

LESS COMMON ABBREVIATIONS

The following abbreviations are also used, though less frequently than the others on these pages.

ad lib.	at pleasure	collyr.	an eyewash	N.F.	National Formulary
add	add (thou)	comp.	compound	non.rep.	do not repeat
agit	shake, stir	cong.; C.	gallon	O.	pint
alt. h.	every other hour	c.c.	with food; with meals	occulent.	eye ointment
a.	before	d.	give (thou); let be given	o.	eye
amp.	ampule	d.	right	o.l.	left eye
ag. dest.	distilled water	dieb. alt.	every other day	o.m.	every morning
aur.; a	ear	emuls.	emulsion	p.a.a.	to be applied to affected
a.l.	left ear	et	and		part
aurist	ear-drops	e.m.p.	in the manner prescribed;	p.r.	per rectum
b.	twice		as directed	pulv.	powder
brach.	the arm	gr.	grain	s.a.	according to the art
BSA	body surface area	lin.	liniment	Sig.	write, label
c.c.	cubic centimeter	lot.	lotion	s.o.s.	if necessary
charts	powder papers; divided	min;	minum	sol.	solution
	powders	m.; M	mix	tinc.; tr.	tincture
cib.; c.	food	n.	at night	troche	lozenge
collun	a nose wash	narist.	nasal drops	tuss.	a cough
collut.	a mouthwash	neb.	a spray		

MEDICAL ABBREVIATIONS

Besides abbreviations used in prescriptions, there are many other abbreviations used in health care.

In addition to the abbreviations on the previous pages, these abbreviations are also important for the pharmacy technician to learn.

The following are a few of the abbreviations with medical significance that health care professionals should know. Some of these abbreviations have multiple meanings. These are the most common.

Name B. Arnold   Date 1/20/99

Room 202.1

Shift	2300-0700	0700-1500	1500-2300
AM Care/HS Care: C-complete, A-assist, S-self, B-bath, P-partial, S-shower	N/A	A-B-P	Backrub-HS
Sleep: G-good, P-poor, N-nap, Inter-interrupted	G-Inter	N/A	N
LOC: Awake, asleep, vague, lethargic, belligerent, nonresp-nonresponsive	Asleep	Awake, alert	Awake, alert
Orientation: D-disoriented (to time, place, etc.) O-oriented	OX3 when awake	OX3	OX3
Activity: B-bedrest, BRP, chair, hoyer, S-self, A-assist—of how many?	N/A	chair-S	chair-S
Ambulation: S-self, A-assist of how many? Walker, Cane, Other, Distance?	N/A	S-W	S-W
Appetite: Percent of food consumed.	N/A	B 50% L 90%	D 80%
Diet Supplement: Type and amt. consumed, HS-snack	N/A	Orange 100%	HS-Ensure 50%
Color: P-pale, F-flushed, D-dusky, Cy-cyanotic, J-jaundice, other, Define.	P	P	P
Skin Condition: W/D-warm & dry, sweating, diaph, cool, clammy, rash, turgor, other.	W/D	W/D	W/D
Turned & Positioned: A-assist, S-self, q2h, other.	S	S	S
Restraints: Type, ✓ - pt. assessed q30 min.	N/A	N/A	N/A
Siderails: Time and number rails Cont=continuous	↑X4	N/A	N/A
Prone to Fall ✓ - in progress	N/A	N/A	N/A

Abbreviations are commonly used in hospitals and other health care settings to make record keeping easier. Note the various abbreviations on the above hospital flow sheet. Also note that these are for a specific hospital and may not be used elsewhere.

AIDS	Acquired immunodeficiency syndrome
AV	Atrial-ventricular
AMI	Acute myocardial infarction
ANS	Autonomic nervous system
BM	Bowel movement
BP	Blood pressure
CA	Cancer
COPD	Chronic obstructive pulmonary disease
CV	Cardiovascular
CVA	Cerebrovascular accident (stroke)
DI	Diabetes insipidus
DOB	Date of birth
DX	Diagnosis
ECG, EKG	Electrocardiogram
GERD	Gastroesophageal reflux disease
GI	Gastrointestinal
H	Hypodermic
HDL	High density lipoprotein
HIV	Human Immunodeficiency virus
IH	Infectious hepatitis
IO, I/O	Fluid intake and output
LDL	Low density lipoprotein
MI	Myocardial infarction
NPO	Nothing by mouth
PUD	Peptic ulcer disease
RBC	Red blood count or red blood cell
T	Temperature
TB	Tuberculosis
U	Units
VD	Venereal disease
WBC	White blood count or white blood cell
WT	Weight
XX	Female sex chromosome
XY	Male sex chromosome

DRUG CLASSIFICATIONS

5

Root	Prefix
Suffix	C.V.

Classification names can be understood by identifying their components.

The same steps in interpreting other medical science terminology can be used to interpret drug classification names.

A classification is a grouping of a number of drugs that have some properties in common.

For example, penicillin, cefoxitine, and ciprofloxacin are used to treat bacterial infections, so they are grouped in a class called anti-infectives.

Each drug has unique properties, but they all share the property of being effective against bacterial infections. So the class name "anti-infective" is created by combing "anti" and "infective" into antiinfective, meaning "against infection." Since much of drug therapy is based on opposing some physiological process in the body, many drugs classes begin with the prefix "anti" or "ant."

THE "AGAINST" CLASS

Some examples of the "anti" class of drugs

antacids	relieves gastritis, ulcer pain, indigestion and heartburn
antianginals	relieves heart pain
anticoagulant	dissolves or prevents blood clots
anticonvulsants	prevents seizures
antidepressants	prevents depression
antidiarrheals	stops diarrhea
antiemetics	prevents nausea and vomiting
antihistamine	blocks the effects of histamine
antihyperlipidemics	lowers high cholesterol levels
antihypertensive	reduces blood pressure
anti-inflammatory	reduces inflammation
antipruritics	prevent or relieves itching
antispasmodics	relieves intestinal cramping
antitussive	relieves coughing by inhibiting cough reflex

OTHER CLASSES

Here are examples of other classification names which can be understood by breaking down the term into its medical terminology components.

de + conges + tant	**decongestant:**	reduces nasal congestion
an + alges + ics	**analgesics:**	without pain, kills pain
hypo + glyc + emics	**hypoglycemics:**	reduce blood sugar levels
hypo + lipid + emics	**hypolipidemics:**	reduce blood lipid (cholesterol) levels
kerat + o + lytics	**keratolytics:**	destroys skin layers such as warts
contra + cep + tives	**contraceptives:**	oral contraceptives, prevent pregnancy
psych + o + tropic	**pyschotropic:**	change mental states
sperm + i + cide	**spermicide:**	formulation that destroys sperm

77

PREFIXES

Root	Prefix
Suffix	C.V.

Below are common prefixes used in medical and pharmaceutical science terminology.

a	without		medi	middle
ambi	both		melan	black
an	without		meso	middle
ante	before		meta	beyond, after, changing
anti	against		micro	small
bi	two or both		mid	middle
brady	slow		mono	one
chlor	green		multi	many
circum	around		neo	new
cirrh	yellow		pan	all
con	with		para	alongside or abnormal
contra	against		peri	around
cyan	blue		polio	gray
dia	across or through		poly	many
dis	separate from or apart		post	after
dys	painful, difficult		pre	before
ec	away or out		pro	before
ecto	outside		pseudo	false
end	within		purpur	purple
epi	upon		quadri	four
erythr	red		re	again or back
eu	good or normal		retro	after
exo	outside		rube	red
heter	different		semi	half
hom	same		sub	below or under
hyper	above or excessive		super	above or excessive
hypo	below or deficient		supra	above or excessive
im	not		sym	with
immun	safe, protected		syn	with
in	not		tachy	fast
infra	below or under		trans	across, through
inter	between		tri	three
intra	within		ultra	beyond or excessive
is	equal		uni	one
leuk	white		xanth	yellow
macro	large		xer	dry

SUFFIXES

Root	Prefix
Suffix	C.V.

Below are common suffixes used in medical and pharmaceutical science terminology.

ac	pertaining to		oi	resembling
al	pertaining to		ole	small
algia	pain		oma	tumor
ar	pertaining to		opia	vision
ary	pertaining to		opsia	vision
asthenia	without strength		osis	abnormal condition
cele	pouching or hernia		osmia	smell
cyesis	pregnancy		ous	pertaining to
cynia	pain		paresis	partial paralysis
eal	pertaining to		pathy	disease
ectasis	expansion or dilation		penia	decrease
ectomy	removal		phagia	swallowing
emia	blood condition		phasia	speech
gram	record		philia	attraction for
graph	recording instrument		phobia	fear
graphy	recording process		plasia	formation
ia	condition of		plegia	paralysis, stroke
iasis	condition, formation of		rrhea	discharge
iatry	treatment		sclerosis	narrowing, constriction
ic	pertaining to		scope	examination instrument
icle	small		scopy	examination
ism	condition of		spasm	involuntary contraction
itis	inflammation		stasis	stop or stand
ium	tissue		tic	pertaining to
lith	stone, calculus		tocia	childbirth, labor
logy	study of		tomy	incision
malacia	softening		toxic	poison
megaly	enlargement		tropic	stimulate
meter	measuring instrument		ula	small
metry	measuring process		y	condition, process

REVIEW

KEY CONCEPTS

✔ Much of medical science terminology is made up of a small number of root words, suffixes and prefixes that originated from either Greek or Latin words.

✔ A prefix is added to the beginning of a root word to clarify its meaning.

✔ The suffix is added to the end of a root word to clarify the meaning.

✔ Combining vowels are used to connect the prefix, root, or suffix parts of the term.

✔ The cardiovascular system distributes blood throughout the body using blood vessels called arteries, capillaries, and veins.

✔ The endocrine system consists of the glands that secrete hormones (chemicals that assist in regulating body functions).

✔ The GI tract contains the organs that are involved in the digestion of foods and the absorption of nutrients.

✔ The integumentary system is the body's first line of defense, acting as a barrier against disease and other hazards.

✔ The lymphatic system is the center of the body's immune system.

✔ Lymphocytes release antibodies that destroy disease cells and provide immunity against them.

✔ The body contains more than 600 muscles which give shape and movement to it.

✔ The nervous system is the body's system of communication. The neuron (nerve cell) is its basic functional unit.

✔ The skeletal system protects soft organs and provides structure and support for the body's organ systems.

✔ The female reproductive system produces hormones (estrogen, progesterone), controls menstruation, and provides for childbearing.

✔ The male reproductive system produces sperm and secretes the hormone testosterone.

✔ The respiratory system brings oxygen into the body through inhalation and expels carbon dioxide gas through exhalation.

✔ The primary organ of the urinary system is the kidney, which filters the blood for unwanted material and makes urine.

✔ The sense of hearing, as well as the maintenance of body equilibrium, is performed by the ear.

SELF TEST

MATCH THE TERMS. *answers are in the back of the book*

a.	arteriosclerosis	g.	myoplasty	m.	bid	s.	q
b.	hyperlipidemia	h.	encephalitis	n.	qid	t.	p.c.
c.	melanocytoma	i.	salpingocyesis	o.	ss	u.	po
d.	hepatoma	j.	prn	p.	au	v.	top.
e.	transdermal	k.	gtt	q.	ung	w.	qd
f.	hematoma	l.	tid	r.	hs		

1. through the skin _____
2. blood tumor _____
3. high fat content in blood _____
4. brain inflammation _____
5. fallopian pregnancy _____
6. hardening of artery _____
7. muscle repair _____
8. black cell tumor _____
9. liver tumor _____
10. ointment _____
11. drop _____
12. twice a day _____

13. three times a day _____
14. four times a day _____
15. as needed _____
16. each ear _____
17. one-half _____
18. at bedtime _____
19. by mouth _____
20. topically, locally _____
21. every day _____
22. after food, after meals _____
23. each, every _____

MATCH THE TERMS. *answers can be checked on page 58*

1. card _____ a. bladder
2. cyst _____ b. blood
3. derma _____ c. bone
4. gastr _____ d. breast
5. hemat _____ e. chest
6. hepat _____ f. ear
7. mast _____ g. eye
8. my _____ h. heart

9. nephr _____ i. vein
10. neur _____ j. liver
11. ocul _____ k. lung
12. oste _____ l. muscle
13. ot _____ m. nerve
14. pector _____ n. skin
15. pneum _____ o. stomach
16. ven _____ p. kidney

MEASUREMENT

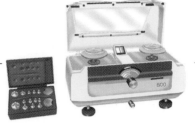

There are a number of measurement systems used in pharmacology, with the metric being the primary one.

Within these systems there are different measurements for weight, volume, and length, as well as for liquids and solids. There are also different measurement systems for temperature. It is often necessary to know how to convert one type of measurement to another.

METRIC SYSTEM

The major system of weights and measures used in medicine is the metric system. It was developed in France in the late 18th century and is based on a decimal system. That is, **different measurement units are related by measures of ten.** Technicians need to know metric measures for both liquids and solids.

Liquids

Liquids (including lotions) are measured by **volume.** The most widely used metric volume measurements are liters or milliliters.

Unit	Symbol	Liquid Conversions		
liter	L	1L	= 10dl	= 1000ml
deciliter	dl	1dl	= 0.1L	= 100ml
milliliter	ml	1ml	= 0.001L	= 0.01dl

Note: deciliters are rarely used, but are included here for reference and to illustrate the decimal relationship of these measures.

Solids

Solids (pills, granules, ointments, etc.) are measured by **weight.**

Unit	Symbol	Solid Conversions		
kilogram	kg	1 kg	= 1,000 g	
gram	g	1 g	= 0.001 kg	= 1000 mg
milligram	mg	1 mg	= 0.001 g	= 1000 mcg
microgram	mcg or μg	1 mcg	= 0.001 mg	= 0.000001 g

 Milliliters are sometimes referred to as *cubic centimeters (cc).* They are not precisely the same but are quite close and are sometimes used interchangeably.

AVOIRDUPOIS SYSTEM

The Avoirdupois system is the system of weight (ounces and pounds) that we commonly use. However, one Avoirdupois unit used in pharmacy is rarely used elsewhere. It is the **grain.**

Unit	symbol	Conversions		
pound	lb	1 lb	=	16 oz
ounce	oz	1 oz	=	437.5 gr
grain	gr	1 gr	=	64.8 mg

THE GRAIN

The grain is the same weight in several different measurement systems: Apothecary, Avoirdupois, and Troy. It is said to have been established as a unit of weight in 1266 by King Henry III of England when he required the English penny to weigh the equivalent of 32 dried grains of wheat. On the metric scale, one grain equals 64.8 milligrams. However, this is often rounded to 65 milligrams and sometimes to 60 milligrams.

APOTHECARY SYSTEM

The Apothecary system is sometimes used in prescriptions, primarily with liquids. It includes the fluid ounce, pint, quart, and gallon. Although there are Apothecary weight units, they are generally not used, with the exception of the grain. The fluid ounce is a volume measure and is different than the weight ounce. It is always indicated by "fl oz."

Unit	symbol	Conversions		
gallon	gal	1 gal	=	4 qt
quart	qt	1 qt	=	2 pt
pint	pt	1 pt	=	16 fl oz
ounce	fl oz	1 fl oz	=	8 fl dr
fluid dram	fl dr	1 fl dr	=	60 min
minim	min or M_x			

Note: drams and minims are rarely used, but are included here for reference.

 conversions the change of one unit of measure into another so that both amounts are equal.

MEASUREMENT (cont'd)

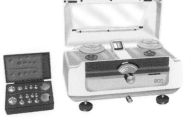

HOUSEHOLD UNITS

The teaspoon and tablespoon are common household measurement units that are regularly used in liquid prescriptions.

Unit	symbol	Conversions
teaspoon	tsp	1tsp = 5ml
tablespoon	tbs	1tbs = 3 tsp = 15ml
cup	cup	1 cup = 8 fl oz

TEMPERATURE

The **Centigrade** scale, which is also called **Celsius**, is used to measure temperature. The relationship of Centigrade (C) to Fahrenheit (F) is:

$$\textbf{F temperature} \quad = \quad (1\tfrac{4}{5} \textbf{ times number of degrees C) + 32}$$

EXAMPLE
$$212°F = 100°C$$
$$\textit{because} \quad \text{a) } 1\tfrac{4}{5} \times 100 = 180$$
$$\textit{and} \quad \text{b) } 180 + 32 = 212$$

$$\textbf{C temperature} \quad = \quad \tfrac{5}{9} \textbf{ x (number of degrees F - 32)}$$

EXAMPLE
$$100°C = 212°F$$
$$\textit{because } \tfrac{5}{9} \times (212\text{-}32) = \tfrac{5}{9} \times 180 = 100$$

Note that the temperature of water freezing is 0°C and 32°F.

CONVERSIONS

Conversions are the change of one unit of measure into another so that both amounts are equal. Following are some commonly used unit conversions.

1 L	=	33.8 fl oz	1 lb	=	453.59 g
1 pt	=	473.167 ml	1 oz	=	28.35 g
1 fl oz	=	29.57ml	1 g	=	15.43 gr
1 kg	=	2.2 lb	1 gr	=	64.8 mg

PERCENTS AND SOLUTIONS

Percentage concentrations refer to a drug's weight per 100 ml if the drug is a solid, or the drug's volume per 100 ml if the drug is a liquid.

$$\text{solid \%} = \frac{\text{weight (gm)}}{100\text{ml}}$$

$$\text{liquid \%} = \frac{\text{volume (ml)}}{100\text{ml}}$$

For example, a 5% dextrose solution contains 5 grams of dextrose (a solid) in 100 ml of solution. A 5% acetic acid solution (common household vinegar) contains 5 ml of acetic acid (a liquid) per 100 ml of solution.

Note that percentage concentrations are applied to other formulations besides solutions. A 10% zinc oxide ointment would have 10 grams of zinc oxide (a solid) in 100 grams of ointment.

MILLIEQUIVALENTS – mEq

Electrolytes are substances that conduct an electrical current and are found in the body's blood, tissue fluids, and cells. Salts are electrolytes and saline solutions are a commonly used electrolyte solution. The concentration of electrolytes in a volume of solution is measured in units called milliequivalents (mEq). They are generally expressed as milliequivalents per milliliter or equivalents per Liter.

Milliequivalents are a unit of measurement specific to each electrolyte. For example, a 0.9% solution of one electrolyte will have a different mEq value than a 0.9% solution of another because mEq values are based on each electrolyte's atomic weight and electron properties. Solutions with different mEq values may be mixed and the new combined mEq value calculated by simply using the ratio and proportion calculation method.

COMMON ELECTROLYTES:

NaCl	Sodium Chloride
$MgSO_4$	Magnesium Sulfate
KCl	Potassium Chloride
K Acetate	Potassium Acetate
Ca Gluconate	Calcium Gluconate
Na Acetate	Sodium Acetate.

MEASUREMENT (cont'd)

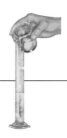

OSMOLES

Another expression for the amount of drug in a solution is the osmole (Osmol). An osmole is equal to the molecular weight of the drug divided by the number of **ions** formed when a drug dissolves in solution.

$$\text{osmole} = \frac{\text{molecular weight}}{\text{ions}}$$

For example, potassium chloride forms two ions when it dissolves in solution. Therefore, 1 Osmol of potassium chloride would be its molecular weight (74.6 grams) divided by two: 37.3 grams. Most drug solution concentrations are expressed as Osmol/liter (written as Osmol/L). Some concentrations are expressed as mOsmol/L. A milliosmole is one-thousandth of an osmole.

MOLARITY

Molarity is an expression of the number of **moles** of a drug in a volume of solution. A mole is the number of grams equal to the molecular weight of the drug.

$$\text{mole} = \text{molecular weight of a drug in grams}$$

The molecular weight is the sum of the atomic weights of all the atoms that make up the molecule. Potassium chloride (KCl) has a molecular weight of 74.6, so one mole of potassium chloride is 74.6 grams.

Concentrations are generally expressed as mole/liter (written as mol/L, or M). A 1M solution of potassium chloride contains 74.6 grams of the drug in 1000 ml (1 liter) of solution. Note: Some molarity concentrations are expressed as millimoles per liter. A millimole is one-thousandth of a mole.

INTERNATIONAL UNITS

Because the potency and purity of drugs from biological sources vary depending on the source, they are measured by **units of activity** rather than by weight. Units may be abbreviated as IU, or U, and are expressed for example as 2,000 U, 1,000,000 U, etc.

Note: Drugs commonly measured in international units include penicillin, insulin, heparin, and some vitamins.

ROMAN NUMERALS

Roman numerals are letters that represent numbers. They were originally developed and used by the Roman Empire. Though arabic numbers are the primary ones we use, Roman numerals are often used to indicate quantities in prescription or order writing. They can be capital or lower case letters, and are:

$ss = \frac{1}{2}$ L or l = 50

I or i = 1   C or c = 100

V or v = 5   D or d = 500

X or x = 10   M or m = 1000

When grouped together, these few letters can express a large range of numbers, using a simple *positional notation.* That means the position of the letters has a mathematical importance, as determined by these rules:

When the second of two letters has a value equal to or smaller than that of the first, their values are to be added.

EXAMPLE:

xx = 20   or   10 plus 10

lxvi = 66   or   50 plus 10 plus 5 plus 1

When the second of two letters has a value greater than that of the first, the smaller is to be subtracted from the larger.

EXAMPLE:

iv = 4   or   1 subtracted from 5

xxxix = 39   or   30 plus (1 subtracted from 10)

 international units units used to measure the activity potential of chemicals from natural sources, including vitamins and drugs such as penicillin.
molecular weight the sum of the atomic weights of one molecule of a substance.
moles the molecular weight of a drug in grams.
osmoles the molecular weight of a drug divided by the number of ions it forms when dissolved in a solution.

CALCULATIONS

RATIO AND PROPORTION

Many of the calculations for dosages and other measurements can be performed using the **ratio and proportion** calculation method.

A ratio states a relationship between two quantities. $\frac{a}{b}$

A proportion contains two equal ratios. $\frac{a}{b} = \frac{c}{d}$

When three of the four quantities in a proportion are known, the value of the fourth (x) can be easily solved. $\frac{x}{b} = \frac{c}{d}$

Example

If there are 125 mg of a substance in a 500 ml solution, and 50 mg is desired, the amount of solution needed can be determined with this equation:

$$\frac{x \text{ ml}}{50 \text{ mg}} = \frac{500 \text{ ml}}{125 \text{ mg}}$$

multiplying both sides by 50 mg gives:

$$x \text{ ml} = \frac{2500 \text{ ml}}{125}$$

solving for x gives:

$$x = 200$$

answer: 200 ml of solution are needed.

USING CALCULATORS

Though many calculations can be done using ratio and proportion, the use of calculators is essential in the correct computation of many dosages. Their answers are precise and provided in decimals. Since it is relatively easy to make entry mistakes on a calculator, always recheck answers. Also, use judgment. If an answer doesn't appear to make sense, check it.

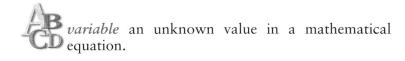 *variable* an unknown value in a mathematical equation.

CALCULATION OF CHILDREN'S DOSES

The average doses in the U.S.P. (United States Pharmacopeia) and other drug reference sources are for adults. Doses for drugs that can be taken by a child are generally not given. When they are not, the adult dose needs to be lowered. One formula for this is:

CLARK'S RULE

$$\frac{\text{weight of child}}{150 \text{ lb}} \times \text{adult dose} = \text{dose for child}$$

150 lbs is considered an average weight for an adult. This is not a very precise way to calculate pediatric doses as there are many factors besides weight which may need to be taken into account: height, age, condition, etc. Another approach is based upon multiplying the adult dose by a ratio of the child's size to that of an average adult:

BODY SURFACE AREA FORMULA

$$\frac{\text{child bsa times adult dose}}{\text{average adult bsa}} = \text{child's dose}$$

The **body surface area** of a person is based on the person's height and weight. It is always given in square meters (m²). 1.73 m² is commonly used as an average bsa for adults. A chart called a **nomogram** has been traditionally used to manually calculate bsa. Body surface area nomograms contain three columns of numbers: height, body surface, and weight. The bsa is identified by the intersection of a line drawn between the weight and height columns with the bsa column, which is in the middle. Now, bsa formulas are generally solved by computer. (There are a number that can be found on the Internet, for example.) For a comparison to the average bsa for adults (1.73 m²), a bsa for a nine year old child that was 44" tall and weighing 50 lbs would be about .92 m².

Because of the many variables, *pediatric doses are generally given by the physician and are stated by kg of body weight (dose/kg).* Since 1 kg = 2.2 lb, a prescribed dose can be calculated by using a proportion equation if the child's body weight is known.

Note: body surface area is often used with chemotherapy doses.

CALCULATIONS (cont'd)

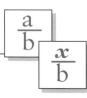

FLOW RATES

In infusion therapy, the flow rate or rate of administration for an IV solution often needs to be calculated. This is done using a ratio and proportion equation. Rates are generally calculated in ml/hour, but calculations are also done in ml/min or gtt/min.

For example, if you have an order for KCl 10mEq and K Acetate 15 mEq in D5W 1000 ml to run at 80 ml/hour, you would determine the administration rate in ml/minute as follows:

$$x \text{ ml} \div 1 \text{ min} = 80 \text{ ml} \div 60 \text{ min}$$

$$x = 80/60 = 1.33$$

To get drops per minute (gtt/min), you must have a conversion rate of drops per ml. For example, if the administration set for the above order delivered 30 drops per ml, you would find the drops per minute as follows:

$$\frac{80 \text{ ml}}{60 \text{ min}} \times \frac{30 \text{ gtt}}{1 \text{ ml}} = \frac{2400 \text{ gtt}}{60 \text{ min}} = 40 \text{ gtt/min}$$

MILLIEQUIVALENT CALCULATIONS

As mentioned previously, performing dosage calculations on solutions with known milliequivalents is simply a matter of applying ratio and proportion. For example, if a solution calls for 5 mEq of an electrolyte that you have in a 1.04 mEq/ml solution, the amount of solution needed is calculated as follows.

$$\textbf{x} \text{ ml} \div 5 \text{ mEq} = 1 \text{ ml} \div 1.04 \text{ mEq}$$

$$\textbf{x} \text{ ml} = 5 \; \cancel{\text{mEq}} \text{ times } \frac{1 \text{ ml}}{1.04 \; \cancel{\text{mEq}}} = \frac{5 \text{ ml}}{1.04} = 4.8 \text{ ml}$$

Answer: 4.8 ml of the solution contains 5 mEq of the electrolyte.

Solutions with different mEq values can also be mixed and the new mEq calculated using ratio and proportion.

MIXING SOLUTIONS – ALLIGATIONS

When mixing solutions of different concentrations, it is possible to calculate the new concentration using ratio and proportion or the **alligation method**. Using this method, if a 95% solution is to be mixed with a 50% solution to create a 70% solution, the amounts of each solution can be determined as follows.

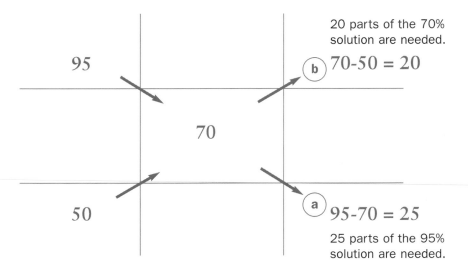

95

70

50

20 parts of the 70% solution are needed.

(b) 70-50 = 20

(a) 95-70 = 25

25 parts of the 95% solution are needed.

a) Determine "**y**" (the amount needed of the weaker solution) by subtracting the desired solution concentration from the concentration with the highest percentage:
$$95\text{-}70 = 25$$

b) Determine "**x**" (the amount needed of the stronger solution) by subtracting the weaker solution concentration from the desired solution concentration:
$$70\text{-}50 = 20$$

c) The **x/y ratio is therefore 20/25,** with x indicating the number of parts of the higher percentage solution and y indicating the number of parts of the lower pecentage solution needed for the mixture.

d) Intepret this as **20 parts of the 95% solution are needed for every 25 of the 50% solution.** (This can also be reduced to four parts of one for every five of the other.)

REVIEW

KEY CONCEPTS

✔ Liquids (including lotions) are measured by volume. The most widely used metric volume measurements are liters or milliliters.

✔ Milliliters are sometimes referred to as cubic centimeters (cc). They are not precisely the same but are quite close and are sometimes used interchangeably.

✔ Solids (pills, granules, ointments, etc.) are measured by weight in grams, milligrams, etc.

✔ The Avoirdupois system is the system of weight (ounces and pounds) that we commonly use. An Avoirdupois unit used in pharmacy that is rarely used elsewhere is the grain.

✔ The Apothecary system is sometimes used in prescriptions, primarily with liquids. It includes the fluid ounce, pint, quart, and gallon. The fluid ounce is a volume measure and is different than the weight ounce. It is always indicated by "fl oz."

✔ The relationship of Centigrade (C) to Fahrenheit (F) is: $F° = (1\frac{4}{5}$ times number of degrees C) + 32°.

✔ Percentage concentrations refer to a drug's weight in grams per 100 ml if the drug is a solid, or the drug's volume in milliliters per 100 ml if the drug is a liquid.

✔ The concentration of electrolytes in a volume of solution is measured in units called milliequivalents (mEq). They are generally expressed as milliequivalents per milliliter.

✔ An osmole is a concentration measurement equal to the molecular weight of the drug divided by the number of ions formed when a drug dissolves in solutions.

✔ Molarity is an expression of the number of moles of a drug in a volume of solution. A mole is the number of grams equal to the molecular weight of the drug.

✔ When three of the four quantities in a proportion equation are known, the value of the fourth (x) can be easily solved.

✔ The average doses in the U.S.P. (United States Pharmacopeia) and other drug reference sources are for adults. Because of the many variables, pediatric doses are generally given by the physician and are stated by kg of body weight (dose/kg).

✔ The body surface area of a person is based on the person's height and weight. It is always given in square meters (m^2). 1.73 m^2 is commonly used as an average bsa for adults.

SELF TEST

answers are in the back of the book

Convert the following:

A. 500 g   = _____ mg   F. 102 kg = _____ lb

B. 10 kg   = _____ g   G. 3.56 kg = _____ g

C. 250 ml = _____ L   H. 473 ml = _____ L

D. 325 mg = _____ g   I. 145 lb = _____ kg

E. 120 mcg = _____ mg   J. 30 kg   = _____ mg

Solve the following in the space beneath the problem:

Temperature Problem

K. Oral Polio Virus Vaccine (Poliovax®) should be stored in a temperature not to exceed 46 degrees Fahrenheit. What is this temperature in Centigrade?

Electrolyte Solution

M. $MgSO_4$ (magnesium sulfate) 10 mEq is ordered for an IV. On hand is a bottle of $MgSO_4$ 4 mEq/ml. How much $MgSO_4$ should be injected into this IV bag?

Liquid Dose

L. A prescription reads for erythromycin 150 mg every six hours for ten days. On hand is erythromycin 250 mg/5 ml. How much erythromycin is needed for one dose?

A Dilution

N. 20% dextrose 500 ml is ordered. On hand is a 1000 ml bag of dextrose 70%. How much of the dextrose 70% is needed to make dextrose 20% 500 ml? How much sterile water should be added?

REVIEW

Choose the correct answer:

O. A solution of halperidol (Haldol®) contains 2 mg /ml of active ingredient. How many grams would be in 473 ml of this solution?

    a.) 9.46 grams
    b.) 0.946 grams
    c.) 0.0946 grams
    d.) 0.00946 grams

P. The physician orders ferrous sulfate 500 mg po qd x 30 days. The available solution is ferrous sulfate 220 mg/5ml 473ml. How many ml of this is required for one dose of the order?

    a.) 5.4 ml
    b.) 8.4 ml
    c.) 11.4 ml
    d.) 13.4 ml

Q. Using the same information in the previous problem, approximately how many ml are required to completely fill the prescription?

    a.) 162 ml
    b.) 252 ml
    c.) 342 ml
    d.) 402 ml

R. The infusion rate of an IV is over twelve hours. The total volume is 800 ml. What would the infusion rate be in ml per minute?

    a.) 66.6 ml / minute
    b.) 6.6 ml / minute
    c.) 0.6 ml / minute
    d.) none of the above

S. How many Kg of dextrose is in 400 ml of a 70% solution of dextrose 1000 ml?

    a.) 280 Kg
    b.) 28 Kg
    c.) 2.8 Kg
    d.) 0.28 Kg

T. An order is written for vancomycin (Vancocin®) 10 mg/Kg 500 ml to be infused over 90 minutes. The patient is five foot eleven inches tall and weighs 165 lb. What dose is needed for this patient?

   a.) 750 mg
   b.) 500 mg
   c.) 250 mg
   d.) 125 mg

U. The doctor orders codeine gr $\frac{1}{4}$. How many milligrams is this?

   a.) 15 mg
   b.) 30 mg
   c.) 60 mg
   d.) none of the above

V. A prescription is written for metronidazole (Flagyl®) 250 mg/5 ml po qid 240 ml. This will have to be compounded using 500 mg tablets. How many tablets are needed to fill this order completely?

   a.) 22 tablets
   b.) 24 tablets
   c.) 42 tablets
   d.) 48 tablets

W. 45 mEq of Ca Gluconate is ordered to be added to an IV bag of D5%W 1000 ml. How many ml of Ca Gluconate 4.4 mEq/ml 50 ml needs to be added to the IV bag?

   a.) 1.2 ml
   b.) 10.2 ml
   c.) 0.12 ml
   d.) 2.4 ml

ROUTES & FORMULATIONS

The way in which the body absorbs and distributes drugs varies with the route of administration.

Drugs are contained in products called **formulations**. There are many drug formulations and many different **routes** to administer them.

Routes are classified as enteral or parenteral.

Oral administration is called **enteral**. Enteral refers to anything involving the **alimentary** tract, i.e., from the mouth to the rectum. This tract is involved with digesting foods, absorbing nutrients, and eliminating unabsorbed wastes. There are three enteral routes: **oral**, **sublingual**, and **rectal**.

Any route other than oral, sublingual, and rectal is considered a parenteral administration route.

The term parenteral means next to, or beside the enteral. It refers to any sites that are outside of or beside the enteral or alimentary tract.

For each route, there are various formulations used to deliver the drug via that route.

Different dosage forms affect onset times, length of action, or concentrations of a drug in the body. Some drugs are formulated in more than one dosage form with each form producing different characteristics in these areas. A consideration for selecting a particular route or dosage form the type of effect desired. A **local effect** occurs when the drug activity is at the site of administration (e.g., eyes, ears, nose, skin). A **systemic effect** occurs when the drug is introduced into the circulatory system by any route of administration and is therefore carried throughout the body.

Route	Dosage Form
Subcutaneous	Solutions
	Suspensions
	Emulsions
	Implants
Vaginal	Solutions
	Ointments
	✳ Creams
	Aerosol foams
	Powders
	✳ Suppositories
	Tablets
	Sponge
	IUDs

✳ most common

FORMULATIONS

Route	Dosage Form
Oral	Tablets
	Capsules
	Bulk Powders
	Solutions
	Suspensions
	Elixirs
	Syrups
Sublingual	Tablets
Rectal	Solutions
	Ointments
	Suppositories
Intraocular	Solutions
	Suspensions
	Ointments
	Inserts
	Contact lenses
Intranasal	Solutions
	Suspensions
	Sprays
	Aerosols
	Inhalers
	Powders
Inhalation	Aerosols
	Powders
Intravenous	Solutions
Intramuscular	Suspensions
Intradermal	Emulsions
Dermal	Solutions
	Suspensions
	Tinctures
	Collodions
	Liniments
	Ointments
	Creams
	Gels
	Lotions
	Pastes
	Plasters
	Powders
	Aerosols
	Transdermal patches

ROUTES

Enteral Routes are in red.
Parenteral routes are in black.
The term is followed by the organ(s) of absorption.

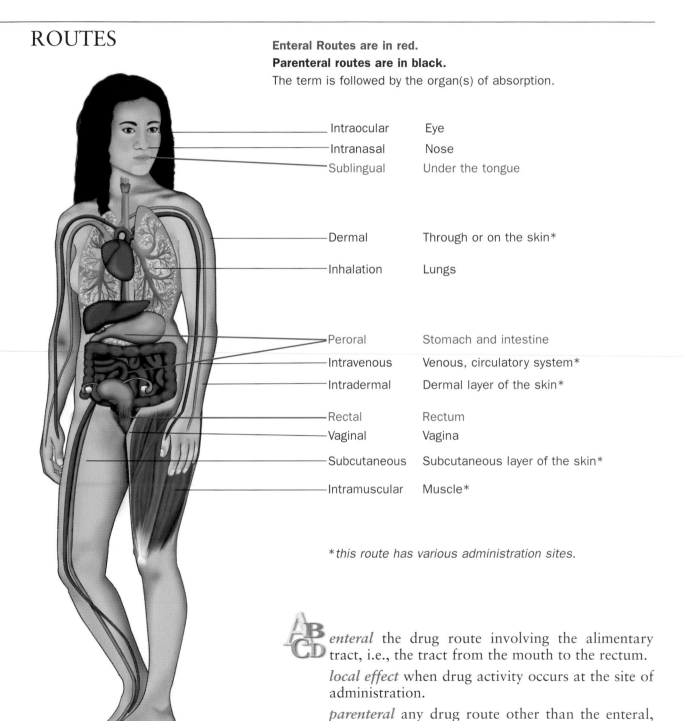

Intraocular	Eye
Intranasal	Nose
Sublingual	Under the tongue
Dermal	Through or on the skin*
Inhalation	Lungs
Peroral	Stomach and intestine
Intravenous	Venous, circulatory system*
Intradermal	Dermal layer of the skin*
Rectal	Rectum
Vaginal	Vagina
Subcutaneous	Subcutaneous layer of the skin*
Intramuscular	Muscle*

this route has various administration sites.

ABCD *enteral* the drug route involving the alimentary tract, i.e., the tract from the mouth to the rectum.

local effect when drug activity occurs at the site of administration.

parenteral any drug route other than the enteral, e.g., intravenous, inhalation, vaginal, etc.

systemic effect the effect caused when a drug is introduced into the circulatory system and carried throughout the body.

ORAL FORMULATIONS

Oral administration is the most frequently used route of administration.

Oral dosage forms are easy to use, carry, and administer. The term used to specify oral administration is **peroral** or **PO** (per os). This indicates that the dosage form is to be swallowed and that absorption will occur primarily in the stomach and the intestine.

When formulations are orally administered, they enter the stomach, which is very acidic.

The stomach has a pH around 1-2. Certain drugs cannot be taken orally because they are **degraded** (chemically changed to a less effective form) or destroyed by stomach acid and intestinal enzymes. Additionally, the absorption of many drugs is affected by the presence of food in the stomach.

Drugs administered by liquid dosage forms generally reach the circulatory system faster than drugs formulated in solid dosage forms.

This is because the processes of **disintegration** and **dissolution** are not required. Oral liquids include solutions, suspensions, syrups, and elixirs. Solid oral dosage forms include tablets, capsules, and bulk powders.

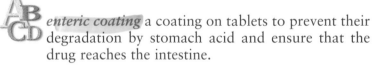

enteric coating a coating on tablets to prevent their degradation by stomach acid and ensure that the drug reaches the intestine.

pH the pH scale measures the *acidity* or the opposite (*alkalinity*) of a substance. 7 is the neutral midpoint of the scale, values below which represent increasing acidity, and above which represent increasing alkalinity.

Most oral dosage forms are intended for systemic effect, but not all. For example, antacids have a local effect confined to the gastrointestinal tract.

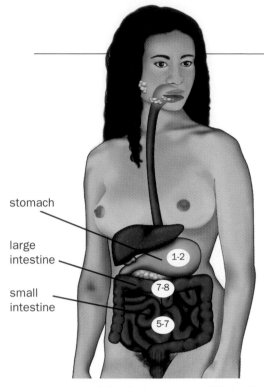

gastrointestinal organs and their pH

Gastrointestinal Action

The disintegration and dissolution of tablets, capsules, and powders generally begins in the stomach, but will continue to occur when the stomach empties into the intestine. **Controlled-release** or **extended-release** formulations are made so that dissolution occurs over a period of hours and provides a longer duration of effect compared to plain tablets. **Enteric coated** tablets serve a different function. They are used when the drug can be degraded by the stomach acid. The enteric coating will not let the tablet disintegrate until it reaches the higher pHs of the intestine.

Inactive Ingredients

Oral formulations contain various ingredients beside the active drug. These include binders, effervescent salts, lubricants, fillers, diluents, and disintegrants. They are added to help in the manufacture of the formulation and to help it disintegrate and dissolve when administered. A sample breakdown of ingredients is illustrated at right. Note, however, that each formulation is different.

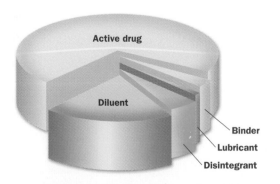

degradation the changing of a drug to a less effective or ineffective form.

adsorb attachment of one chemical to another.

SOLID FORMULATIONS

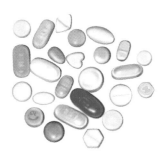

Tablets are hard formulations in which the drug and other ingredients are machine compressed under high pressure into a shape. Tablets vary in size, weight, hardness, thickness, and disintegration and dissolution characteristics depending upon their intended use. Most tablets are manufactured for peroral use, and many are coated to give an identifying color or logo on the formulation. **Sugar-coated** tablets are coated with a sweet glaze. **Film-coated** tablets are coated with a non-sweet coating. **Multiple compressed** tablets contain one drug in an inner layer and another drug (or the same drug) compressed at a lower pressure over it as an outer layer. They are used when a rapid release is desired for one drug (the outer layer) and a slower release is desired for the other drug (the inner layer). Other popular tablets are **chewable** and **effervescent.**

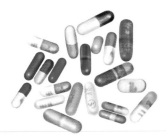

Capsules contain the drug and the other ingredients packaged in a gelatin shell. There are several capsule sizes. The capsule size used in any formulation is based on the amount of material to be placed inside the capsule. The gelatin shell dissolves in the stomach and releases the contents of the capsule. The freed contents must still undergo disintegration and dissolution before the drug is absorbed into the circulatory system. There are some capsule formulations that contain liquid instead of powders inside the gelatin shell. These are called "soft" capsules or "soft-gel" capsules. The active drug is already dissolved in the liquid.

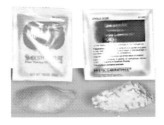

Bulk powders (e.g., Goody's BC powders) contain the active drug in a small powder paper or foil envelope. The patient empties the envelope into a glass of water or juice and drinks the contents. Most of the drug and ingredients dissolve in the water before the patient takes it.

LIQUID FORMULATIONS

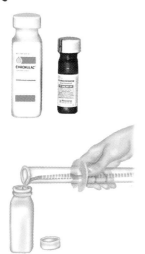

Solutions are made up of one or more solvents containing one or more dissolved substances. A solvent is a liquid which can dissolve another substance to form a solution. Solutions, elixirs, and syrups contain the drug and other ingredients already dissolved in the liquid. Elixirs are sweetened water and alcohol solutions that are generally less thick or viscous than water. Syrups are generally sugar-based solutions which are more viscous than water.

Suspensions are formulations where the drug cannot completely dissolve in the liquid. The drug particles are suspended in the liquid formulation. When suspensions are administered, the particles must dissolve before the drug is absorbed into the circulatory system. There are some suspensions that are intended for local activity: (e.g., activated charcoal, kaolin). These suspensions are orally administered to **adsorb** excessive intestinal fluid. In these suspensions, the particles will not dissolve.

SUBLINGUAL

The mouth is the route of administration for certain drugs where a rapid action is desired.

Formulations used in the mouth are generally fast dissolving uncoated tablets which contain highly water soluble drugs. These tablets are placed under the tongue (**sublingual** administration). When the drug is released from the tablet, it is quickly absorbed into the circulatory system since the membranes lining the mouth are very thin and there is an rich blood supply to the mouth.

Nitroglycerin is the best known example of a sublingual tablet formulation.

Nitroglycerin is sublingually administered since it is degraded in the stomach and intestine. Nitroglycerin is also available in a **translingual aerosol** that permits a patient to spray droplets of nitroglycerin under the tongue. There are also some steroid sex hormones that are sublingually administered.

Sublingual administration has certain limitations.

For various reasons (including the condition of the mouth, the patient, etc.), other routes of administration are considered more convenient for many drugs that would otherwise be candidates for sublingual administration. An additional consideration is that holding a drug in the mouth for almost any period of time is unpleasant since most drugs have a bitter taste.

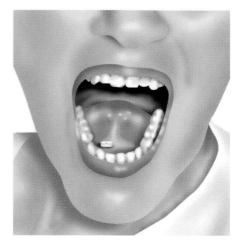

Using Sublingual Tablets

Sublingual tablets are highly water soluble, so patients should first take a sip of water to wet their mouth if it is dry.

The tablet is then placed far under the tongue and the mouth is closed and must remain closed until the tablet dissolves and is absorbed. No food or beverages can be taken until the drug is fully absorbed.

sublingual under the tongue.
water soluble the property of a substance being able to dissolve in water.

RECTAL

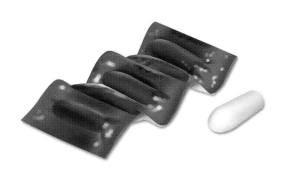

Suppositories

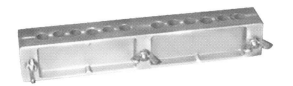

Mold used for making suppositories

Drugs are administered via the rectum either for a local effect or to bypass degradation caused by oral administration.

Local effects may include the soothing of inflamed hemorrhoidal tissues, promoting laxation, and enemas. Rectal administration for systemic activity is preferred when the drug is destroyed by stomach acid or intestinal enzymes, or if oral administration is unavailable (if the patient is vomiting, unconscious or incapable of swallowing oral formulations). Rectal administration is used to achieve a variety of systemic effects, including: asthma control, anti-nausea, antimotion sickness, and anti-infective.

The most common rectal administration forms are suppositories, solutions, and ointments.

Suppositories are semi-solid dosage forms that dissolve or melt when inserted into the rectum. Suppositories are manufactured in a variety of shapes and are used in other routes of administration such as vaginal or urethral. Most rectal solutions are used as enemas or cleansing solutions. Ointments are intended to be spread around the anal opening and are most often used to treat inflamed hemorrhoidal tissues.

Rectal dosage forms have certain significant disadvantages.

They are not preferred by most patients. They are inconvenient. Moreover, rectal absorption of most drugs is frequently erratic and unpredictable.

Enemas

Enemas create an urge to defecate due to the injection of fluid into the rectum. A **cleansing** enema injects water or a cleansing solution. A **retention** enema injects an oil that is held in the rectum to soften the stool. Frequent use of enemas is discouraged as it can can have significant adverse effects.

 enema a solution injected into the rectum that creates the urge to defecate.

hemorrhoid painful swollen veins in the anal/rectal area, generally caused by strained bowel movements from hard stools.

PARENTERAL ROUTES

Parenteral routes of administration are used for a variety of reasons.

If an orally administered drug is poorly absorbed, or is degraded by stomach acid or intestinal enzymes, then a parenteral route may be indicated. Parenteral routes are also preferred when a rapid drug response is desired, as in an emergency situation. Parenteral routes of administration are also useful when a patient is uncooperative, unconscious, or otherwise unable to take a drug by an enteral route.

There are disadvantages of formulations given by parenteral routes.

One is cost. Most parenterals are more expensive than enteral route formulations. Another is that injection parenterals require skilled personnel to administer them. An additional disadvantage is that once a parenteral drug is administered, it is most difficult to remove the dose if there is an adverse or toxic reaction. Finally, parenteral administration by injection has risks associated with invading the body with a needle (infection, thrombus, etc.).

Several parenteral routes require a needle and some type of propelling device (syringe, pump, gravity fed bag) to administer a drug.

These routes of administration are the **intravenous, intramuscular, intradermal,** and **subcutaneous.** These injectable routes have several characteristics in common. The formulations that can be used with injectables are limited to **solutions, suspensions,** and **emulsions.** Any other dosage formulation cannot pass through the syringe. These formulations must be **sterile** (bacteria-free) since they are placed in direct contact with the internal body fluids or tissues where infection can easily occur. The pH of the formulation must also be carefully maintained. This is commonly done by adding ingredients to the formulation as a **buffer** system. A fourth characteristic is that limited volumes of formulation can be injected. Too great an injection volume can cause pain and cell death (necrosis).

PARENTERALS

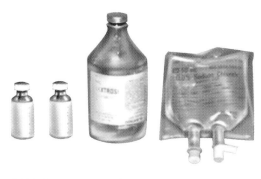

Which Parenteral?

Besides meaning any route other than oral, sublingual, and rectal, "parenteral" is commonly used to describe drugs administered through syringes. It is also used to describe the various bottles, vials, and bags used in preparing and delivering solutions for intravenous administration. It is possible to say that parenterals are prepared and parenterally administered at parenteral sites. As a result, extreme care must be taken when using the word parenteral so that the intended meaning is clear to all.

necrosis the death of cells.

sterile a sterile condition is one which is free of *all* microorganisms, both harmful and harmless.

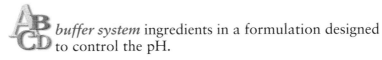
buffer system ingredients in a formulation designed to control the pH.

INJECTION ROUTES

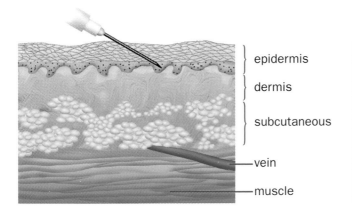

epidermis
dermis
subcutaneous
vein
muscle

Intradermal

Intradermal injections are administered into the top layer of the skin at a slight angle using short needles.

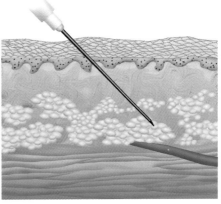

Subcutaneous

Subcutaneous injections are administered to the subcutaneous tissue of the skin using 3/8 inch to 1inch needles.

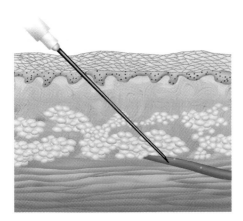

Intravenous

Intravenous injections are administered directly into veins.

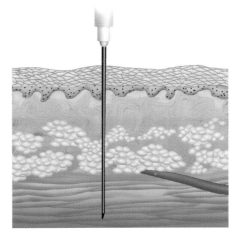

Intramuscular

Intramuscular injections are administered into muscle tissue using one to one-and-a-half inch needles.

INTRAVENOUS FORMULATIONS

Intravenous dosage forms are administered directly into a vein and therefore the blood supply.

Solutions are the most common formulation intravenously administered. Most solutions are **aqueous** (water based), but they may also have glycols, alcohols, or other non-aqueous solvents in them.

Injectable suspensions are difficult to formulate because they must possess syringeability and injectability.

Syringeability refers to the ease with which the suspension can be drawn from a container into a syringe. **Injectability** refers to the properties of the suspension while being injected, properties such as flow evenness, freedom from clogging, etc.

Emulsions are formulations that contain both aqueous and non-aqueous (oil) components.

Fat emulsions and total parenteral nutrition (TPN) emulsions are used to provide triglycerides, fatty acids, and calories for patients who cannot absorb them from the gastrointestinal tract.

Dry powder formulations are also manufactured for intravenous use, but they must be reconstituted with a suitable solvent to make a liquid formulation.

Some drugs are not stable in liquid form, and so these drugs are put into the powder form and reconstituted just prior to use. There are several solvents that might be used to reconstitute the dry powders. The appropriate solvent is indicated in the product information insert. The most common solvents are Sterile Water for Injection USP, Bacteriostatic Water for Injection USP, Sodium Chloride Injection USP, and Ringer's Injection USP.

COMPLICATIONS

There are a number of complications that can occur from intravenous administration. Some have already been mentioned: **sterility, excessive volumes, maintaining pH.** Additional complications are thrombosis, phlebitis, air emboli, and particulate material.

➡ **Thrombus** (blood clot) formation can result from many factors: extremes in solution pH, particulate material, irritant properties of the drug, needle or **catheter trauma,** and selection of too small a vein for the volume of solution injected.

➡ **Phlebitis,** or inflammation of the vein, can be caused by the same factors that cause thrombosis.

➡ **Air emboli** occur when air is introduced into the vein. The human body is generally not harmed by very small amounts of air injected into the venous system, but *air injected into the veins can be fatal,* and it is necessary to remove all air bubbles from formulation and administration sets before use.

➡ **Particulate material** can include small pieces of glass that chip from the formulation vial or rubber that comes from the rubber closure on injection vials. Although great care is taken to eliminate the presence of particulate material, a final filter in the administration line just before entering the venous system is an important precaution.

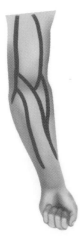

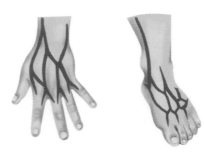

Intravenous Sites

Several sites on the body are used to intravenously administer drugs: the veins of the antecubital area (in front of the elbow), the back of the hand, and some of the larger veins in the foot. On some occasions, a vein must be exposed by a surgical cut.

aqueous water based.

solvent a liquid that dissolves another substance in it.

trauma an injury.

DEVICES

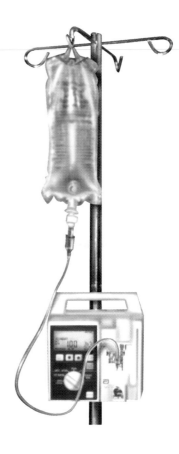

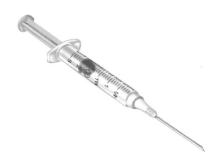

Syringes

Simple syringe and needle setups can be used to inject formulations over a short period of time (generally up to about 2 minutes). There are a variety of syringe sizes and needle sizes; syringe size is selected based on the volume of the formulation to inject. The needle size is generally based on the route of administration being used (IV, IM, SC, ID). Needle sizes of 16G to 20G are commonly used for intravenous injections. Some products come from the manufacturer already assembled and prefilled.

Infusion

Infusion is the gradual intravenous injection of a volume of fluid into a patient. The fluid consists of a primary fluid and whatever drug(s) are prescribed. The primary fluid is generally a large volume (500 ml to 1000 ml) bag or bottle of electrolyte solution such as D5W (dextrose 5% in water) or 1/2NS (one-half normal saline, 0.45% sodium chloride in water). It is intravenously infused at a rate of 2 ml to 3 ml per minute. The fluid bag has an administration set that includes an injection port between the bag and the needle. A simple syringe and needle may be used to inject a drug through the injection port into the primary fluid, or a second small plastic bag containing the drug can be **piggybacked** onto the primary fluid administration set.

Infusion Pumps

Administration devices that were dependent upon gravity have been shown to have a variable delivery rate. To ensure a constant delivery rate, controlled rate infusion pumps are used. Beginning in the late 1980s, patients were allowed to operate these pumps for occasional self-administration of analgesics. The term **patient-controlled analgesia (PCA)** was coined to describe this. PCA devices can provide either on-demand dosing or a constant infusion rate of drug as well as the on-demand feature.

INTRAMUSCULAR

Drugs are often given by the intramuscular route to patients unable to take them by oral administration. This route is also used for drugs that are poorly absorbed from the gastrointestinal tract. It is generally considered less hazardous and easier to use than the intravenous route. However, patients experience more pain from intramuscular administration than intravenous administration.

Intramuscular (IM) injections are made into the muscle fibers that are under the subcutaneous layer of the skin.

Needles used for the injections are generally 1 inch to 1.5 inches long, and are generally 19 to 22 gauge in size. The principal sites of injection are the **gluteal** (buttocks), **deltoid** (upper arm), and **vastus lateralis** (thigh) muscles. When giving intramuscular injections into the gluteus maximus, one must be aware of the thickness of gluteal fat, particularly in female patients and an appropriate size needle must be used. Otherwise, the injection will not reach the muscle.

The site of injection should be as far as possible from major nerves and blood vessels to avoid nerve damage and accidental intravenous administration.

Injuries that can occur following intramuscular injection are abscesses, cysts, embolism, hematoma, skin sloughing, and scar formation. To avoid injury, when a series of injections are given, the injection site is changed or rotated. Generally only limited volumes can be given by intramuscular injection: 2 ml in the deltoid and thigh muscles, and up to 5 ml in the gluteus maximus.

Intramuscular injections generally result in lower but longer lasting blood concentrations than after intravenous administration.

Part of the reason is that intramuscular injections require an absorption step, which delays the time to peak concentrations. Also, when a formulation is injected, a **depot** forms inside the muscle tissue where the drug deposits. Absorption from this depot is dependent on many factors such as muscle exercise, particle size of the drug, and the salt form of the drug used in the formulation.

FORMULATIONS

Drugs for intramuscular injection are formulated as:

➥ solutions;
➥ suspensions;
➥ **colloids** in aqueous and oleaginous (oil-based) solvents;
➥ oil-in-water **emulsions;**
➥ water-in-oil emulsions.

Colloids and suspensions both contain insoluble particles in solution, but the particles in colloids are about 100 times smaller than those in suspensions.

Emulsions are mixtures of two liquids, generally oil and water, which do not dissolve into each other. One liquid is spread through the other by mixing or shaking and the use of a stabilizing substance called an **emulsifier**.

Different salt forms of the drug may also be used to take advantage of a slower dissolution rate or a lower solubility.

All these things can be varied to achieve the desired absorption rate. In general, aqueous solutions have a faster absorption rate than oleagineous solutions. Both of these have a faster absorption rate than colloids or suspensions.

INJECTION SITES

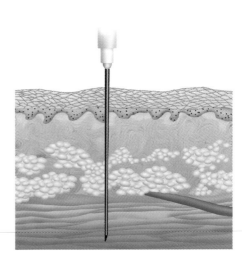

When administering intramuscular injections, it is necessary to adjust for any layers of body fat (especially in the gluteal area) and to use a size of needle that will penetrate to the muscle.

Z-Tract Injection

This is a technique used for medications that stain the skin (e.g., iron dextran injection) or irritate tissues (e.g., diazepam). The skin is pulled to one side prior to injection. Then the needle is inserted and the injection is performed. Once the needle is removed, the skin is released so that the injection points in the skin and muscle are no longer aligned. This keeps the drug from entering the subcutaneous tissue and staining or irritating the skin. A Z-track injection is generally 2 to 3 inches deep.

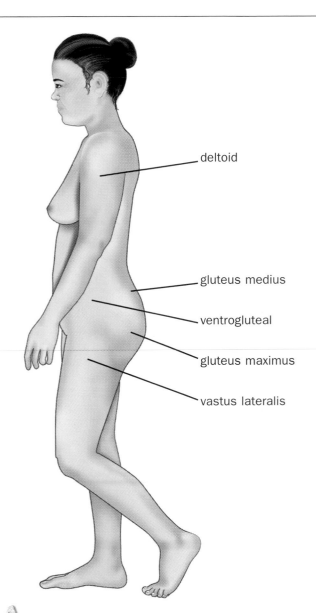

deltoid

gluteus medius

ventrogluteal

gluteus maximus

vastus lateralis

ABCD *colloids* particles up to a hundred times smaller than that those in suspensions that are, however, likewise suspended in a solution.

emulsions mixture of two liquids that do not dissolve into each other in which one liquid is spread through the other by mixing and use of a stabilizer.

 Intramuscular injections are generally more painful than intravenous.

SUBCUTANEOUS

Can be pronounced both ways

The subcutaneous (SC, SQ) route is a versatile route of administration that can be used for both short term and very long term therapies.

The injection of a drug or the **implantation** of a device beneath the surface of the skin is made in the loose tissues of the upper arm, the front of the thigh, and the lower portion of the abdomen. The upper back also can be used as a site of subcutaneous administration. The site of injection is usually rotated when injections are given frequently. The maximum amount of medication that can be subcutaneously injected is about 2 ml. Needles are generally 3/8 to 1 inch in length and 24 to 28 gauge.

Absorption of drugs from the subcutaneous tissue is influenced by the same factors that determine the rate of absorption from intramuscular sites.

However, there are fewer blood vessels in the subcutaneous tissue than in muscle, and absorption may be slower than with intramuscular administration. On the other hand, absorption after subcutaneous administration is generally more rapid and predictable than after oral administration. There are several ways to change the absorption rate. Using heat, or massaging the site have been found to increase absorption rates of many drugs. Also, there are various drugs that have been shown to increase absorption rate. By contrast, epinephrine decreases blood flow, which in turn decreases the absorption rate.

Many different solution and suspension formulations are given subcutaneously, but insulin is the most important drug routinely administered by this route.

Insulin comes in many different formulations each having a characteristic rate of absorption. The rate is controlled by the same factors used for intramuscular formulations: slowly soluble salt forms, suspensions versus solutions, differences in particle size, viscosity (thickness) of the injection form, etc.

In spite of the advantages of this route of administration, there are some precautions to observe.

Drugs which are irritating or in very **viscous** (thick) suspensions may produce serious adverse effects (including abscesses and necrosis) and be painful to the patient.

INJECTION SITES

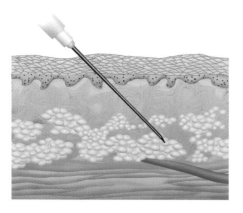

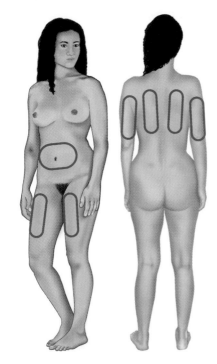

Subcutaneous injection sites are:
➡ lower abdomen;
➡ front of thigh;
➡ upper back;
➡ back of upper arm.

 viscosity the thickness of a liquid.

INTRADERMAL

IMPLANTS

One of the most popular ways to achieve very long term drug release is to place the drug in a delivery system or device that is implanted into the body tissue. The subcutaneous tissue is the ideal tissue for implantation of such devices. Implantation generally requires a surgical procedure or a specialized injection device. The fact that the device will be in constant contact with the subcutaneous tissue requires that the device materials be **biocompatible,** i.e., not irritating, and won't promote infection or sterile abscess. An advantage of the subcutaneous tissue for the site of implantation is that the device can be easily removed if necessary.

There are many devices that are used in subcutaneous implantation. Norplant® are silicone rods that provide contraception for up to five years. Several pellet formulations (Oreton®, Percorten®) are also available, as well as a mini-pump (Alzet®) which can deliver drug solutions for up to twenty-one days, as well as other devices.

Sometimes **ports** and **pumps** are placed in subcutaneous tissue and an attached delivery catheter is placed in a vein, cavity, artery, or CNS system. This allows for the injection of intravenous fluids, total parenteral nutrition (TPN) solutions, chemotherapy agents, or antibiotics.

Intradermal injections involve small volumes that are injected into the top layer of skin.

They are used for diagnostic reasons, desensitization, or immunization. Their effects are generally local rather than systemic.

An intradermal injection forms a *wheal*, or raised blister-like area, from which the drug will slowly be absorbed into the dermis.

The dermis is the layer of the skin just beneath the epidermis. It contains more blood vessels than the epidermis but fewer than most other injection sites. As a result, absorption is gradual.

The usual site for intradermal injections is the rear of the forearm.

Needles are usually 3/8 inches long and 25 to 26 gauge. For this route of administration, 0.1 ml of solution is the maximum volume that can be administered.

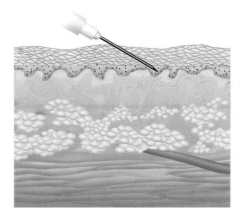

cross-section of an intradermal injection

 biocompatibility not irritating or infection or abscess causing to body tissue.

wheal a raised blister-like area on the skin, as caused by an intradermal injection.

on test = applications.

OPHTHALMIC FORMULATIONS

Drugs are administered to the eye for local treatment of various eye conditions and for anesthesia.

Formulations used include aqueous solutions, aqueous suspensions, ointments, and implants. *Every ophthalmic product must be manufactured to be sterile in its final container.* Also, because of the sensitivity of the eye, various elements of the formulation, including pH and viscosity, must be carefully controlled.

A major problem of ophthalmic administration is the immediate loss of a dose by natural spillage from the eye.

The normal volume of tears in the eye is estimated to be 7 microliters, and if blinking occurs, the eye can hold up to 10 microliters without spillage. The normal commercial eyedropper dispenses 50 microliters of solution. As a result, *more than half of a dose will be expelled from the eye by overflow.* The ideal volume of drug solution to administer would be 5 to 10 microliters. However, microliter dosing eye droppers are not generally available to patients.

Other problems include lacrimal (tear) drainage and too rapid absorption by the eyelid lining.

Tears wash the eyeball as they flow from the **lacrimal gland** across the eye and drain into the **lacrimal canalicula** (tear ducts). In man, the rate of tear production is approximately 2 microliters per minute, and so the entire tear volume in the eye turns over every 2 to 3 minutes. This rapid washing and turnover accounts for loss of an ophthalmic dose in a relatively short period of time. It can also cause systemic absorption because the drug drains into the lacrimal sac and is then emptied into the gastrointestinal tract. A similar and frequently occurring problem is caused by absorption of the drug into the **conjunctiva** (eyelid lining). The drug is then rapidly carried away from the eye by the circulatory system.

OPHTHALMIC ADMINISTRATION

lacrimal gland

canalicula

lacrimal sac

anatomy of the eye

Administration Considerations

➡ The eye is highly sensitive, requiring careful formulation for sterility, pH, viscosity, etc. to avoid irritation.

➡ The eye only holds a very small volume of liquid (7-10 microliters), so most eyedropper doses are lost through overflow.

➡ Systemic absorption can occur from drainage through the tear ducts or absorption through the eyelid.

R Ophthalmic administration is used to deliver a drug on the eye, into the eye, or onto the conjunctiva. Drug penetration into the eye (**transcorneal transport**) is not considered an effective process as it is estimated that only one-tenth of a dose penetrates into the eye.

ABCD *ophthalmic* related to the eye.

lacrimal gland the gland that produces tears for the eye.

lacrimal canalicula the tear ducts.

conjunctiva the eyelid lining.

transcorneal transport drug transfer into the eye.

Drops -
1. Never touch dropper to eye
2. Wash hands before + after
3. Put # of drops suggested.

Most ophthalmic solutions and suspensions are dispensed in eye dropper bottles.

Because of the problems of this route, patients must be shown how to properly instill the drops in their eyes, and every effort should be made to emphasize the need for instilling only one drop, not two or three.

To maintain longer contact between the drug and the surrounding tissue, suspensions, ointments, and inserts have been developed.

Ophthalmic suspensions are aqueous, with the particle size kept to a minimum to prevent irritation of the eye. Ointments tend to keep the drug in contact with the eye longer than suspensions. Most ophthalmic ointment bases are a mixture of mineral oil and white petrolatum and have a melting point close to body temperature. But ointments tend to blur patient vision as they remain viscous and are not removed easily by the tear fluid. Therefore, ointments are generally used at night as additional therapy to eye drops used during the day.

There are three types of devices commonly used to deliver ophthalmic dosages: hydrogel (soft) contact lenses, non-erodible inserts, and soluble inserts.

Hydrogel contact lenses are placed in a solution containing a drug such as an antibiotic, and the lenses absorb some of the drug solution. The lenses are then placed in the eye and the drug will release from the lenses over a period of time. **Ocusert®** is a non-erodible ocular insert designed to deliver pilocarpine at a controlled rate for up to 7 days. The insert is placed between the eyeball and the lower eyelid. With the Ocusert, patients use a fraction of the amount of pilocarpine they would with drop therapy. The biggest disadvantage of the insert is its tendency to float on the eyeball, particularly in the morning after waking. Soluble ophthalmic drug inserts are dried solutions that have been fashioned into a film or rod. These solid inserts are placed between the eyeball and the lower eyelid, and as they absorb tears, they slowly erode away. **Lacrisert®** is a soluble insert used in the treatment of moderate to severe **dry eye syndrome.**

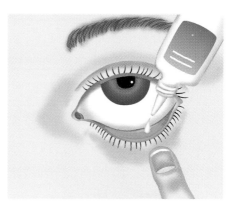
using an eye dropper

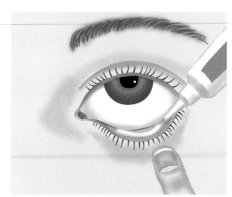
using an ointment — tend to blur vision

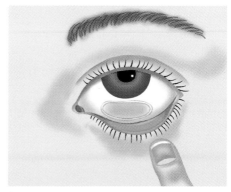
Ocusert

Rx Ophthalmic ointment tubes are typically small, holding approximately 3.5 g of ointment and fitted with narrow gauge tips which permit the extrusion of narrow bands of ointment.

INTRANASAL FORMULATIONS

The adult nasal cavity has a capacity of about 20 ml, a very large surface area for absorption, and a very rich blood supply.

The formulations used for intranasal administration are primarily used for their decongestant activity on the **nasal mucosa,** the cellular lining of the nose. The drugs that are typically used are decongestants, antihistamines, and corticosteroids.

The intranasal absorption of some drugs produces blood concentrations similar to when the drug is intravenously administered.

Because of this, intranasal administration is being investigated as a possible route of administration for insulin in the treatment of diabetes mellitus and for glucagon in the treatment of hypoglycemia. Intranasal administration also serves as a possible alternate route for drugs that are seriously degraded or poorly absorbed by oral administration.

Intranasal formulations include solutions, suspensions, sprays, aerosols, and inhalers.

Each product is formulated so it will not irritate the mucosa. Generally solutions or suspensions are administered by drops or as a fine mist from a nasal spray or aerosol container. Nasal sprays are preferred to drops because drops are more likely to drain into the back of the mouth and throat and be swallowed. A plastic spray bottle that is gently squeezed is used to issue a spray. A nasal inhaler is a tube which is inserted into the nostril opening. The tube contains a material that is saturated with the drug. As the patient inhales, the drug is vaporized and pulled into the nasal cavity.

DEVICES

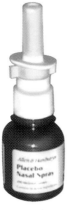

nasal spray

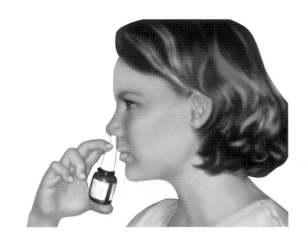

using a nasal spray

nasal mucosa the cellular lining of the nose.

nasal cavity the cavity behind the nose and above the roof of the mouth that filters air and moves mucous and inhaled contaminants outward and away from the lungs.

nasal inhaler a device which contains a drug that is vaporized by inhalation.

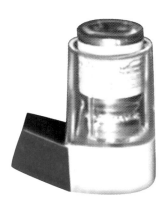

nasal aerosol

There are three ways a dosage can be lost following nasal administration.

The nasal lining contains enzymes which can metabolize and degrade some drugs. In addition, normal mucous flow, which protects the lungs by moving mucus and inhaled contaminants away from the lungs and out the nostril, will carry dosage with it as well. Finally, nasal administration often causes amounts of the drug to be swallowed. In some cases, enough drug will be swallowed to be equal to an oral dose. This may lead to a systemic effect from the drug even though it is intranasally administered.

Intranasal dosage forms should not be used for prolonged periods.

This may lead to chronic swelling (**edema**) of the nasal mucosa which aggravates the symptoms the dosage forms were intended to relieve. As a result, intranasal administration should be for short periods of time (no longer than 3 to 5 days). Patients should be advised not to exceed the recommended dosage and frequency of use.

Insufflator

In instances where a powder is to be intranasally administered, an insufflator is used. Squeezing the rubber bulb causes a turbulence within the powder reservoir, forcing some of the powder into the air stream and out of the device. Insufflators are also used in inhalation administration.

✱ on test.

Ways Intranasal Dosage Is Lost

✔ enzymes in the mucosa metabolize certain drugs.

✔ normal mucous flow removes dosage.

✔ amounts of the drug are swallowed.

 Because it can lead to irritation and swelling, intranasal administration is generally kept to limited volumes for short periods of time.

INHALATION FORMULATIONS

Inhalation dosage forms are intended to deliver drugs to the pulmonary system (lungs).

The lungs have a large surface area for absorption and a rich blood supply. This route avoids the problems of degradation and poor absorption found with the oral route. However, there is enough inconsistency in the absorption of drugs from the lungs that this route is not considered an alternative to intravenous administration.

Gaseous or volatile anesthetics are the most important drugs administered via this route.

Other drugs administered affect lung function, act as bronchodilators (bronchial tube decongestants), or treat allergic symptoms. Examples of drugs administered by this route are **adrenocorticoid steroids** (beclomethasone), **bronchodilators** (epinephrine, isoproterenol, metaproterenol, albuterol), and **antiallergics** (cromolyn).

Most of the inhalation dosage forms are aerosols that depend on the power of compressed or liquefied gas to expel the drug from the container.

Aerosols are easy to use, and have no danger of contamination. However, they are not very effective in delivering a drug to the respiratory tract. This is not due to poor aerosol design, but to the physical barriers of the airway and lungs that any inhalation dosage form must overcome to be effective.

Particle size is the critical factor with these dosage forms.

Large particles (about 20 microns) hit in the back of the mouth and throat and are eventually swallowed rather than inhaled. Particles from 1 to 10 microns reach the bronchioles. Smaller particles (0.6 micron) penetrate to the alveolar sacs of the lungs where absorption is rapid, but retention is limited since a large fraction of the dose is exhaled. The particles that reach the alveolar sacs and remain there are responsible for providing systemic effects. Breathing patterns and the depth of breathing also play important roles in the delivery of inhaled aerosols into the lung.

ABSORPTION

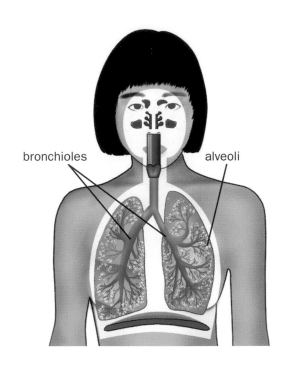

bronchioles   alveoli

For an inhalation dosage form to reach the alveoli of the lungs, it has to pass through a series of twists, turns, and increasingly smaller passageways as it travels from the mouth to the lungs. When the drug reaches the alveoli, it will be absorbed directly into the circulatory system. Because of the difficult route, varying amounts of inhalation dosages are swallowed and wind up in the gastrointestinal system.

inspiration breathing in.

alveolar sacs (alveoli) the small sacs of specialized tissue that transfer oxygen out of inspired air into the blood and carbon dioxide out of the blood and into the air for expiration.

DEVICES

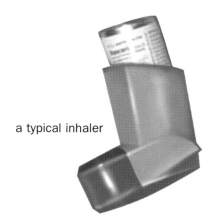

a typical inhaler

Metered Dose Inhalers

Aerosols to administer powerful drugs use special metering valves that deliver a fixed dose when the aerosol is activated. These are called metered dose inhalers. The amount of drug released with each activation is regulated by a valve that has a fixed capacity or dimensions.

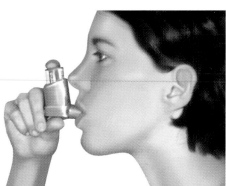

using an inhaler

Adapters and Spacers

Coordination is required on the part of the patient between breathing in (**inspiration**) and activation of the aerosol. Extender devices or spacers have been developed to assist patients who cannot coordinate these two processes. The spacer goes between the aerosol's mouthpiece and the patient's mouth. The spacer allows the patient to separate activation of the aerosol from inhalation by 3 to 5 seconds.

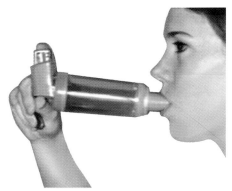

using an inhaler with spacer

Powder Inhalers

Some drugs are administered in powder form using a special inhalation device such as a **Rotahaler.** The device automatically releases the drug when the user inhales. The powdered drug is supplied in hard gelatin capsules that are placed in the inhaler. The patient squeezes the inhaler to pierce the capsule and release the powder. When the patient inhales from the device, the powder is mixed with the inspired air by a small propeller and is then delivered to the lungs with the inspired air.

Some patients may not be able to use inhaled powders and humid conditions may also make inhaling powder difficult.

DERMAL FORMULATIONS

The skin is the largest and heaviest organ in the body and accounts for about 17% of a person's weight.

It forms a barrier that protects the underlying organ systems from trauma, temperature, humidity, harmful penetrations, moisture, radiation, and micro-organisms. Dosage forms that are applied to the skin are called **dermal** or **percutaneous** forms.

Most dermal dosage forms are used for local (topical) effects on or within the skin.

Formulations are used as protectants, lubricants, emollients, or drying agents, or for the specific effect of the drug present. Examples of treatments using dermal formulations include minor skin infections, itching, burns, diaper rash, insect stings and bites, athlete's foot, corns, calluses, warts, dandruff, acne, psoriasis, and eczema.

Dermal administration has a number of advantages.

It provides an ease of administration not found in other routes, and usage by patients is generally good. It can also provide continuous drug adminis-tration. In addition, dermal formulations can be easily removed if necessary. The major disadvantage of this route of administration is that the amount of drug that can be absorbed will be limited to about 2 mg/day. This is often a significant limitation if the route is being considered for systemic therapy.

Basic rules of dermal absorption:
- More drug is absorbed when the formula-tion is applied to a larger surface area.
- Formulations or dressings that increase the hydration of the skin generally improve absorption.
- The greater the amount of rubbing in (inunction) of the formulation, the greater the absorption.
- The longer the formulation remains in con-tact with the skin, the greater will be the absorption.

ABCD

percutaneous the absorption of drugs through the skin, often for a systemic effect.

topical applied for local effect, usually to the skin.

hydrates absorbs water.

THE SKIN

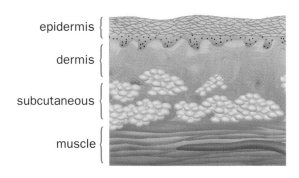

epidermis {
dermis {
subcutaneous {
muscle {

The skin is composed of three layers of tissue:
- epidermis;
- dermis;
- subcutaneous tissue.

The skin is generally 3-5 millimeters thick, though it is thicker in the palms and soles of the feet and thinner in the eyelids and genitals. Within the skin are several other elements: hair follicles, sebaceous glands, sweat glands, and nails.

The outer layer of skin is called the **stratum corneum**. In normal skin, the cells of this layer are continually replaced by new cells from underneath. As new cells develop, they displace the outer cells that have died. The turnover time from cell devel-opment to shedding of the dead cells (**sloughing**) is about 21 days.

The skin's outer layer is a barrier to drug penetration. It is about 10 micrometers thick, but can swell to approximately three times that by absorbing as much as five times its weight in water. When the stratum corneum absorbs water (**hydrates**), it becomes easier for drugs to penetrate. For that reason, certain dressings are designed to do this. Also, some skin conditions such as eczema and psoriasis can hydrate the stratum corneum and increase the absorption of some drugs.

FORMULATIONS

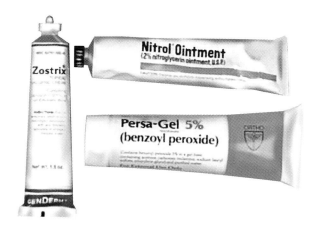

Ointments, Creams, Gels, and Lotions

Ointments, creams, gels, and lotions are the most popular dermal formulations. Physically, they appear to be very similar in consistency and texture, but there are differences. **Ointments** have drugs that have been incorporated into a base. There are several different types of bases ranging from petrolatum to polyethylene glycols. **Creams** are semisolid emulsions, and are less viscous and lighter in texture than ointments. Creams have an added feature in that they vanish or disappear with rubbing. **Gels** are dispersions of solid drugs in a jelly-like liquid vehicle. **Lotions** are suspensions of solid drugs in an aqueous vehicle.

Solutions, Tinctures, Collodions, and Liniments

Dermal **solutions** and **tinctures** are generally used as anti-infective agents. *Solutions are aqueous and tinctures are alcoholic.* Both are generally dispensed in small volumes, and should be packaged in containers that make them convenient to use. Dropper bottles (glass bottles with an applicator tip) are most often used. Examples of solutions and tinctures are Coal Tar Solution, Hydrogen Peroxide, Povidone-Iodine, Iodine Tincture, and Compound Benzoin Tincture.

Collodions are liquid preparations of pyroxylin dissolved in a solvent mixture of alcohol and ether. Pyroxylin looks like raw cotton and is slowly but completely soluble in the solvent mixture. When applied to the skin, the solvent rapidly evaporates, leaving a protective film on the skin that contains a thin layer of the drug. **Liniments** are alcoholic or oleaginous solutions generally applied by rubbing.

Pastes, Powders, Plasters

Pastes are generally used for their protective action and for their ability to absorb discharges from skin lesions. Pastes contain more solid material than ointments, and are stiffer and less penetrating. Medicinal **powders** are a mixture of drug and an inert (inactive) base such as talcum or corn starch. Powders have different dusting and covering capability. **Plasters** are solid or semisolid adhesive masses that are spread on a suitable backing material. They provide prolonged contact at the site of application. Some of the common backing materials used are paper, cotton, felt, linen, muslin, silk, and moleskin. The backing is cut into different shapes appropriate to cover the body surface area.

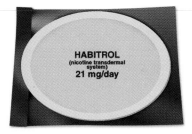

Transdermal Patches, Tapes, and Gauzes.

Transdermal systems (patches, tapes, and gauzes) *deliver drugs through the skin for a systemic effect.* The systems can be divided into two kinds: those that control the rate of drug delivery to the skin, and those that allow the skin to control the rate of absorption. The first type is for powerful drugs that must have their absorption rate controlled by a device. The second type is for less powerful drugs. The largest problems with transdermal patches are skin sensitivity experienced by some patients, and technical difficulties associated with the adhesiveness of the systems to different skin types and under various conditions.

Aerosols

Percutaneous aerosols are generally used to apply anesthetic and antibiotic dosages for local effect.

VAGINAL FORMULATIONS

Vaginal administration has many of the same characteristics found with other parenteral routes of administration.

It avoids the degradation that occurs with oral administration; doses can be retrieved if necessary; and it has the potential of long term drug absorption. However, vaginal administration leads to variable absorption since the vagina is a physiologically and anatomically dynamic organ with pH and absorption characteristics changing over time. Another disadvantage of this route is that administration of a formulation during menstruation could predispose the patient to **Toxic Shock Syndrome.** There is also a tendency of some dosage forms to be expelled after insertion into the vagina.

Formulations for this route of administration are: solutions, powders for solutions, ointments, creams, aerosol foams, suppositories, tablets, contraceptive sponges and IUDs.

Powders are used to prepare solutions for vaginal douches used to cleanse the vagina. The powders are supplied either as bulk or unit packages and are dissolved in a prescribed amount of water prior to use. Most douche powders are used for their hygienic effects, but a few contain antibiotics.

Vaginal administration gives the opportunity for long term administration.

This potential has been explored in the area of contraception protection using **intrauterine devices (IUDs).** The first IUD was developed in 1970 and was effective for 21 days. The vaginal ring was worn until the onset of menstruation, removed during menstruation, and then reinserted for another 21 days. Several IUDs have been marketed since that time, including the Progestasert.

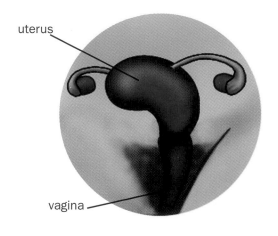

uterus

vagina

The Vagina

The vagina is a cylinder-like organ that leads from the cervix and uterus to an external opening. It is used for intercourse, the release of menstrual fluids, and as the lower portion of the birth canal.

Toxic Shock Syndrome (TSS)

Toxic shock syndrome is a rare and potentially fatal disease that results from a severe bacterial infection of the blood. In women, it can be caused when bacteria natural to the vagina move into the bloodstream. Though primarily associated with the use of super-absorbency tampons, it has also been associated with various vaginal dosage forms. Its symptoms include a high fever, nausea, skin rash, faintness and muscle ache. It is treated with antibiotics and other medicines.

Suppositories

Vaginal suppositories are employed as contraceptives, feminine hygiene antiseptics, bacterial antibiotics, or to restore the vaginal mucosa. Vaginal suppositories are inserted high in the vaginal tract with the aid of a special 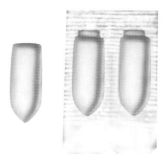 applicator. The suppositories are usually globe, egg, or cone-shaped and weigh about 5 grams.

Suppositories are made from a variety of bases. Cocoa butter is a popular oleaginous base, but is difficult to formulate as a suppository. Glycerinated gelatin (glycerin and gelatin) is excellent for prolonged local effects since it softens slowly. However, **polyethylene glycols** (polyols or **PEGs**) are the most popular of all bases. They dissolve when inserted into a body cavity, so the base does not need to be formulated to melt at body temperature. This allows convenient storage without refrigeration. They also do not melt in the fingers while being inserted, nor do they leak from the vaginal opening.

Ointments, creams, and aerosol foams

Vaginal ointments, creams, and aerosol foams typically contain antibiotics, estrogenic hormonal substances, and contraceptive agents.

Creams and foams are placed into a special applicator tube, and the tube is then inserted high in the vaginal tract. The applicator plunger is depressed and the formulation is deposited.

IUD

The progestasert IUD (intrauterine device) releases an average of 60 micrograms of progesterone per day for a period of one year. This IUD is replaced annually to maintain contraception.

Tablets

Vaginal tablets, also called inserts, have the same activity and are inserted in the same manner as vaginal suppositories. Patients should be instructed to dip the tablet into water before insertion. Also, because tablets are generally used at bedtime and can be messy if the formulation is an oleaginous base, it should be recommended to patients that they wear a sanitary napkin to protect nightwear and bed linens. These same instructions should be given to patients receiving vaginal suppositories.

Contraceptive Sponge

A unique formulation for vaginal administration is the contraceptive sponge. Though it was voluntarily removed from the U.S. market by the manufacturer, it is marketed elsewhere and may be marketed in the U.S. again. The sponge is made of polyurethane and contains a spermicidal agent. Contraception occurs by the action of the drug and the physical blockage of the cervix by the sponge. The sponge is designed to provide contraceptive protection for a 24 hour period. Before its removal from the market, the sponge was found to have occasional removal problems after use and a few cases of toxic shock were associated with it.

 contraceptive device or formulation designed to prevent pregnancy.

IUD an intrauterine contraceptive device that is placed in the uterus for a prolonged period of time.

REVIEW

KEY CONCEPTS

✔ The way in which the body absorbs and distributes drugs varies with the route of administration.

✔ A local effect occurs when the drug activity is at the site of administration (e.g., eyes, ears, nose, skin). A systemic effect occurs when the drug is introduced into the circulatory system.

✔ Enteral refers to anything involving the tract from the mouth to the rectum. There are three enteral routes: oral, sublingual, and rectal. Oral administration is the most frequently used.

✔ The stomach has a pH around 1-2. Certain drugs cannot be taken orally because they are degraded or destroyed by stomach acid and intestinal enzymes.

✔ Drugs administered by liquid dosage forms generally reach the circulatory system faster than drugs formulated in solid dosage forms.

✔ Oral formulations contain various ingredients beside the active drug. These inactive ingredients include binders, effervescent salts, lubricants, fillers, diluents, and disintegrants.

✔ Formulations used in the mouth are generally fast dissolving uncoated tablets which contain highly water soluble drugs.

✔ The most common rectal administration forms are suppositories, solutions, and ointments.

✔ Any route other than oral, sublingual, and rectal is considered a parenteral administration route. These routes are often preferred when oral administration causes drug degradation or when a rapid drug response is desired, as in an emergency situation.

✔ The parenteral routes requiring a needle are intravenous, intramuscular, intradermal, and subcutaneous. These solutions must be sterile (bacteria-free), have an appropriate pH, and be limited in volume.

✔ Intravenous dosage forms are administered directly into a vein (and the blood supply).

✔ Most solutions are aqueous (water based), but they may also have glycols, alcohols, or other non-aqueous solvents in them.

✔ Fat emulsions and TPN emulsions are used to provide triglycerides, fatty acids, and calories for patients who cannot absorb them from the gastrointestinal tract.

✔ Infusion is the gradual intravenous injection of a volume of fluid into a patient.

✔ Intramuscular injections generally result in lower but longer lasting blood concentrations than after intravenous administration.

✔ The subcutaneous (SC, SQ) route can be used for both short term and very long term therapies. Insulin is the most important drug routinely administered by this route.

✔ Intradermal injections involve small volumes that are injected into the top layer of skin.

✔ Every ophthalmic product must be manufactured to be sterile in its final container.

✔ Inhalation dosage forms are intended to deliver drugs to the pulmonary system (lungs).

✔ Most dermal dosage forms are used for local (topical) effects on or within the skin.

✔ A potential side effect of vaginal administration is Toxic Shock Syndrome.

SELF TEST

aqueous	a condition which is free of all microorganisms.
buffer system	a device which contains a drug that is vaporized by inhalation.
degradation	a liquid that dissolves another substance in it.
emulsions	absorbs water.
hydrates	an injury.
local effect	applied for local effect, usually to the skin.
nasal inhaler	ingredients in a formulation designed to control the pH.
nasal mucosa	mixture of two liquids that do not dissolve into each other.
ophthalmic	the absorption of drugs through the skin, often for a systemic effect.
percutaneous	related to the eye.
solvent	the cellular lining of the nose.
sterile	the changing of a drug to a less effective or ineffective form.
sublingual	the property of a substance being able to dissolve in water.
systemic effect	the thickness of a liquid.
topical	under the tongue
trauma	water based.
viscosity	when a drug is introduced into the circulatory system.
water soluble	when drug activity is at the site of administration.

CHOOSE THE BEST ANSWER. *answers are in the back of the book*

1. Which of the pH values listed below indicates a substance may be alkaline?
   a. pH 1-2
   b. pH 3-4
   c. pH 5-6
   d. pH 7-8

2. Which of the following routes is least likely to give a systemic effect?
   a. oral (po)
   b. sublingual (sl)
   c. rectal (pr)
   d. intradermal (id)

3. Which pathway would the use of a metered dose inhaler (MDI) follow?
   a. mouth, trachea, alveoli, bronchioles
   b. mouth, bronchioles, trachea, alveoli
   c. mouth, trachea, bronchioles, alveoli
   d. none of the above

4. The Norplant® device is made of cylindrical silicone rods that slowly release progesterone to provide contraception for up to 5 years. The method of implantation for these rods is:
   a. intradermal
   b. subcutaneous
   c. intramuscular
   d. intrathecal

PARENTERAL SOLUTIONS

In intravenous therapy, there are special requirements for how formulations are packaged and how they are administered.

In Chapter 7, *Routes and Formulations*, the methods by which parenteral formulations are administered were reviewed. This chapter will review how the parenteral solutions that are administered by injection and infusion are prepared and packaged.

Intravenous solutions are packaged as two types of products: *large volume parenteral* (LVP) solutions and *small volume parenteral* (SVP) solutions.

LVP solutions are typically bags or bottles containing larger volumes of intravenous solutions. Common uses of LVP solutions without additives include: correction of electrolyte and fluid balance disturbances, nutrition, and vehicles for administering other drugs.

SVP solutions are generally contained in ampules or vials.

Their contents are withdrawn by syringe and either added to an LVP container or injected directly into the patient. SVP solutions are administered directly into the patient by several routes and for reasons that include inability to take oral medications, degradation of some drugs by the gastrointestinal tract, and when rapid and/or continuous action is required (see Chapter 7, *Routes and Formulations*).

PARENTERAL SOLUTIONS

Because intravenous products are administered directly into the bloodstream, there are a number of special considerations and precautions that must be taken.

✔ **Solutions for injection must be sterile, that is, free from bacteria and other microorganisms.**

Techniques that maintain sterile conditions and prevent contamination must be followed. These are called **aseptic techniques.**

✔ **Solutions must be free of all visible particulate material.**

Examples of such contaminants are glass, rubber cores from vials, cloth or cotton fibers, metal, and plastic. Undissolved particles of an active drug may be present in intravenous suspensions, but no contaminants should be present.

Inspections

Intravenous solutions should always be visually inspected before use. Formulated or admixed solutions should be inspected after compounding. Visual inspection can show two of the six characteristics of parenteral solutions: particulate material and stability (if lack of stability is indicated by precipitation or crystallization in the solution). Inspection is generally performed against a brightly lit white background.

Visual inspection cannot reveal anything about the sterility, pH, osmolality, presence of pyrogens, or chemical degradation of the drug. Special equipment and skilled personnel are needed to determine these factors. Since sterilty cannot be determined visually, good **aseptic technique** must be used when dealing with parenteral solutions.

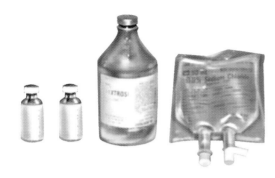

✔ All intravenous solutions must be pyrogen-free.

Intravenous solutions can cause **pyretic** (fever) reactions if they contain pyrogens. Pyrogens are chemicals that are produced by microorganisms. They are soluble in water and are not removed by sterilizing or filtering the solution.

✔ The solution must be stable for its intended use.

Most admixtures are prepared hours in advance of when they are to be administered. So the stability of a particular drug in a particular intravenous solution must be factored into the admixture preparation. This information is generally available in a number of reference sources.

✔ The pH of intravenous solution should not vary significantly from physiological pH, about 7.4.

Sometimes, other factors may be more important, such as when acidic or alkaline solutions are needed to increase drug solubility or used as a therapeutic treatment themselves.

✔ Intravenous solutions should be formulated to have an osmolarity similar to that of blood.

Osmotic pressure is the characteristic of a solution determined by the number of dissolved particles in it (see page 86). This is measured in terms of **osmoles** (Osmol) or **milliosmoles** (mOsmol) per liter and referred to as **osmolarity**. Blood has an osmolarity of approximately 300 mOsmol per liter. Both 0.9% sodium chloride solution and 5% dextrose solution have a similar osmolarity. When a solution has an osmolarity equivalent to that of blood, it is **isotonic** to blood, i.e., it will have the same osmotic pressure as blood.

Intravenous solutions that have greater osmolarity than blood are called **hypertonic** to it, and those with lower osmolarity, **hypotonic.** Both may cause damage to red blood cells, pain, and tissue irritation. However, it is at times necessary to administer such solutions. In these cases, the solutions are usually given slowly through large, free flowing veins to minimize the reactions.

 aseptic techniques techniques that maintain sterile condition.

pyrogens chemicals produced by microorganisms that can cause *pyretic* (fever) reactions in patients.

osmolarity the number of Osmoles per liter of solution (a measure of the amount of dissolved particles).

isotonic when one solution has an osmolarity equivalent to another.

hypertonic when a solution has a greater osmolarity than another.

hypotonic when a solution has a lesser osmolarity than another.

LVP SOLUTIONS

Large volume parenteral (LVP) solutions are intravenous solutions packaged in containers holding 100 ml or more.

There are three types of containers: glass bottle with an air vent tube, glass bottle without an air vent tube, and plastic bags. Plastic bags are available in different sizes. The most common sizes are 50, 100, 250, 500, and 1,000 ml. The top of the bag has a flap with a hole in it to hang the bag on an administration pole. At the other end of the bag are two ports of about the same length. One is the administration set port, and the other is the medication port. Graduation marks to indicate the volume of solution in the bag are on its front. They are marked at 25 ml to 100 ml intervals depending on the overall size of the bag.

The administration set port has a plastic cover on it to maintain the sterility of the bag.

The cover is easily removed. Solution will not drip out of the bag through this port because of a plastic diaphragm inside the port. When the spike of the administration set is inserted into the port, the diaphragm is punctured, and the solution will flow out of the bag into the administration set. This inner diaphragm cannot be resealed once punctured.

The medication port is covered by a protective rubber tip.

Drugs are added to the LVP solution through this port using a needle and syringe. There is an inner plastic diaphragm about one half inch inside the port, just like the administration set port. This inner diaphragm is also not self-sealing when punctured by a needle, but the protective rubber tip prevents solutions from leaking from the bag once the diaphragm is punctured. The plastic bag system is not vented to outside air. It collapses as the solution is administered, so a vacuum is not created inside.

Piggybacks

Medications are often administered with piggybacks, which are small volumes of fluid (usually 50-100 ml) infused into the administration set of an LVP solution. Piggybacks are typically infused over a period of thirty to sixty minutes. Some medications are also administered directly into a **volume control chamber**, which is a container in the administration line that holds measured amounts of solution from the IV bag.

ADMINISTRATION

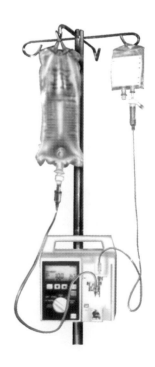

Administration Set

The basic method to administer a LVP solution is to use an administration set. The set contains a spiked plastic device to pierce a **port** on the IV container.

This connects to a **sight** or **drip chamber** that may be used to set the **flow rate**, the rate ordered by the physician at which the solution is to be administered to the patient (generally measured in ml/hour). A clamp pinching the tubing also regulates flow. The line then leads to a rubber injection port to which a needle may be attached or to an **infusion pump** which will control the flow rate.

DEVICES

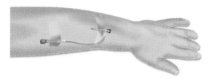

Heparin Lock

In some instances, a patient may not have a primary LVP solution, yet must receive piggyback medications. This is done through a heparin lock, which is a short piece of tubing attached to a needle or intravenous catheter. When the tubing is not being used for the piggyback, heparin is used to fill the tubing. This drug prevents blood from clotting in the tube.

Other Devices

Infusion pumps, syringe pumps, and **ambulatory pumps** are devices used to administer LVP solutions and control flow rates.

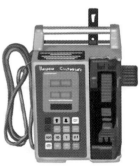

Administration sets are threaded through infusion pumps, and the pumps control the gravity flow. Syringe pumps expel solutions from a syringe into an administration set such as a heparin lock. An ambulatory pump is about the size of a hand. It allows patients to have some freedom of movement compared to being restricted to an infusion pump attached to an administration pole. Infusion pumps have made the infusion process much more accurate and easier to administer and have been a major factor in the growth of home infusion.

Plastic bags have advantages not found with glass bottles.

They do not break. They weigh less. They take up less storage space, and they take up much less disposal space. As a result, glass LVP solution bottles are rarely used.

Some drugs and solutions may not be used with plastic because they interact with it.

In these cases, glass IV bottles are used. They are packaged with a vacuum, sealed by a solid rubber closure, and the closure is held in place by an aluminum band. Graduation marks are along the sides of the bottle and are usually spaced every 20 to 50 ml. The solution bottle is hung on an administration pole in an inverted position using the aluminum or plastic band on the bottom of the bottle.

Solutions flow from the containers to the patient through the administration set.

For solutions to flow out of a glass container, air must be able to enter the container to relieve the vacuum as the solution leaves. Some bottles have air tubes built into the rubber closure for this. Some bottles do not, and then an administration set with a filtered airway in the spike must be used.

Common LVP Solutions

Many different intravenous solutions are commercially available. However, four solutions are commonly used either as LVP solutions or as the primary part of an admixture solution. The solutions are:

➥ **sodium chloride solution,**
➥ **dextrose solution,**
➥ **Ringer's solution,**
➥ **Lactated Ringer's solution.**

Various combinations of different strengths of sodium chloride and dextrose solutions are also available, e.g., 5% dextrose and 0.45% sodium chloride, or 5% dextrose and 0.2% sodium chloride.

 flow rate the rate (in ml/hour or ml/minute) at which the solution is administered to the patient.

heparin lock an injection device which uses heparin to keep blood from clotting in the device.

piggybacks small volume solution added to an LVP.

infusion the slow continuous introduction of a solution into the blood stream.

SVP SOLUTIONS

Small volume parenteral (SVP) solutions are usually 100 ml or less and are primarily used as vehicles for delivering medications.

When a drug is added to a parenteral solution, the drug is referred to as the additive, and the final mixture is referred to as the **admixture**.

The phrase "small volume parenterals" can also refer to formulations packaged for parenteral administration: ampules, vials, and prefilled syringes.

Liquid drugs are supplied in prefilled syringes, heat-sealed ampules, or in glass vials sealed with a rubber closure. Powdered drugs are supplied in vials and must be reconstituted (dissolved in a suitable solvent) before being added to the intravenous solution.

Ampules are sealed glass containers with a neck that must be snapped off.

Most ampules are weakened around the base of the neck for easy breaking. These will have a colored band around the base of the neck. Some ampules, however, must first be scored and weakened with a file or the top may shatter. It is useful to wrap a gauze pad around the top of the ampule when opening. This will provide some protection to the fingers if the ampule shatters and will also reduce the possibility of glass splinters becoming airborne. A 5 micron (µm) **filter needle** should be used when withdrawing the contents of an ampule, since glass particles may have fallen inside when the top was snapped off. The filter needle should be removed and replaced with the regular needle before injecting the drug into any solution.

ADDING SVPs TO LVPs

Generally the LVP solution is used as a continuous infusion because of its large volume and slow infusion rates. SVP solutions can be introduced into the on-going LVP infusion by injecting the SVP into the rubber injection port or the volume control chamber of the administration set. However, most often the medication is introduced into the LVP solution, or into a minibag and used as a piggyback.

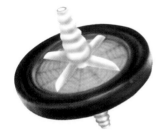

Filters

A filter similar to the one above is often placed between the syringe and needle before the medication is introduced into the bottle or bag. Double ended filtered needles are also used to transfer solutions from a vial directly into a bottle or bag. This eliminates the need of using a syringe.

admixture the resulting solution when a drug is added to a parenteral solution.

lyophilized freeze-dried.

diluent a liquid that dilutes a substance or solution.

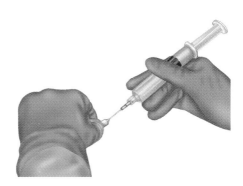

Using a Needle and Syringe to Add a Drug to an LVP:

1. Remove the protective covering from the LVP package.

2. Assemble the needle and syringe.

3. If the drug in the SVP is in powder form, reconstitute it with the recommended diluent.

4. Swab the SVP with an alcohol swab and draw the necessary volume of drug solution.

5. Swab the medication port of the LVP with an alcohol swab.

6. Insert the needle into the medication port and through the inner diaphragm. The medication port should be fully extended to minimize the chance of going through the side of the port.

7. Inject the SVP solution

8. Remove the needle.

9. Shake and inspect the admixture.

Drugs and other additives to intravenous solutions are packaged in vials.

They are available either in liquid form or as **lyophilized** (freeze dried) powders. Powders must be reconstituted with a suitable solution (**diluent**) before use. Vials are made of glass or plastic and have a rubber stopper through which a needle is inserted to withdraw or add to the contents. Before withdrawing solution from a vial, an equal volume of air is usually drawn up in the syringe and injected into the vial. Some medications are packaged under pressure or can produce gas (and pressure) upon reconstitution. In such cases, air is not injected into the vial before withdrawing the solution.

Vials may be prepared for single-dose or multidose use.

Single-dose vials do not contain preservatives and should be discarded after one use. Multidose vials contain a preservative to inhibit bacterial contamination once the vial has been used. Also, the rubber closure will reseal on a multidose vial. These vials can be used for a number of doses of variable volume.

There are two varieties of prefilled syringes.

One type, a cartridge type package, is a single syringe and needle unit which is to be placed in a special holder before use. Once the syringe and needle unit is used, they are discarded but the holder can be used again with a new unit. Another type of prefilled syringe consists of a glass tube closed at both ends with rubber stoppers. The prefilled tube is placed into a specially designed syringe that has a needle attached to it. After using this type of prefilled syringe, all of the pieces are discarded.

Ready to mix systems

Ready-to-mix systems consist of a specially designed minibag with an adapter for attaching a drug vial. The admixing takes place just prior to administration. The major advantages of ready-to-mix systems include a significant reduction in waste and lower potential for medication error because the drug vial remains attached to the minibag and can be rechecked if necessary. However, the systems do cost more, and there is the potential that the system will not be properly activated so that the patient receives only the diluent or a partial dose.

SYRINGES

The basic parts of a syringe are the barrel, plunger, and tip.

The barrel is a tube that is open at one end and tapers into a hollow tip at the other end. The plunger is a piston-type rod with a slightly cone-shaped stopper that passes inside the barrel of the syringe. The tip of the syringe provides the point of attachment for a needle. The volume of solution inside a syringe is indicated by graduation lines on the barrel. Graduation lines may be in milliliters or fractions of a milliliter, depending on the capacity of the syringe. The larger the capacity, the larger the interval between graduation lines. Special purpose syringes, such as **insulin syringes**, have graduation lines in both milliliters and insulin units to reflect their intended use.

There are several common types of syringe tips.

Slip-Tip® tips allow the needle to be held on the syringe by friction. The needle is reasonably secure, but it may slip off if not properly attached or if considerable pressure is used. **Luer-lock®** tips have a collar with grooves that lock the needle in place. **Eccentric** tips, which are off-center, are used when the needle must be parallel to the plane of injection such as in an intradermal injection.

Syringes come in sizes ranging from 1 to 60 ml.

As a rule, the syringe size is the next size larger than the volume to be measured. For example, a 3 ml syringe should be selected to measure 2.3 ml, or a 5 ml syringe to measure 3.8 ml. In this way, the graduation marks on the syringe will be in the smallest possible amounts for the volume measured. Syringes should not be filled to capacity because the plunger can be easily dislodged.

SYRINGES

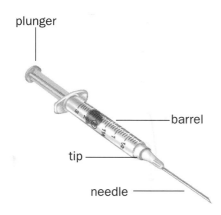

A syringe with graduation marks

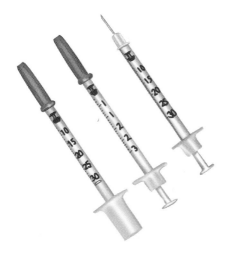

Insulin syringes, with and without needle and barrel caps.

Measuring Volume

The volume of solution in a syringe is measured to the edge of the plunger's stopper while the syringe is held upright and all the air has been removed from the syringe.

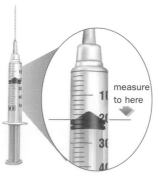

measure to here

Disposable needles should always be used when preparing admixtures as they are presterilized and individually wrapped to maintain sterility.

NEEDLES

Components

A needle has three parts: the **hub**, the **shaft**, and the **bevel**. The hub is at one end of the needle and is the part that attaches to the syringe. It is designed for quick and easy attachment and removal. The shaft is the long, slender stem of the needle that is beveled at one end to form a point called the "bevel." The hollow bore of the needle shaft is known as the **lumen**.

Sizes

Needle sizes are indicated by length and **gauge**. The length of a needle is measured in inches from where the shaft meets the hub to the tip of the bevel. Needle lengths range from 3/8 inch to three and a half inches. Some special use needles are even longer. The gauge of a needle, used to designate the size of the lumen, ranges from 27 (the smallest) to 13 (the largest). *In other words, the higher the gauge number, the smaller is the lumen.*

Needle sizes are chosen based on both the viscosity of the parenteral solution and the type of rubber closure on the container. Needles with a relatively small lumens can be used for most solutions. However, some viscous solutions require large lumens. One problem with this, however, is that large needles are more likely to damage the rubber closures of solution containers, causing particles to fall into the container and contaminate the solution. This is called **"coring."** As a result, small gauge needles are used if the rubber closure can be easily cored.

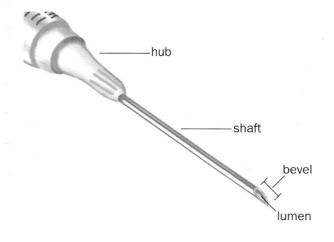

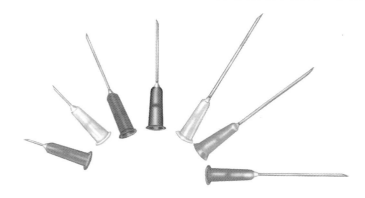

different size needles

bevel an angled surface, as with the tip of a needle.

gauge a measurement—with needles, the higher the gauge, the thinner the lumen.

lumen the hollow center of a needle.

coring when a needle damages the rubber closure of a parenteral container, causing fragments of the closure to fall into the container and contaminate its contents.

FILTERS

Filters are often used to remove contaminating particles from solutions.

They can be attached at the end of a syringe or can be part of the needle. They are divided into two basic groups: **depth filters** and **membrane filters.** Depth filters work by passing the solution through twisting channels that trap particles. A membrane filter looks like paper and consists of many small pores of a uniform size that trap particles larger than the pores. Filters have a wide range of pore sizes. Common ones are 0.22, 0.45, 1, 5, or 10 μm (microns).

MEMBRANE FILTERS

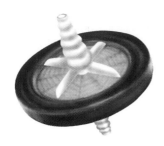

a membrane filter

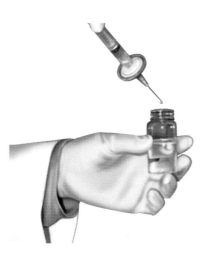

a membrane filter attached to a syringe

Membrane filters are intended to filter a solution only as it is expelled from a syringe.

1. A regular needle is attached to the syringe.

2. The solution is pulled into the syringe.

3. Air bubbles are removed from the syringe.

4. The needle is removed from the syringe.

5. A membrane filter is then attached to the syringe.

6. Another needle is placed on the end of the filter.

7. Air is eliminated from the filter chamber by holding the syringe in a vertical position so that the needle is pointing upward. The air in the filter chamber is then expelled by slowly pushing in the plunger. Air must be expelled before the filter becomes wet; otherwise, the air will not pass through the filter. Do not pull back on the plunger when the membrane filter is being used because the filter may rupture.

8. Once air has been expelled, pressure should be slowly and continuously applied to push the solution through the filter.

DEPTH FILTERS

The depth filter is rigid enough so the solution may be filtered either as it is pulled into or expelled from the syringe, but not both ways in the same procedure. If the drug solution is to be filtered as the solution is pulled into the syringe, the following steps are used:

1. The filter needle is attached to the syringe.

2. The solution is pulled into the syringe.

3. The filter needle is removed.

4. A new needle is attached to the syringe.

5. The solution is expelled from the syringe.

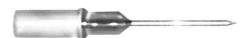

The depth filter is inside the clear hub of this filter needle.

FINAL FILTERS

A filter that filters a solution immediately before it enters the patient's vein is called a **final filter**. Some administration sets contain final filters as components. Some filters are designed to be attached to administration sets and serve as final filters.

 membrane filter a filter that attaches to a syringe and filters solution through a membrane as the solution is expelled from the syringe.

depth filter a filter placed inside a needle hub that can filter solutions being drawn in or expelled, but not both.

final filter a filter that filters solution immediately before it enters a patient's vein.

LAMINAR FLOW HOODS

Microorganisms invisible to the eye are present in natural air and on most surfaces, even those that appear clean.

Unless aseptic technique is used to prepare parenteral solutions, contamination can easily occur from the environment in which the product is being prepared or from the person preparing it.

The best way to reduce the environmental risk is to use a laminar flow hood which establishes and maintains an ultraclean work area.

Room air is drawn into a horizontal hood and passed through a prefilter to remove relatively large contaminants such as dust and lint. The air is then channeled through a high efficiency particulate air (HEPA) filter that removes particles larger than 0.3 μm (microns). The purified air then flows over the work surface in parallel lines at a uniform velocity (i.e., laminar flow). The constant flow of air from the hood prevents room air from entering the work area and removes contaminants introduced into the work area by material or personnel.

The surfaces of the hood's work area are clean, not sterile.

Therefore, it is necessary to use techniques which maintain the sterilty of all sterile items. These are called **aseptic techniques.** They apply to the technician, the laminar flow hood, and all substances and materials involved in the procedure.

A B C D *aseptic techniques* techniques that maintain the sterile condition.

laminar flow continuous movement at a stable rate in one direction.

HEPA filter a high efficiency particulate air filter.

Types of Laminar Flow Hoods

There are two models of laminar flow hoods: the console model and the bench model. The console model sits on the floor and the work area ranges in width from 3 to 8 feet. The bench (counter top) model is also available in several different sizes. In this model, room air enters at the top of the unit and is channeled downward through the HEPA filter and out horizontally across the work surface.

SAFE PRACTICES

Positioning of material and working inside a hood aseptically requires training, practice, and attention to details.

✔ **Never sneeze, cough, talk directly into a hood.**

✔ **Close doors or windows.** Breezes can disrupt the air flow sufficiently to contaminate the work area.

✔ **Perform all work at least 6 inches inside the hood** to derive the benefits of the laminar air flow. Laminar flow air begins to mix with outside air near the edge of the hood.

✔ **Maintain a direct, open path between the filter and the area inside the hood.**

✔ **Place nonsterile objects, such as solution containers or your hands, downstream from sterile ones.** Particles blown off these objects can contaminate anything downstream from them.

✔ **Do not put large objects at the back of the work area next to the filter.** They will disrupt air flow.

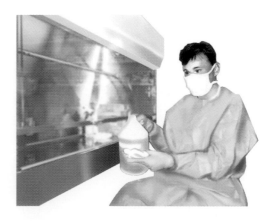

AIR FLOW

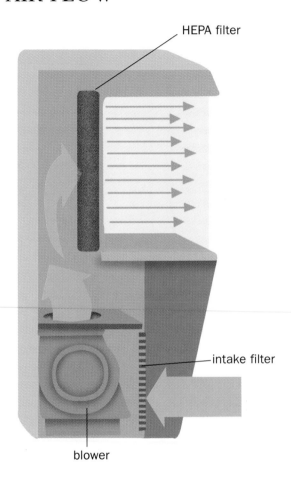

HEPA filter

intake filter

blower

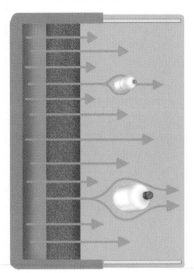

view from above

The illustration at left shows how the laminar air flow hood draws in air through its filters and channels it outward over the work surface.

The illustration above shows how air is channeled around objects on the work surface. Note that there is a "dead" area behind the large container.

BIOLOGICAL SAFETY HOODS

Biological safety hoods protect both personnel and the environment from contamination. It is used in the preparation of hazardous drugs. A biological safety cabinet functions by passing air through a HEPA filter and directing it down toward the work area. As the air approaches the work surface, it is pulled through vents at the front, back, and sides of the hood. A major portion of the air is recirculated back into the cabinet and a minor portion passes through a secondary HEPA filter and is exhausted into the room.

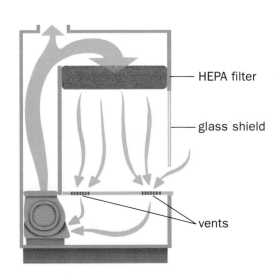

HEPA filter

glass shield

vents

ASEPTIC TECHNIQUE

Personnel involved with admixing parenteral solutions must use good aseptic technique.

Aseptic techniques are the sum total of methods and manipulations required to minimize the contamination of sterile products. Contamination can be from microorganisms and/or particulate material. Working in a laminar flow hood does not, by itself, guarantee aseptic technique. The guidelines on these pages must also be followed, along with any facility and manufacturer guidelines that apply.

Turn On Flow Hood

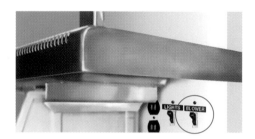

✔ Turn the laminar flow hood on and let it operate for at least 30 minutes before use in order to produce a particle free environment. Maintain a designated "clean" area around the hood.

Clothing and Barriers

✔ Wear clean lint-free garments or **barrier** clothing, including gowns, hair covers, and a mask.
✔ Wear **sterile gloves.**
✔ Follow facility or manufacturer guidelines for putting on and removing barrier clothing. Unless barriers are put on properly, they can easily become contaminated.

Cleaning Flow Hood

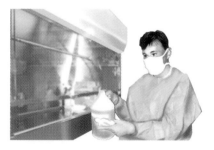

✔ Clean the inside of the hood with a suitable disinfectant such as 70% isopropyl alcoho. Cleaning is started with long side-to-side motions on the back surface of the hood working from top to bottom.
✔ Then the sides of the hood are cleaned using back-to-front motions again working from the top to the bottom of each side.
✔ Then the surface of the hood is cleaned using back-to-front motions.

Collect Supplies

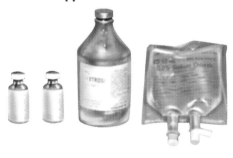

✔ Assemble all necessary supplies checking each for expiration dates and particulate material.
✔ Plastic solution containers should be squeezed to check for leaks.
✔ Use only presterilized needles, syringes, and filters. Check the protective covering of each to verify they are intact.

Wash hands

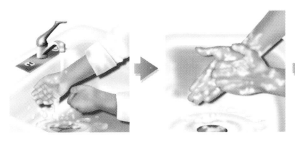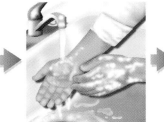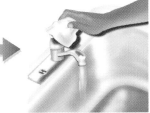

✔ Remove all jewelry and scrub hands and arms to the elbows with a suitable antibacterial agent.

✔ Stand far enough away from the sink so clothing does not come in contact with it.

✔ Turn on water. Wet hands and forearms thoroughly. Keep hands pointed downward.

✔ Scrub hands vigorously with an antibacterial soap.

✔ Work soap under fingernails by rubbing them against the palm of the other hand.

✔ Interlace the fingers and scrub the spaces between the fingers.

✔ Wash wrists and arms up to the elbows.

✔ Thoroughly rinse the soap from hands and arms.

✔ Dry hands and forearms thoroughly using a nonshedding paper towel.

✔ Use a dry paper towel to turn off the water faucet.

✔ After hands are washed, avoid touching clothes, face, hair, or any other potentially contaminated object in the area.

Position Supplies for Use

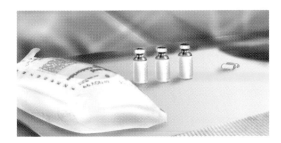

✔ Place supplies on a sterile cloth with smaller supplies closer to the HEPA filter and larger supplies further away from the filter.

✔ Space supplies to maximize laminar flow.

Sterilize Puncture Surfaces

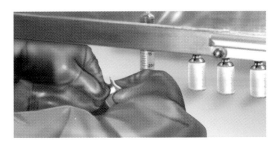

✔ Swab all surfaces that require entry (puncture) with an alcohol wipe. Avoid excess alcohol or lint that might be carried into the solution.

 Sterile supplies often have instructions for use as well as expiration dates. Always follow such instructions along with any facility or manufacturer instructions.

WORKING WITH VIALS

There are two types of parenteral vials that are used in making admixtures.

One contains the drug in solution. The other contains a powder that must be dissolved in a diluent to make a solution. In either case, a needle will be used to penetrate the rubber closure on the vial. To prevent coring and other problems, the techniques on these pages should be followed whenever you are transferring medications from vials.

CORING

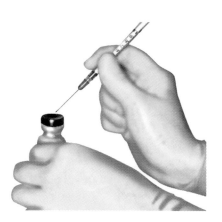

To prevent coring, follow these steps:

✔ Place the vial on a flat surface and position the needle point on the surface of the rubber closure so that the bevel is facing upward and the needle is at about a 45 to 60 degree angle to the closure surface.

✔ Put downward pressure on the needle while gradually bringing the needle up to an upright position. Just before penetration is complete, the needle should be at a vertical (90 degree) angle.

✔ Before the needle is withdrawn from the vial, the drug solution in the needle and the tip of the syringe should be cleared by drawing additional air into the syringe.

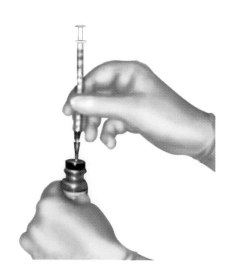

vial a small glass or plastic container with a rubber closure sealing the contents in the container.

coring when a needle damages the rubber closure of a parenteral container, causing fragments of the closure to fall into the container and contaminate its contents.

VIAL WITH SOLUTION

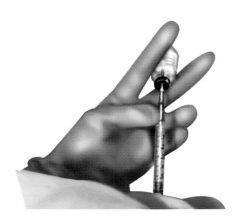

✔ Draw into the syringe a volume of air equal to the volume of drug to be withdrawn. This will offset the pressure in the vial and help in withdrawing the solution.

✔ Penetrate the vial without coring and inject the air.

✔ Turn the vial upside down. Using one hand to hold the vial and the barrel of the syringe, pull back on the plunger with the other hand to fill the syringe. Fill the syringe with a slight excess.

✔ Tap the syringe to allow air bubbles to come to the top of the syringe. Press the plunger to push air and excess solution into the vial.

✔ Withdraw the needle from the vial and transfer the solution into the intravenous bag or bottle, minimizing coring.

VIAL WITH POWDER

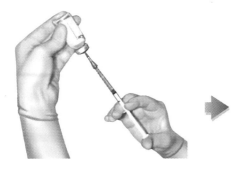 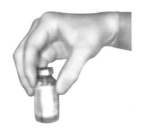 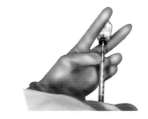

✔ Determine the correct volume of diluent and withdraw it from its vial following the steps outlined above (Vial with Solution).

✔ Inject the diluent into the medication vial.

✔ Once the diluent is added, withdraw a volume of air equal to the volume of diluent added. This lowers the chance that aerosol droplets will be sprayed when the needle is withdrawn.

✔ Unless shaking is not recommended, swirl the vial until the drug is dissolved.

✔ Using a new needle and syringe, perform the steps above for "Vial with Solution" again.

✔ Transfer the reconstituted solution into the final container.

WORKING WITH AMPULES

Ampules are always broken open at the neck.

Ampules have a colored stripe around the neck if they are prescored to indicate the neck has been weakened by the manufacturer to facilitate opening. Some ampules are not prescored by the manufacturer, and the neck must first be weakened (scored) with a fine file.

TO OPEN AN AMPULE

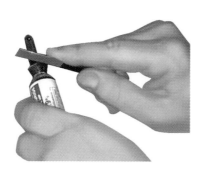 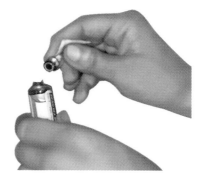

✔ If the ampule is not pre-scored, use a fine file to lightly score the neck at its narrowest point. Do not file all the way through the glass.

✔ Hold the ampule upright and tap the top to settle the solution in the ampule.

✔ Swab the neck of the ampule with an alcohol swab.

✔ Wrap a gauze pad around the neck of the ampule. Grasp the top of the ampule with the thumb and index finger of one hand. Grasp the bottom with the other hand.

✔ Quickly snap the ampule moving your hands outward and away. If the ampule does not snap easily, rotate it slightly and try again.

✔ Inspect the opened ampule for glass particles that may have fallen inside.

Note: Hands may be clean but are never sterile. Once they touch a sterile surface, it is no longer sterile. The outside surface of the above ampule would no longer be sterile. In situations where all surfaces must be sterile, hands would be gloved.

 ampules sealed glass containers with an elongated neck that must be snapped off.
sharps needles, jagged glass or metal objects, or any items that might puncture or cut the skin.

TRANSFERRING SOLUTION

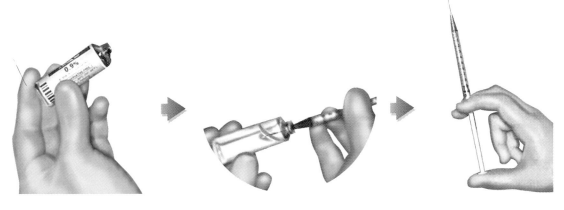

✔ Hold the ampule at about a 20-degree angle.

✔ Insert the needle into the ampule. Avoid touching the opening of the ampule with the needle point.

✔ Position the needle in the solution. Place its beveled edge against the side of the ampule to avoid pulling glass particles into the syringe.

✔ Withdraw solution but keep needle submerged to avoid withdrawing air into the syringe.

✔ Withdraw needle from ampule and remove all air bubbles from the syringe.

✔ Transfer the solution to the final container through a filter needle or membrane filter.

DISPOSAL

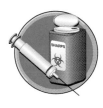

Discarded gloves, needles, syringes, ampules, vials, and prefilled syringes used in preparing parenterals pose a source of contamination and must be disposed of properly. In many health care facilities and other locations, such containers often have a label with **"Sharps"** on it, indicating objects that might puncture or cut the skin of anyone who handles them.

✔ Always separate sharps from other refuse for disposal.

✔ Receptacles that are easy to identify and are leakproof, punctureproof, and sealable should be used exclusively for this type of hazardous waste.

✔ Excess solutions should be returned to their original vial, an empty vial, or some other suitable closed container.

SPECIAL SOLUTIONS

TOTAL PARENTERAL NUTRITION SOLUTIONS

Total parenteral nutrition (TPN) solutions are complex admixtures used to provide nutritional support to patients who are unable to take in adequate nutrients through their digestive tract. These admixtures are composed of dextrose, fat, protein, electrolytes, vitamins, and trace elements. They are hypertonic solutions. Base parenteral nutrition solutions are available in 2,000 and 3,000 ml sizes. The base solution consists of:

➡ an amino acid solution (a source of protein);
➡ a dextrose solution (a source of carbohydrate calories).

These solutions, sometimes referred to as **macronutrients,** make up most of the volume of a parenteral nutrition solution. Several electrolytes, trace elements, and multiple vitamins (together referred to as **micronutrients**) may be added to the base solution to meet individual patient requirements. Common electrolyte additives include sodium chloride (or acetate), potassium chloride (or acetate), calcium gluconate, magnesium sulfate, and sodium (or potassium) phosphate. Multiple vitamin preparations containing both water-soluble and fat-soluble vitamins are usually added on a daily basis. A trace element product containing zinc, copper, manganese, selenium, and chromium may be added.

Intravenous fat (lipid) emulsion is required as a source of essential fatty acids. It is also used as a concentrated source of calories. Fat provides nine calories per gram, compared to 3.4 calories per gram provided by dextrose. Intravenous fat emulsion may be admixed into the parenteral nutrition solution with amino acids and dextrose, or piggybacked into the administration line. When intravenous fat emulsion is admixed with a TPN base solution, the resulting solution is referred to as a **total nutrient admixture (TNA)**.

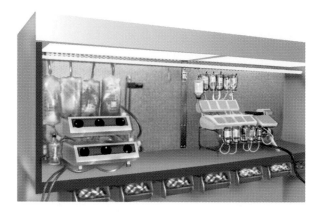

TPN preparation system

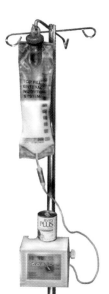

Administration

TPN solutions are generally (though not always) administered via the subclavian vein under the collar bone over 8 to 24 hours. Slow administration using this vein minimizes the adverse effects that may occur with such a hypertonic solution. The subclavian vein is large and close to the heart, so the solution is diluted rapidly by the large volume of blood in the heart.

To assure accurate delivery, nutrition solutions are almost always administered with an intravenous infusion pump. Parenteral nutrition solutions are commonly administered through an in-line filter in the administration set positioned as close to the patient as possible. However, intravenous fat emulsions, either alone or as part of a TPN solution, can be administered through an in-line filter only if it has a pore size of 1.2 micron or larger. An alternative is to piggyback the intravenous fat emulsion into the primary line below the in-line filter.

macronutrients amino acids and dextrose in the base parenteral nutrition solution.

micronutrients electrolytes, vitamins, and trace elements added to a base parenteral nutrition solution.

DIALYSIS SOLUTIONS

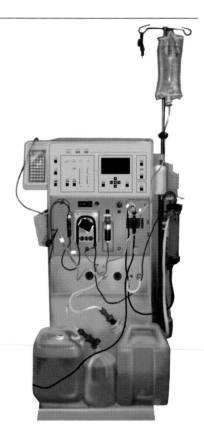

Dialysis refers to the passage of small particles through membranes. This is caused by **osmosis,** the action in which a drug in a solution of a higher concentration will move through a **permeable** membrane (one that can be penetrated) to a solution of a lower concentration.

Like irrigation solutions, dialysis solutions are not administered into the venous system and are supplied in containers larger than 1000 ml capacity. **Peritoneal dialysis solutions** are used by patients who do not have functioning kidneys. The solution is administered directly into the **peritoneal cavity (**the cavity between the abdominal lining and the internal organs) to remove toxic substances, excess body waste, and serum electrolytes through osmosis. *These solutions are hypertonic to blood so the water will not move into the circulatory system.*

Peritoneal solutions are administered several times a day. The solution is permitted to flow into the abdominal cavity, and then remains in the cavity for 30 to 90 minutes. It is then drained by a siphon into discharge bottles. This procedure is repeated many times a day and may use up to 50 liters of solution.

IRRIGATION SOLUTIONS

Irrigation solutions are not administered directly into the venous system but are subject to the same stringent controls as intravenous fluids. They are packaged in containers that are larger than 1000 ml capacity and are designed to empty rapidly. **Surgical irrigating solutions** (splash solutions) are used to:

➡ bathe and moisten body tissues,
➡ moisten dressings,
➡ wash instruments.

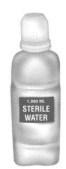

They are typically Sodium Chloride for Irrigation or Sterile Water for Irrigation. **Urologic solutions** are used during operations to:

➡ maintain tissue integrity,
➡ remove blood to maintain a clear field of vision.

Sterile Water for Irrigation, 1.5% glycine, and 3% sorbital solutions are commonly used because they are **non-hemolytic (**do not damage blood cells).

osmosis the action in which drug in a higher concentration solution passes through a permeable membrane to a lower concentration solution.

dialysis movement of particles in a solution through permeable membranes.

REVIEW

KEY CONCEPTS

✔ Parenteral solutions are packaged as two types of products: large volume parenteral (LVP) solutions and small volume parenteral (SVP) solutions.

✔ LVP solutions are typically bags or bottles containing larger volumes of intravenous solutions. SVP solutions are generally contained in ampules or vials.

✔ Solutions for injection must be sterile, free of all visible particulate material, pyrogen-free, stable for their intended use, have a pH around 7.4, and in most (but not all) cases isotonic.

✔ The flow rate is the rate at which the solution is administered to the patient.

✔ Piggybacks are small volumes of fluid (usually 50-100 ml) infused into the administration set of an LVP solution.

✔ Infusion pumps, syringe pumps, and ambulatory pumps are devices used to administer LVP solutions and control flow rates.

✔ When a drug is added to a parenteral solution, the drug is referred to as the additive, and the final mixture is referred to as the admixture.

✔ The volume of solution in a syringe is measured to the edge of the plunger's stopper while the syringe is held upright and all air has been removed from the syringe.

✔ Syringes come in sizes ranging from 1 to 60 ml. As a rule, a syringe size is used that is one size larger than the volume to be measured.

✔ Needle sizes are indicated by length and gauge. The higher the gauge number, the smaller is the lumen (the hollow bore of the needle shaft). Large needles may be needed with highly viscous solutions but are more likely to cause coring.

✔ Syringe filters are often used to remove contaminating particles from solutions.

✔ A laminar flow hood establishes and maintains an ultraclean work area for the preparation of IV admixtures.

✔ Aseptic techniques maintain the sterilty of all sterile items and are used in preparing IV admixtures.

✔ Biological safety hoods are used in the preparation of hazardous drugs and protect both personnel and the environment from contamination.

✔ Parenteral nutrition solutions are complex admixtures composed of dextrose, fat, protein, electrolytes, vitamins, and trace elements. They are hypertonic solutions. Most of the volume of TPN solutions is made up of macronutrients: amino acid solution (a source of protein) and a dextrose solution (a source of carbohydrate calories).

✔ Peritoneal dialysis solutions are used by patients who do not have functioning kidneys to remove toxic substances, excess body waste, and serum electrolytes through osmosis.

SELF TEST

MATCH THE TERMS. *answers can be checked in the glossary*

admixture

aseptic techniques

bevel

dialysis

diluent

gauge

HEPA filter

hypertonic

hypotonic

ion

isotonic

osmolality

pyrogens

a characteristic of a solution determined by the number of dissolved particles in it.

when a solution has a lesser osmolarity than another.

a high efficiency particulate air filter.

a liquid that dilutes a substance or solution.

a needle measurement–the higher the gauge, the thinner the lumen.

when one solution has an osmolarity equivalent to another.

an angled surface, as with the tip of a needle.

chemicals produced by microorganisms that can cause fever reactions in patients.

molecular particles that carry electric charges.

movement of particles in a solution through permeable membranes.

techniques that maintain sterile condition.

the resulting solution when a drug is added to a parenteral solution.

when a solution has a greater osmolarity than another.

CHOOSE THE BEST ANSWER. *answers are in the back of the book*

1. An intravenous solution that is formulated to have an osmolality similar to that of blood is
   a. isotonic to it
   b. hypotonic to it
   c. hypertonic to it
   d. none of the above

2. If 2.4 ml of diluent is used to reconstitute a vial of medication, what size of syringe should be used?
   a. 20 ml
   b. 10 ml
   c. 5 ml
   d. 3 ml

3. When using a laminar flow hood, the user should work inside the hood at least
   a. two inches
   b. four inches
   c. six inches
   d. eight inches

4. Of the following needles, which size of needle is most likely to cause coring?
   a. 13 G
   b. 16 G
   c. 20 G
   d. 23 G

DRUG NAMES & CLASSES

When a drug compound is first synthesized or isolated, it is known by its atomic composition: the types and numbers of atoms contained in it. For example, the compound $C_{14}H_{19}Cl_2NO_2$ has 14 carbon atoms, 19 hydrogen atoms, 2 chlorine atoms, 1 nitrogen atom, and 2 oxygen atoms. Besides being awkward to pronounce, this kind of identification does not really describe the structure of the molecule.

A drug's name begins with a chemical name that describes its structure and its components.

These names identify a specific compound, but they are long and complicated and not useful for general communication. As a result, highly specific chemical names are shortened to less descriptive but more easily pronounceable ones.

While a potential drug is under development, the developer gives it a code number or a "suggested nonproprietary name."

Once a suggested nonproprietary name is officially approved, it becomes the generic name of the drug compound. Many pharmaceutical companies will assign code numbers to their compounds in the earliest development stages, and then a suggested nonproprietary name if the compound shows promise of being effective as a drug. At that point, the sponsor will apply for a proprietary or trademark name from both the U.S. Patent Office and foreign agencies. If approved, the proprietary name will have the ® symbol next to it when used in interstate commerce.

When a drug is under patent protection, it has one nonproprietary name and one proprietary or brand name, and both of these belong to the sponsor.

When a drug goes off-patent, other companies may market the same compound under their own brand names. For example, ampicillin is a generic drug that has been off patent for many years. It is available as Polycillin®, Principen®, D-Amp®, Omnipen®, or Totacillin®. Each name is a brand name used by a different company. But Viagra® (which has the generic name sildenafil) is available only under one brand name because the compound is still under patent protection. The point to remember is that there is only one nonproprietary (generic) name for a drug, but it may be sold under many different brand names once its patent protection has expired.

WHAT'S IN A NAME

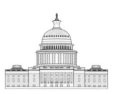

USAN

The United States Adopted Names Council (USAN) designates non-proprietary names for drugs. This council was organized in the early 1960s at the joint recommendation of the American Medical Association and the United States Pharmacopeial (USP) Convention. Other organizations, the American Pharmaceutical Association and the FDA, were included in the Council during the latter part of the 1960s. There are publications that list "official" nonproprietary and proprietary names, drug code designations, empirical names, chemical names, and show molecular structures. The USP Dictionary of USAN and International Drug Names is such a reference.

Applying for a name

To apply for a name, the sponsoring company initiates a request for a name. The USAN and the sponsor will arrive at a "Proposed USAN" that is suitable to both. This proposed name is then submitted for consideration to US and foreign drug regulatory agencies. When approved by these different agencies, the name becomes the "official" name of the drug. The USAN guidelines for names include that the name should:

➡ be short and distinctive in sound and spelling and not be such that it is easily confused with existing names;
➡ indicate the general pharmacological or therapeutic class into which the substance falls or the general chemical nature of the substance if the latter is associated with the specific pharmacological activity;
➡ embody the syllable or syllables characteristic of a related group of compounds.

D rug classes are group names for drugs that have similar activities or are used for the same type of diseases and disorders.

The assignment of a drug to a drug class is proposed when the sponsor makes an application to the USAN Council for an adopted name. The USAN Council and the sponsor then agree to a pharmacological or therapeutic classification. Unlike the generic and brand names, this classification is not an "official" one, however, and the drug may be listed in different classifications by different sources. For example, drugs classified one way in this chapter may appear in other classifications in other reference works.

There are common stems or syllables that are used to identify the different drug classes.

The USAN Council approves the stems and syllables and recommends using them in making new nonproprietary names. There are always new stems and syllables being approved by the Council, so the list is ever changing. On this page is a list of some common stems and syllables and the drug class associated with them.

STEMS & CLASSES

Following are the USAN approved stems and the drug classes associated with them.

Stem	Drug Class
-alol	Combined alpha and beta blockers
-andr-	Androgens
-anserin	Serotonin 5-HT$_2$ receptor antagonists
-arabine	Antineoplastics (arabinofuranosyl derivatives)
-ase	Enzymes
-azepam	Antianxiety agents (diazepam type)
-azosin	Antihypertensives (prazosin type)
-bactam	Beta-lactamase inhibitors
-bamate	Tranquilizers/antiepileptics
-barb	Barbituric acid derivatives
-butazone	Anti-inflammatory analgesics (phenylbutazone type)
-caine	Local anesthetics
-cef	Cephalosporins
-cillin	Penicillins
-conazole	Anti-fungals (miconazole type)
-cort-	Cortisone derivatives
-curium	Neuromuscular blocking agents
-cycline	Antibiotics (tetracycline type)
-dralazine	Antihypertensives (hydrazine-phthalazines)
-erg-	Ergot alkaloid derivatives
estr-	Estrogens
-fibrate	Antihyperlipidemics
-flurane	Inhalation anesthetics
-gest-	Progestins
-irudin	Anticoagulants (hirudin type)
-leukin	Interleukin-2 derivatives
-lukast	Leukotriene antagonists
-mab	Monoclonal antibodies
-mantadine	Antivirals
-monam	Monobactam antibiotics
-mustine	Antineoplastics
-mycin	Antibiotics
-olol	Beta-blockers (propranolol type)
-olone	Steroids
-oxacin	Antibiotics (quinolone derivatives)
-pamide	Diuretics (sulfamoylbenzoic acid derivatives)

Stem	Drug Class
-pamil	Coronary vasodilators
-parin	Heparin derivatives
-peridol	Antipsychotics (haloperidol type)
-poetin	Erythropoietins
-pramine	Antidepressants (imipramine type)
-pred	Prednisone derivatives
-pril	Antihypertensives (ACE inhibitors)
-profen	Anti-inflammatory/analgesic agents (ibuprofen type)
-rubicin	Antineoplastic antibiotics (daunorubicin type)
-sartan	Angiotensin II receptor antagonists
-sertron	Serotonin 5-HT$_3$ receptor antagonists
-sulfa	Antibiotics (sulfonamide derivatives)
-terol	Bronchodilators (phenethylamine derivatives)
-thiazide	Diuretics (thiazide derivatives)
-tiazem	Calcium channel blockers (diltiazem derivatives)
-tocin	Oxytocin derivatives
-trexate	Antimetabolites (folic acid derivatives)
-triptyline	Antidepressants
-vastatin	Antihyperlipidemics (HMG-CoA inhibitors)

CLASSIFICATION SCHEMES

There are various systems for classifying drugs: by disorder, body system affected, type of receptor acted on, type of action, etc. This text uses common classifications, but it is important to recognize that there is no standard classification system used in medicine.

A number of classifications are based on whether they influence the parasympathetic or sympathetic nervous system.

Most organs in the body are influenced by both the parasympathetic and sympathetic nervous systems. These systems generally stimulate opposing responses, which balances their effects and results in a normal state of **homeostasis**. Drugs that act on the parasympathetic system are called **cholinergic** because acetylcholine is the **neurotransmitter** of this system. Drugs that act on the sympathetic nervous system are called **adrenergic,** because the neurotransmitters for this system (norepinepherine and epinepherine) are secreted from the adrenal glands.

Many classifications are also named for the type of interaction with the receptor.

Agonist or **antagonist** interaction is the primary basis for classification (i.e., cholinergic antagonist, etc.), but drugs may be classified based on specific receptor characteristics. For example, adrenergic receptor responses may be categorized as alpha (α) and beta (β).

Classification schemes have grown significantly as different types of receptors have been discovered.

Each new type of receptor has been found to be responsible for a specific pharmacological effect. As drugs designed to interact with these receptors are developed the complexity of classifications increases.

There are also other factors that complicate classifications schemes.

One factor for drugs that affect the autonomic nervous system is the use of prefixes or suffixes such as **blocker**, **-lytic**, or **anti-** to mean antagonist, and **mimetic** to mean agonist. Another factor is the presence of neurotransmitters other than acetylcholine, norepinephrine, and epinephrine. These include serotonin, dopamine, histamine, gamma-amino butyric acid (GABA), etc. Each has subtypes, and each has agonists and antagonists that act by a variety of mechanisms.

CLASSIFICATIONS

Classification schemes for drugs can be highly complex. They can also vary greatly and any combination of terms or nomenclature schemes might be used. The classifications used in this text should provide insight into how and why the drugs in them are used, but are not the only way to classify these drugs.

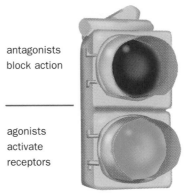

antagonists block action

_____

agonists activate receptors

blocker another term for an antagonist drug, because antagonists block the action of neurotransmitters.

homeostasis the state of equilibrium of the body.

mimetic another term for an agonist, because agonists imitate or "mimic" the action of the neurotransmitter.

neurotransmitter substances that carry the impulses from one neuron to another.

The primary classifications used in this text are:

Analgesics
  Salicylates
  NSAIDs
  Acetaminophen
  Opiate Type
Anesthetics
  Local
  General
Anti-infectives
  Antibiotic (Antimicrobial)
  Antiviral
  Antifungal
  Antimycobacterial
  Antiprotozoal
  Antihelminthic
Antineoplastic Agents
  Antimetabolites
  Alkylating Agents
  Plant Alkaloids
  Hormonal
Cardiovascular Agents
  Antianginal
  Antiarrhythmic
  Antihypertensive
  Vasopressors
  Antihyperlipidemic
  Thrombolytic
  Anticoagulant
Dermatological Agents
Electrolytes
Dermatologicals
Gastrointestinal Agents
  Enzymes
  Antidiarrheals
  Antiemetics
  Antacid / Antiulcer
  Laxatives and Stool Softeners

Hematological Agents
  Coagulation Enhancers
  Hematopoietic Agents
  Hemostatic Agents
Hormones & Modifiers
  Adrenal
  Antidiabetic
  Thyroid & Parathyroid
  Estrogen
  Contraceptive
  Androgen
  Pituitary
Immunobiologic Agents
  Vaccines
  Immune Globulins
Musculoskeletal Agents
Neurological Agents
  Antiparkinsonian
  Antialzheimer's
  Antiepileptic
  Antimigraine
Ophthalmic Agents
  Antiglaucoma agents
  Other Ophthalmics
Psychotropic Agents
  Antianxiety
  Antidepressants
  Antipsychotics
  Hypnotics
  Drug Dependency
Respiratory Agents
  Antihistamines
  Decongestants
  Antitussives
  Mucolytics
  Expectorants
  Bronchodilators
  Anti-inflammatory

LOOKALIKE / SOUNDALIKE

It is important to recognize that a number of drugs have similar sounding or looking names, but very different properties.

Besides similarity, one of the primary problems with accuracy in drug name identification is that prescriptions are still largely written by hand. However, it is also true that there are many ways drug names may be miscommunicated (by mispronunciation, typos, etc.). Therefore, the identification of a drug should be verified as many ways as possible.

Accuracy in handling and using drugs is essential.

Confusing one drug with another can lead to terrible, sometimes fatal consequences. It is critical to make certain that you have the name correct when involved in any aspect of the prescription process. At right is a list of drugs that can be mistaken for one another either by their sound or how they appear when written. There are many others, but this should illustrate the need for accuracy in drug names.

IDENTIFYING DRUG NAMES

At right is a list of drug names that might be easily misread, mispronounced, or otherwise mistaken for each other. Note that this is only a sample and that there are many other drugs with similar looking or sounding names.

Identifying Forms

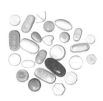

Frequent handling of a drug will help you to remember its physical characteristics (size, shape, color, markings, etc.), and this can be a valuable skill in the safe handling of drugs. It should be noted, however, that the most important step in identifying drugs is identifying the correct name. All drug information from the manufacturer to the prescriber, pharmacist, and ultimately the user is based upon communicating the correct name of the drug.

Acetazolamide	Acetohexamide	Hydralazine	Hydroxyzine
Alfentanil	Fentanyl, Sufentanil	Hydrochlorothiazide	Hydroflumethiazide
Amitriptyline	Aminophylline	Hydrocortisone	Hydrocodone
Atenolol	Albuterol	Kanamycin	Garamycin®, Gentamicin
Azathioprine	Azatadine		
Baclofen	Bactroban®, Beclovent®	Lisinopril	Fosinopril
Bupropion	Buspirone	Magnesium Sulfate	Manganese Sulfate
Calcitonin	Calcitriol	Methicillin	Mezlocillin
Captopril	Capitrol®	Metolazone	Metaxalone
Cefamandole	Cefmetazole	Metoprolol	Metaproterenol
Cefonicid	Cefobid®	Nifedipine	Nicardipine
Cefotaxime	Ceftizoxime	Oxymorphone	Oxymetholone
Cefoxitin	Cefotaxime	Pancuronium	Pipecuronium
Ceftizoxime	Ceftazidime	Pentobarbital	Phenobarbital
Cephalexin	Cephalothin	Phenytoin	Mephenytoin
Chlorpropamide	Chlorpromazine	Pramoxine	Pralidoxime
Clomiphene	Clomipramine	Prazosin	Prednisone
Clonazepam	Clofazimine	Prednisone	Prednisolone
Clorazepate	Clofibrate	Primidone	Prednisone
Clotrimazole	Co-trimoxazole	Proparacaine	Propoxyphene
Cyclosporine	Cycloserine	Quazepam	Oxazepam
Dexamethasone	Desoximetasone	Reserpine	Risperidone
Digoxin	Digitoxin	Ribavirin	Riboflavin
Diphenhydramine	Dimenhydrinate	Ritodrine	Ranitidine
Dopamine	Dobutamine	Sucralfate	Salsalate
Doxazosin	Doxorubicin	Sulfadiazine	Sulfasalazine
Doxepin	Doxapram, Doxidan®	Sulfamethizole	Sulfamethoxazole
Dronabinol	Droperidol	Terbutaline	Tolbutamide
Dyclonine	Dicyclomine	Terconazole	Tioconazole
Encainide	Flecainide	Testoderm®	Estraderm®
Enflurane	Isoflurane	Thyrar®	Thyrolar®
Etidronate	Etretinate	Thyrolar®	Theolair®
Flunisolide	Fluocinonide	Timolol	Atenolol
Glyburide	Glipizide	Tolazamide	Tolbutamide
Guanadrel	Gonadorelin	Torsemide	Furosemide
Guanethidine	Guanidine	Tretinoin	Trientine
Guanfacine	Guaifenesin, Guanidine	Triamterene	Trimipramine
Halcinonide	Halcion®	Vincristine	Vinblastine

REVIEW

KEY CONCEPTS

✔ A drug's name begins with a chemical name that describes its structure and its components.

✔ While a potential drug is under development, the developer gives it a code number or a "suggested nonproprietary name." The United States Adopted Names Council (USAN) designates nonproprietary names for drugs.

✔ Drug manufacturers apply for a proprietary or trademark names from both the U.S. Patent Office and foreign regulatory agencies. If approved, the proprietary name will have the ® symbol next to it when used in interstate commerce.

✔ When a drug is under patent protection, it has one nonproprietary name and one proprietary or brand name, and both of these belong to the sponsor.

✔ A drug has only one nonproprietary (generic) name, but may be sold under many different brand names once its patent protection has expired.

✔ The assignment of a drug to a drug class is proposed when the sponsor makes an application to the USAN Council for an adopted name. The USAN Council and the sponsor then agree to a pharmacological or therapeutic classification. Unlike generic and brand names, this classification is not an official one, and the drug may be listed in different classifications by different sources.

✔ There are various systems used for classifying drugs: by disorder, body system affected, type of receptor acted on, type of action, etc.

✔ Drugs that act on the parasympathetic nervous system are called cholinergic.

✔ Drugs that act on the sympathetic nervous system are called adrenergic.

✔ Agonist or antagonist interaction is another basis for classification (i.e., cholinergic antagonist, etc.), and drugs may be further classified based on specific receptor characteristics.

✔ Prefixes or suffixes such as blocker, -lytic, or anti- indicates an antagonist, and mimetic indicates an agonist.

✔ Homeostasis is the state of equilibrium of the body.

✔ Neurotransmitters are substances that carry the impulses from one neuron to another.

✔ It is important to recognize that a number of drugs have similar sounding or looking names, but very different properties. Confusing one drug with another can lead to terrible, sometimes fatal consequences.

SELF TEST

MATCH THE STEMS FROM THE CHOICES AT RIGHT.   *answers can be checked in the back of the book*

1. -andr-	Androgen	~~Steroids~~
2. -ase	enzymes	~~Progestins~~
3. -azepam	antianxiety agents	~~Prednisone~~ derivatives
4. -azosin	Antihypertensives	~~Penicillins~~
5. -caine	local anesthetics	~~Oxytocin~~ derivatives
6. -cef	Cephalosporins	Monoclonal antibodies
7. -cillin	penicillins	~~Local anesthetics~~
8. -conazole	anti-fungals	~~Estrogens~~
9. -cort-	Cortisone derivatives	~~Enzymes~~
10. -cycline	Antibiotics	~~Cortisone derivatives~~
11. estr-	estrogens	~~Coronary vasodilators~~
12. -gest-	Progestins	Cephalosporins
13. -mab	~~steroids~~ monoclonal antibodies	Calcium channel blockers (diltiazem derivatives)
14. -olone	steroids	~~Antimetabolites (folic acid derivatives)~~
15. -oxacin	Antibiotics (quinolone)	Antihypertensives (ACE inhibitors)
16. -pamil	coronary vasodilators	Antihypertensives
17. -pred	prednisone derivatives	Antihyperlipidemics (HMG-CoA inhibitors)
18. -pril	Antihypertensives (ACE)	~~Anti-fungals~~
19. -sulfa	antibiotics (sulfonamide)	Antidepressants
20. -tiazem	Calcium Channel Blockers	Antibiotics (sulfonamide derivatives)
21. -tocin	oxytocin derivatives	Antibiotics (quinolone derivatives)
22. -trexate	Antimetabolites	~~Antibiotics~~
23. -triptyline	Antidepressants	Antianxiety agents
24. -vastatin	coronary vasodilators Antihyperlipidemics	~~Androgens~~

ANALGESICS

Analgesic drugs create a state in which the pain from a painful medical condition is not felt.

Once pain has signaled the presence of a medical condition, its usefulness is generally complete and in most cases it can be safely blocked with the use of an analgesic.

There are several types of analgesics.

Two groups are used for mild to moderate pain, the non-steroidal anti-inflammatory drugs (NSAIDs) and the salicylates. Acetaminophen is also a popular agent for treating mild to moderate pain that some consider an NSAID but others do not.

Opiate-type narcotic analgesics are used for severe pain.

The naturally occurring opiates (morphine and codeine) and the synthetic opioids such as meperidine and propoxyphene are called "narcotic analgesics" and have a high abuse potential. In this chapter, we'll explore the types of analgesics and identify and describe common drug examples of each group.

 analgesia a state in which pain is not felt even though a painful condition exists.

anti-pyretic reduces fever.

The Transmission of Pain

Nerve fibers carry pain impulses from the body's receptor sites through the spinal cord and up to the thalamus and cerebral cortex. The cerebral cortex is the ridge-like neural tissue that covers the brain's hemispheres. Analgesics are thought to depress the thalamus and interfere with the transmission of pain impulses. In addition, the brain's interpretation of pain may be altered with the use of these drugs.

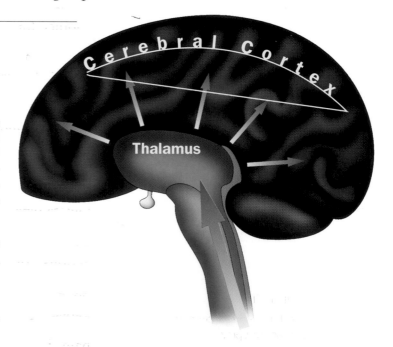

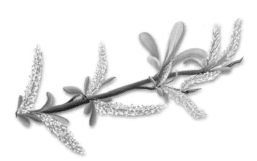

the white willow, a source of salicylic acid

Salicylates

➡ Relieve mild to moderate pain.

➡ Anti-inflammatory.

➡ Anti-pyretic.

Acetaminophen

➡ Relieves mild to moderate pain.

➡ Anti-pyretic.

NSAIDs

➡ More potent than salicylates.

➡ Relieve mild to moderate pain.

➡ Anti-inflammatory.

➡ Anti-pyretic.

Opiate-type

➡ For severe pain.

➡ Addicting.

Opiate-type Drugs & the Brain

Three specific receptors in the brain have been identified to react to opiate and opioid drugs:

➡ Mu (μ): produces euphoria, respiratory depression and physical dependence.

➡ Kappa (κ): produces analgesia,

➡ Sigma (σ): produces dysphoria and hallucinations.

An extract of willow bark, salicylic acid has been used to relieve pain for thousands of years.

Hippocrates and other ancient physicians used plants such as gaultheria and the poplar tree to obtain natural salicylates. Today, non-addicting analgesic products such as aspirin (acetylsalicylic acid) and methyl salicylate are widely used. Salicylates, acting both centrally and peripherally, are found effective as mild to moderate pain relievers, anti-inflammatory medications and fever reducers (antipyretics).

The action of non-steroidal anti-inflammatory drugs (NSAIDs) is both analgesic and anti-inflammatory.

They are generally more potent than the salicylates and serve to relieve mild to moderate pain, reduce fever and treat rheumatic symptoms. At higher doses, NSAIDs inhibit the synthesis of **prostaglandins**, a chief contributor to the inflammation process. As a result, inflammation is slowed or reduced. The effect of lower doses is analgesic. The selection and dosing of these drugs is very patient specific as one NSAID may be more effective than another for any given patient. NSAIDs may also have an antipyretic quality by which they reduce fever. The temperature regulating brain center is the hypothalamus and it is believed that some NSAIDs affect select areas of the hypothalamus to increase vasodilation, sweating, and encourage excess heat loss. Common drugs in this category include ibuprofen and naproxen.

Taken from the poppy plant, Papaver Somniferum, opium was also used in ancient times to relieve pain.

Opiate-type and opioid narcotics of today have been found to affect the CNS by reducing the awareness and perception of pain. They mimic the actions of the body's natural narcotic-like substances called endorphins. The narcotic analgesics do not eradicate the pain, but rather alter the patient's perception of it. Therefore, these drugs are thought to be most helpful if given before the severe pain is present. Common naturally occurring opiate-type drugs include morphine and codeine, while common opioid drugs include meperidine and propoxyphene.

ANALGESICS

Acetylsalicylic Acid (Aspirin)

Action and Indication

This drug functions as an antipyretic, analgesic, anti-inflammatory, and antithrombotic agent. It is used to treat fever, inflammation, and mild to moderate pain, and as preventive therapy for heart attack or stroke. Acetylsalicylic acid works as an anticoagulant by inhibiting the process of platelet aggregation.

Dosage

For minor pain or fever, 325- 650 mg every 4-6 hours. For prevention of stroke or heart attack, 325 mg 1-2 times daily. This medication is also available in enteric coated tablets to help avoid the potential GI side effects.

Route

GI upset.

Side Effects

GI upset including ulcers and bleeding, nausea/vomiting, heartburn

Warnings

Caution must be used in patients taking anticoagulants. Special caution should be used if prescribing aspirin for children. There is a direct cause and effect relationship between children with the Varicella Virus (Chicken Pox) and Reye's Syndrome, a potentially fatal reaction for children with the virus who have taken aspirin products.

Special Patient Teaching Considerations

Parents of children with flu-like or Chicken Pox symptoms *should not give their children aspirin*. Also, adults with GI history of ulcers or blood coagulation problems need to notify their physician before taking this drug.

 Reye's Syndrome a potentially fatal reaction to aspirin in children having Chicken Pox.

Methyl Salicylate (Ben Gay®, Deep-Heat®)

Action and Indication

A topical anti-inflammatory agent which causes irritation below the surface of the skin therefore increasing blood flow to the application site.

Dosage

One application of ointment to cover the affected site every 4-6 hours. If pain or discomfort continues after a few days, notify the physician.

Route

Topical.

Side Effects

A local allergic skin reaction may occur. Patients sensitive to salicylate products should consult their physician before using this ointment.

Warnings

This product is for topical use only. Ingestion could be harmful or fatal. Sensitivity to salicylate products needs to be known and disclosed.

Special Patient Teaching Considerations

Use this product as directed. If in doubt as to your reaction to salicylates, consult your physician first.

ANALGESICS

Acetaminophen (Tylenol®)

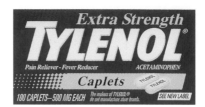

Tylenol®
Courtesy of McNeill-PPC

NSAID or not?

Though some sources classify acetaminophen as an NSAID, others do not, because it does not inhibit the synthesis of prostaglandins, and so does not have an anti-inflammatory effect.

Acetaminophen with Codeine

This combination drug is a narcotic analgesic used to treat moderate to severe pain. The acetaminophen acts to reduce fever and as an analgesic. Codeine increases the analgesic effect and may produce drowsiness, shock, and/or a worsening of asthma.

Alcohol should not be consumed while taking this medication. Although strengths for children and the elderly are available, caution should be used for these populations. A recommended regular adult dosage may range from 15-60 mg of codeine with 300-1000 mg of acetaminophen every 6 hours. The suggested maximum is 360 mg of codeine and 4000 mg of acetaminophen in a 24 hour period. This drug is available in tablet and elixir form.

Note: Caution is used regarding the amount of codeine as tolerance to codeine varies from patient to patient.

Action and Indication

Acetaminophen is an agent that raises the threshold of pain, relieves painful response, and acts on the hypothalamus for an antipyretic effect.

Dosage

This is a common medication recommended for use by children as well as adults. Regular strength for adults is 325 mg and extra strength is 500 mg. These strengths may be taken as two tablets or caplets every 4 hours, depending on the severity of the pain or fever. For children, the dose is titrated depending on their age and is offered as a liquid suspension or chewable tablet. An example of a dose for children 2-3 years old would be 160 mg or 1 tsp every 4 hours with a maximum of 5 doses over a 24 hour period.

Route

PO tablets, caplets, or liquid elixir.

Side Effects

Acetaminophen is relatively free of side effects, although an allergic response could occur (hives, rash, difficulty breathing). Liver toxicity can occur if abused or overdosed. Signs of overdose may include nausea/vomiting, diaphoresis (sweating), and anorexia.

Warnings

When acetaminophen is taken in combination with other selected drugs (alcohol, phenytoin, and warfarin), the effects of either could be altered.

Special Patient Teaching Considerations

Do not take this drug if also consuming alcohol due to the risk of liver toxicity. If the targeted pain or fever persists for several days, consult the physician immediately as the illness could be of a serious nature.

Ibuprofen (Motrin®)

Action and Indication

This **NSAID** is used to treat inflammation and fever. Stronger doses requiring a physician's order may be indicated for rheumatoid arthritis and moderate muscle or menstrual pain.

Dosage

For mild to moderate pain, 400-600 mg every 4-6 hours. For more severe events, such as rheumatoid or osteoarthritis, 1200-2400 mg per day could be given in 3-4 divided doses. Children's dosages are calculated according to their body weight. An example for children's fever reduction may be 5 mg per 2.2 lb of weight for a fever of 101°F to 102.5°F and 10 mg per 2.2 lb of weight for a fever over 102.5°.

Route

PO tablets or liquid suspension.

Side Effects

GI upset, bleeding or ulceration, fluid retention, edema and elevated liver enzymes.

Warnings

Use caution in patients with history of GI bleeding or ulceration, pregnancy, or who are elderly. Drugs such as lithium, warfarin, or aspirin when taken in combination with ibuprofen could cause an alteration in effect. Interaction with lithium may also lead to lithium toxicity. There have been several reports of kidney disease with doses exceeding 2400 mg/day.

Special Patient Teaching Considerations

Notify the physician if the patient is pregnant, breastfeeding or experiences GI symptoms.

Ibuprofen tablets
Courtesy of Par Pharmaceutical

ANALGESICS

Nabumetone (Relafen®)

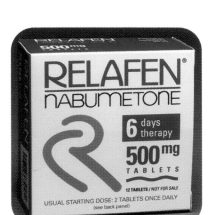

Relafen®
(nabumetone)
Courtesy of Smith, Kline, Beecham

Action and Indication

Relafen is an **NSAID** that is used to treat cases of both rheumatoid and osteoarthritis.

Dosage

500 mg-1000 mg to start, with a possible increase to 2000 mg daily. The larger amounts may be divided into 2 doses. Usually this medication is taken at bedtime.

Route

PO tablets.

Side Effects

GI effects such as abdominal pain and diarrhea. Stomach ulceration and bleeding may also occur. Other side effects include fluid retention, kidney dysfunction, and prolonged bleeding time.

Warnings

Contraindicated for patients with history of allergy to salicylates or NSAIDs. Due to the possibility of fluid retention, use with caution in patients with congestive heart failure or hypertension. This drug is not recommended for pregnant women.

Special Patient Teaching Considerations

Watch for signs or symptoms of gastric ulcers or bleeding. Take this medication with food. Avoid bright sunlight while taking Relafen.

COX-2 Inhibitors

A recent new group of NSAIDs is the cyclooxygenase-2 enzyme (COX-2) inhibitor. COX-2 inhibitors have been found to be effective in treating the pain of arthritis. The COX-2 enzyme is thought to play a role in causing arthritis pain and inflammation and COX-2 inhibitors block it. Celecoxib (Celebrex®) and rofecoxib (Vioxx®) are popular COX-2 inhibitors. Note: Celexcoxib is contraindicated for patients with a known sulfa drug allergy and both agents are contraindicated for patients with an allergic reaction to salicylates or NSAIDs.

Naproxen (Naprosyn®)

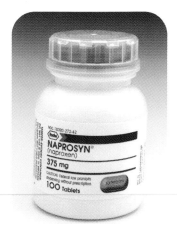

Naprosyn®
(naproxen)
Courtesy of Roche

Action and Indication

This **NSAID** is often prescribed in cases of rheumatoid arthritis, tendinitis, bursitis, menstrual cramps, or other types of mild to moderate pain. This agent will block the synthesis of prostaglandins to decrease pain and swelling.

Dosage

250-500 mg twice per day for mild to moderate complaints. For more acute conditions, 750-1000 mg per day may be ordered. For children, the dosage is calculated according to body weight and medical history. In elderly patients, it is prudent to use the lowest effective dose.

Route

PO tablets or liquid suspension. The tablets may be enteric coated to protect against gastric irritation.

Side Effects

Abdominal pain, bruising, itching, nausea, and constipation.

Warnings

Patient's history should not include GI bleeding or ulceration, known allergy to salicylates or NSAIDs, pregnancy, liver or kidney disease, or prolonged bleeding time. Naproxen should not be used at the same time as naproxen sodium.

Special Patient Teaching Considerations

Notify the physician should any of the above named side effects occur. Naprosyn may also cause the patient to become drowsy and less alert. Therefore machinery operation or hazardous activity should be avoided.

ANALGESICS

Oxaprozin (Daypro®)

Action and Indication

Indicated in the treatment of arthritic inflammation and pain relief. This **NSAID** is a long acting analgesic with antipyretic properties and it inhibits prostaglandin synthesis.

Dosage

This medication is recommended for use in adults at a dose of 1200 mg once daily. Oxaprozin is dispensed in 600 mg caplets and the suggested maximum daily dose is 1800 mg.

Route

PO caplets.

Side Effects

GI effects such as abdominal pain, nausea, diarrhea, and possible depression and/or confusion.

Warnings

Caution should be used in patients with a history of liver or kidney dysfunction, hypertension, heart disease, and anticoagulant therapy usage. This agent is contraindicated for patients with an allergic asthmatic reaction to salicylates or NSAIDs. Consider blood counts to assess for anemia following extended use of this drug. Note: Oxaprozin may cause fluid retention.

Special Patient Teaching Considerations

Prior to an invasive procedure, notify your surgeon of oxaprozin use as it may increase bleeding time. Avoid prolonged exposure to sunlight and taking aspirin while taking this agent.

Tramadol Hydrochloride (Ultram®)

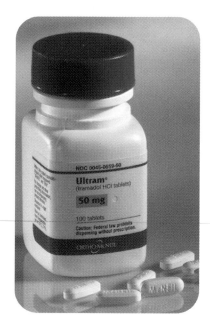

Ultram®
(tramadol hydrochloride)
Courtesy of Ortho-McNeil
Pharmaceutical Company

Action and Indication

Ultram is a synthetic analgesic that acts to inhibit reuptake of serotonin and norepinephrine. While not a narcotic, it also has an opioid effect, and is used in cases of moderate to severe pain.

Dosage

50-100 mg every 4-6 hours, not to exceed 400 mg daily. For the elderly and those with liver or kidney dysfunction, the dosage may be decreased.

Route

PO tablets.

Side Effects

Anxiety, confusion, urinary problems, drowsiness, abdominal pain, and general malaise.

Warnings

Some patients experience serious allergic reactions to this drug. Concurrent use of CNS depressants or monoamine oxidase inhibitors (MAOIs) could produce serious drug interactions and potentiations. Use caution in patients with a history of head injury and liver/kidney dysfunction.

Special Patient Teaching Considerations

Do not drink alcohol while taking this drug. Also avoid operation of dangerous machinery and activities which are hazardous and/or require optimal mental alertness. This drug is not recommended for use in children.

Not an NSAID

ANALGESICS

Hydrocodone Bitartrate + Acetaminophen (Vicodin®, Lorcet®, various)

Percocet-canadian version

Action and Indication

This **narcotic analgesic** is used in cases of moderate to severe pain as well as cough.

Dosage

This product should not be used in children. The active ingredients vary with the formulation and the formulation varies with the severity of pain. An example of an adult dosage might be 1 tablet of 7.5 mg acetaminophen and 500 mg of hydrocodone every 4-6 hours, with a maximum of 6 tablets in 24 hours.

Side Effects

Nausea, vomiting, dizziness, and possible sedation.

Warnings

Use caution in patients with history of head injury, liver, kidney, lung or thyroid disease. Use judiciously in the elderly.

Special Patient Teaching Considerations

This medication causes drowsiness and caution should be used if operating dangerous machinery or participating in activities involving mental alertness. Avoid the use of alcohol and antianxiety agents, antidepressants, and some antihistamines while taking this drug.

Morphine Sulfate (various)

Action and Indication

A **narcotic analgesic** that is generally the drug of choice for severe pain and in cases of a myocardial infarction because it decreases the heart's oxygen demand. This agonist will interact with several receptors in the brain to create pain relief, euphoria, stuporous sleep-like state, and possible dependence. Note: MS Contin® is a controlled drug which contains morphine and is used if patients require morphine for a longer duration.

Dosage

Initially, morphine may be given IV, IM or PO, and the dosage varies with the route chosen. For example, 2 mg might be given IV, 5-10 mg SQ or IM, and 10-30 mg PO. For maintenance, these dosages may be given every 3-4 hours. This drug may also be given rectally at a suggested dose of 10-20 mg every 3-4 hours. MS Contin® may be given every 8-12 hours in a dose of 15-30 mg PO.

Route

PO, SQ, IM, IV, or rectal.

Side Effects

Both morphine and MS Contin® may cause respiratory depression, hypotension, nausea/vomiting, urinary retention, constipation, and sedation.

Warnings

This narcotic is potentially dangerous as it could cause death due to over sedation or respiratory depression. Tolerance varies greatly among individuals. Each patient needs to be assessed individually and their dosage chosen. Patients must be monitored frequently. If MS Contin® is given PO, do not crush tablets as it could cause release of high doses of this drug.

Special Patient Teaching Considerations

Side effects must be reported to the physician immediately. *Caution: This drug may be addictive and dangerous.*

ANALGESICS

Meperidine Hydrochloride (Demerol®)

Action and Indication

A **synthetic opioid** used to treat moderate to severe pain. This drug will effect analgesia by reacting with selected receptor sites in the brain.

Dosage

PO 50-150 mg every 3-4 hours; IM 25-100 mg every 3-4 hours; and IV 5-10 mg every 5 min, prn.

Route

PO tablet or liquid syrup; IM, or IV.

Side Effects

Drowsiness, hypotension, sweating, possible respiratory depression, tremors, and seizure activity.

Warnings

Patients who have recently taken or are taking monoamine oxidase inhibitors (MAOIs) should not take this drug. Harmful or fatal reactions could occur. Should be used with caution in patients with history of renal failure.

Special Patient Teaching Considerations

Notify a doctor if the patient is presently taking or has recently taken any antidepressant drugs or has experienced renal failure. If taking liquid meperidine, doses should be taken in a half glass of water. Note that this medication may cause drowsiness and that while taking this drug the patient should not participate in activities requiring a high degree of alertness.

Propoxyphene Hydrochloride (Darvon®)

Action and Indication
This is a **mild narcotic analgesic** that is used for treatment of mild to moderate pain. It may be more effective when used in combination with NSAIDs.

Dosage
65 mg every 3-4 hours, PO.

Route
PO capsules.

Side Effects
Dizziness, nausea/vomiting, drowsiness.

Warnings
It is possible to build up a dependence on this drug over a period of time. Caution should be used in patients with history of liver or kidney failure or allergies to propoxyphene. Note: The Darvon-65 compound contains aspirin and caffeine. Darvocet-N is a combination agent of propoxyphene and acetaminophen. Good pain control has been reported with Darvocet-N 100, every 4 hours, prn.

Special Patient Teaching Considerations
Although this is a mild narcotic, it still has sedative-like qualities and care should be taken during normal daily activities. For patients taking the Darvon-65 compound, note the aspirin and caffeine components and notify the physician of any allergies to aspirin or cardiovascular conditions that could be affected by the caffeine.

DRUG CHART

Generic Name	Trade Name	Route	Generic Name	Trade Name	Route
NSAIDs					
Diclofenac	Voltaren	PO, Eye	Naproxen	Aleve	PO
	Cataflam	PO		Anaprox	PO
	Various	PO		Naprelan	PO
Diclofenac / Misoprostol	Arthrotec	PO		Naprosyn	PO
Diflunisal	Dolobid	PO		Various	PO
	Various	PO	Oxaprozin	Daypro	PO
Etodolac	Lodine	PO	Piroxicam	Feldene	PO
	Various	PO		Various	PO
Fenoprofen	Nalfon	PO	Sulindac	Clinoril	PO
	Various	PO		Various	PO
Flurbiprofen	Ansaid	PO	Tolmetin	Tolectin	PO
	Ocufen	Eye		Various	PO
	Various	PO			
Hydrocodone / Ibuprofen	Vicoprofen	PO			
Ibuprofen	Advil	PO	**Salicylates**		
	Excedrin IB	PO	Salicylate Salts	Trilisate	PO
	Motrin IB	PO		Various	PO
	Nuprin	PO	Salsalate	Disalcid	PO
	Various	PO		Various	PO
Indomethacin	Indocin	PO	Aspirin/Carisoprodol	Soma Compound	PO
	Various	PO	(a compound)	Various	PO
Ketoprofen	Actron	PO			
	Orudis	PO			
	Oruvail	PO			
	Various	PO			
Ketoralac	Acular	Eye			
	Toradol	PO, Inj.			
	Various	PO			
Meclofenamate	Meclomen	PO			
	Ponstel	PO			
	Various	PO			
Nabumetone	Relafen	PO			

 Trade (brand) names are registered trademarks of
the drug manufacturer.

GENERIC NAME	TRADE NAME	ROUTE	GENERIC NAME	TRADE NAME	ROUTE
NARCOTIC ANALGESICS					
Acetaminophen / Codeine	Tylenol with Codeine	PO	Methadone	Dolophine	PO
	Various	PO		Various	PO
Acetaminophen / Hydrocodone	Anexsia	PO	Morphine	MS Contin	PO
	Lorcet	PO		Duramorph	Inj.
	Lortab	PO		Various	PO, Inj.
	Vicodin	PO	Nalbuphine	Nubain	Inj.
	Various	PO	Oxycodone	Percolone	PO
Acetaminophen / Oxycodone	Percocet	PO		Roxicodone	PO
	Tylox	PO		Various	PO
	Various	PO	Propoxyphene	Darvon	PO
Acetaminophen/Propoxyphene	Darvocet-N	PO		Various	PO
	Various	PO			
Aspirin / Oxycodone	Percodan	PO			
	Various	PO	**OTHER**		
Butorphanol	Stadol	Nasal, Inj.	Acetaminophen	Tylenol	PO, Supp.
	Various	Inj.		Various	PO, Supp.
Codeine	Codeine	PO	Acetaminophen + Butalbital + Caffeine	Esgic	PO
	Various	PO		Fioricet	PO
Fentanyl	Duragesic	PO		Various	PO
	Sublimaze	Inj.	Aspirin + Butalbital + Caffeine	Fiorinal	PO
	Oralet	PO, Lozenge		Butalbital Compound	PO
	Actiq	PO, Transmucosal		Various	PO
Hydrocodone	Various	PO	Phenazopyridine	Pyridium	PO
Hydromorphone	Dilaudid	PO		Various	PO
	Various	PO	Tramadol	Ultram	PO
Meperidine	Demerol	PO, Inj.			
	Various	PO, Inj.			

 Note that the generic names indicated in these charts are listed without the complete compound name of the drug, e.g., propoxyphene rather than propoxyphene hydrochloride (its salt form). This is done in an effort to simplify recognition. In many cases, knowing and using the specific chemical compound is highly important.

REVIEW

KEY CONCEPTS

✔ Analgesic drugs create a state in which the pain from a painful medical condition is not felt.

✔ Analgesics are thought to depress the thalamus and interfere with the transmission of pain impulses.

✔ Two groups are used for mild to moderate pain, the non-steroidal anti-inflammatory drugs (NSAIDs) and the salicylates.

✔ Acetaminophen is a popular agent for treating mild to moderate pain. Some sources classify acetaminophen as an NSAID, but others do not because it does not inhibit the synthesis of prostaglandins, and so does not have an anti-inflammatory effect.

✔ Opiate-type narcotic analgesics are used for severe pain. They act on Kappa (κ) receptors in the brain to produce analgesia. The naturally occurring opiates (morphine and codeine) and the synthetic opioids such as meperidine and propoxyphene are called "narcotic analgesics" and have a high abuse potential.

✔ NSAIDs and salicylates are also anti-pyretic. That is, they reduce fever.

✔ An extract of willow bark, salicylic acid has been used to relieve pain for thousands of years.

✔ The action of non-steroidal anti-inflammatory drugs (NSAIDs) is both analgesic and anti-inflammatory.

✔ Acetaminophen with codeine is a narcotic analgesic combination drug used to treat moderate to severe pain. Caution is used regarding the amount of codeine as tolerance to codeine varies from patient to patient.

✔ In addition to its analgesic and pyretic effects, acetylsalicylic acid works as an anticoagulant by inhibiting the process of platelet aggregation.

✔ At higher doses, NSAIDs inhibit the synthesis of prostaglandins, a chief contributor to the inflammation process. As a result, inflammation is slowed or reduced.

✔ Selection and dosing of NSAIDs is patient specific as one NSAID may be more effective than another for any given patient.

✔ Opiate-type and opioid narcotics affect the CNS to reduce the perception of pain. They mimic the actions of the body's natural narcotic-like substances called endorphins.

✔ Reye's Syndrome is a potentially fatal reaction to aspirin in children that have Chicken Pox.

✔ A new group of NSAID for treating arthritis are the COX-2 inhibitors which block the COX-2 enzyme that is thought to play a role in causing arthritis pain and inflammation.

SELF TEST

MATCH THE GENERIC AND TRADE NAMES.

answers are in the back of the book

1. Acetaminophen _____   Actron

2. Diclofenac _____   Advil

3. Ibuprofen _____   Aleve

4. Indomethacin _____   Darvon

5. Ketoprofen _____   Daypro

6. Meperidine _____   Demerol

7. Morphine _____   Indocin

8. Nabumetone _____   MS Contin

9. Naproxen _____   Relafen

10. Oxaprozin _____   Tylenol

11. Propoxyphene _____   Ultram

12. Tramadol _____   Voltaren

CHOOSE THE BEST ANSWER.

answers are in the back of the book

1. Of the following receptor sites, which one (when stimulated) produces analgesia?
   a. Mu
   b. Kappa
   c. Sigma
   d. Beta

2. NSAID's work by inhibiting which one of the following chemical mediators, resulting in the reduction of inflammation?
   a. leukotrienes
   b. substance P
   c. prostaglandins
   d. histamine

3. Of the following drugs, which one is considered an NSAID?
   a. acetaminophen
   b. aspirin
   c. morphine
   d. naproxen

4. Opiates are drugs that are derived from the poppy plant and have a high abuse potential. Of the following drugs which is an opiate?
   a. acetaminophen
   b. aspirin
   c. morphine
   d. naproxen

ANESTHETIC AGENTS

Anesthetics cause an absence of sensation or pain.

They are classified into two groups: local and general.

Local anesthetics block pain conduction from peripheral nerves to the central nervous system without causing a loss of consciousness.

They do this by allowing the nerve's membrane to stabilize in a resting position and not respond to painful stimuli. Cocaine is credited by some sources as the first recognized local anesthetic, but it has a limited use today (i.e., topical application in eye and nasal surgery) and is a Schedule II substance.

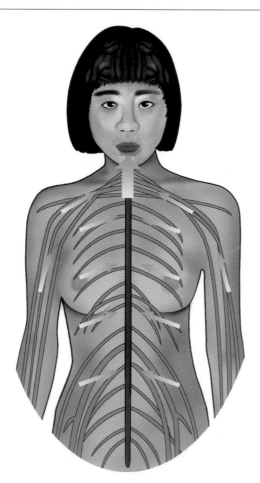

Blocking Pain

Pain is conducted from its local site through the Peripheral Nervous System (blue) to the Central Nervous System (red). Local anesthetics block pain conduction to the CNS, but do not affect the CNS, so the patient remains conscious. General anesthetics block pain sensation by depressing the CNS, causing unconsciousness.

LOCAL ANESTHETICS

Indications

Common indications for local anesthetics include:

➡ dental work or discomfort (topical or injection);

➡ birth pain (spinal, epidural or caudal IV);

➡ sunburn, hemorrhoids and skin irritations (topical).

Groups

Local anesthetics can be grouped by chemical structure as follows:

➡ **Esters** – metabolized by enzymes found in the blood or skin, short to moderate duration of effectiveness. Examples include: procaine, benzocaine, butamben, and tetracaine.

➡ **Amides** – metabolized in the liver and therefore longer acting. Examples include: lidocaine, procainamide, bupivacaine, and dibucaine.

➡ **Others** - those agents suitable for patients with allergies to esthers or amides. Examples are dyclonine and pramoxine.

ABCD *surgical anesthesia* the stage of anesthesia in which surgery can be safely conducted.

medullary paralysis an overdose of anesthesia that paralyzes the respiratory and heart centers of the medulla, leading to death.

GENERAL ANESTHESIA

The Four Stages

There are four stages of general anesthesia:

Stage I – Analgesia

Euphoria with loss of pain and consciousness.

Stage II – Excitement

Increase in sympathetic nervous system effects such as blood pressure, heart and respiratory rate.

Stage III – Surgical Anesthesia

The stage in which surgery can safely be conducted. There are four levels of surgical anesthesia, with the higher numbered levels producing deeper anesthesia and more serious systemic effects.

Stage IV – Medullary Paralysis

An overdose of anesthesia can compromise the respiratory and heart centers of the brain's medulla and cause death.

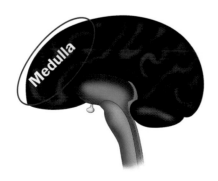

General anesthetics depress the CNS (central nervous system) to the level of unconsciousness.

The first general anesthetic, nitrous oxide (laughing gas), was developed about 150 years ago. The vapors ethyl ether and chloroform followed soon after. However, these products were found to have many safety concerns and less hazardous agents have been subsequently developed.

General anesthetics are generally classified according to their route of administration: *inhalation* or *intravenous* (*IV*).

IV anesthesia often produces a more pleasant, smoother and quicker onset than the inhaled anesthetics. A combination of various agents is widely used to avoid undesired side effects and produce the best effects of general anesthesia.

General anesthesia is administered by a medical doctor called an anesthesiologist.

The desired level of general anesthesia can be controlled by balancing the amount of anesthesia the patient receives with the amount their lungs eliminate through exhalation. In ceasing the administration of anesthesia, the process will reverse and the level of anesthesia lighten.

In addition to the anesthetic drug choice, adjunctive drugs such as analgesics, atropine-like drugs, and anti-infectives may also be used.

This is to prevent certain negative side effects (those that occur from too much of one anesthetic), potentiate other desired effects (such as pain relief and reduced amount of anesthesia), cause the drying of secretions (preventing aspiration during surgery), or act to prevent infections (post-op). The safety, comfort, and general well being of the patient are of utmost concern when an anesthesiologist chooses the anesthetic or combination of anesthetics that are the most appropriately indicated for a particular case.

Inhalation Anesthetics

Examples of inhalation anesthetics include:

➡ nitrous oxide,

➡ ether,

➡ halothane, and

➡ desflurane.

Intravenous Anesthetics

IV anesthetics include:

➡ midazolam,

➡ diazepam,

➡ fentanyl, and

➡ alfentanil.

ANESTHETIC AGENTS

Common Local Anesthetics

Procaine (Novocain®)

Given as an injection, 1-2% and 10% solutions, duration of 15 – 30 minutes.

Tetracaine (Pontocaine®)

Given as an injection, 0.2, 0.3 and 1% solutions, duration of 2-3 hours.

Bupivacaine (Marcaine®)

Given as an injection, 0.25 - 0.75% solution, duration of 2-4 hours.

Dibucaine (Nupercaine®)

Given as an injection, 0.25% solution, duration of 3-4 hours.

Side Effects

The potential side effects for all the above local anesthetics are the same: local skin irritation at injection site and possible allergic response.

Common General Anesthetics

Nitrous Oxide

A gaseous inhalation anesthetic, used as an induction. It does not cause skeletal relaxation. However it does provide a risk of hypoxemia (decreased oxygenation of the blood). This agent is nonexplosive.

Halothane (Fluothane®)

A volatile liquid inhalation anesthetic, used for maintenance. Moderate muscle relaxation may occur. This agent does not produce respiratory tract irritation and it may be given with a combination of nitrous oxide and oxygen.

Midazolam (Versed®)

An injectable anesthetic, used for pre-op sedation and induction. This short acting agent effects a state of conscious sedation, but when used for induction may cause loss of consciousness in 1-2 minutes.

Fentanyl Citrate and Droperidol (Innovar®)

An injectable anesthetic, used for induction. The combination of these drugs causes neuroleptanalgesia which is characterized by reduced motor activity, serious analgesia and overall quietness. Actual complete loss of consciousness may not occur if using this anesthetic solely.

Recovery

Following a patient to the PARR (post anesthesia recovery room), health care personnel:

➥ monitor vital signs every 5 - 15 minutes (as stability will dictate);

➥ assess respiratory status (O_2 use is often indicated), skin color and condition;

➥ monitor IV lines, CVP (central venous pressure) monitors and lines, catheters, drainage tubes, dressings, casts;

➥ assess level of consciousness and alertness;

➥ monitor positioning to avoid aspiration and side effect occurrence (e.g., nausea/vomiting, dizziness).

The surgeon is often in nearby attendance should an event of concern occur.

DRUG CHART

Generic Name	Trade Name	Route	Generic Name	Trade Name	Route
General			**Local**		
Nitrous Oxide	Various	Inhalation	Bupivacaine	Marcaine	Injectable
Enflurane	Enthrane	Inhalation	Etidocaine	Duranest	Injectable
Halothane	Fluothane	Inhalation	Mepivacaine	Carbocaine	Injectable
Isoflurane	Forane	Inhalation		Various	Injectable
	Various	Inhalation	Prilocaine	Citanest	Injectable
Methoxyflurane	Penthrane	Inhalation	Chloroprocaine	Nesacaine	Injectable
Sevoflurane	Ultane	Inhalation		Various	Injectable
Droperidol	Inapsine	Intravenous	Cocaine	Various	Topical
	Various	Intravenous	Procaine	Novocain	Injectable
Etomidate	Amidate	Intravenous	Propoxycaine	Propoxycaine	Injectable
Ketamine	Ketalar	Intravenous	Tetracaine	Pontocaine	Inj, Eye, Loz.
Propofol	Diprivan	Intravenous	Benzocaine	Americaine	Top., various
			Lidocaine	Xylocaine	Inj., Topical
Barbiturate					
Methohexital	Brevital	Intravenous			
Thiopental	Pentothal	Intravenous			
Benzodiazepine					
Diazepam	Valium	Intravenous			
	Various	Intravenous			
Midazolam	Versed	Intravenous			
Opiate					
Sufentanil	Sufenta	Intravenous			
Fentanyl	Sublimaze	Intravenous			

KEY CONCEPTS

✔ Anesthetics cause an absence of sensation or pain.

✔ Local anesthetics block pain conduction from peripheral nerves to the central nervous system without causing a loss of consciousness.

✔ Cocaine is credited by some sources as the first recognized local anesthetic, but it has a limited use today (i.e., topical application in eye and nasal surgery) and is a Schedule II substance.

✔ General anesthetics depress the CNS (central nervous system) to the level of unconsciousness. They are generally classified according to their route of administration: inhalation or intravenous (IV).

✔ A combination of various agents is widely used to avoid undesired side effects and produce the best effects of general anesthesia.

✔ The desired level of general anesthesia can be controlled by balancing the amount of anesthesia the patient receives with the amount their lungs eliminate through exhalation. In ceasing the administration of anesthesia, the process will reverse and the level of anesthesia lighten.

✔ Surgical anesthesia is the stage of anesthesia in which surgery can be safely conducted.

✔ Medullary paralysis occurs from an overdose of anesthesia that paralyzes the respiratory and heart centers of the medulla, leading to death.

✔ Examples of inhalation anesthetics include: nitrous oxide, ether, halothane, and desflurane.

✔ IV anesthetics include: midazolam, diazepam, fentanyl, and alfentanil.

CHOOSE THE BEST ANSWER.

answers are in the back of the book

1. Of the following four stages of general anesthesia, which stage should an individual be in before a surgical procedure can begin?
   a. Stage I
   b. Stage II
   c. Stage III
   d. Stage IV

2. Which of the following general anesthetics would be given IV?
   a. nitrous Oxide
   b. ether
   c. halothane
   d. midazolam

3. Common indications for local anesthesia include:
   a. dental work
   b. birth pain
   c. hemorrhoids
   d. all of the above

4. Which local anesthetic listed has the shortest duration of action?
   a. Marcaine®
   b. Novocaine®
   c. Nupercaine®
   d. Pontocaine®

ANTI-INFECTIVES

Anti-infectives treat disease produced by microorganisms such as bacteria, viruses, fungi, protozoa, and parasitic worms. Historically, natural chemicals from the earth such as mercury and molds have been used to treat infections, but it wasn't until Paul Ehrlich synthesized hundreds of chemicals in the 1930's, that a chemotherapeutic approach was widely used. There are now a large number of naturally occurring, semi-synthetic and synthetic drugs and vaccines available for treatments of infectious diseases.

In this chapter, *antibiotics (antimicrobials)*, *antivirals* and *antifungals* will be discussed and explored.

Other forms of anti-infectives include: *antimycobacterials* (agents that treat tuberculosis, leprosy and the MAC complex in AIDS); *antiprotozoals* (agents that treat malaria, vaginitis and sleeping sickness); and *antihelminthics* (agents that treat parasitic worms in the GI tract). Metronidazole, a stand alone miscellaneous antibacterial and antiprotozoal agent, is also included in the drug chart. (Note: vaccines and other immunity causing agents are discussed in chapter 20.)

ANTIBIOTICS

Early discovery of antibiotics comes from Sir Alexander Fleming and his work isolating the naturally occurring **penicillin**. In the latter 1930's, a team from Oxford reinvestigated this research and developed potent extracts which were important in fighting infections during WWII. Since this time, synthetic penicllins (e.g., ampicillin) and the first semisynthetic penicillin, carbenicillin, have been introduced.

Other forms of antibiotics include:

➡ **cephalosporins** (cefazolin, cefoxitin, ceftibuten, cefepime, etc.)

➡ **tetracyclines** (tetracycline, doxycycline, etc.);

➡ **sulfonamides** (sulfasoxazole, sulfamylon, etc.).

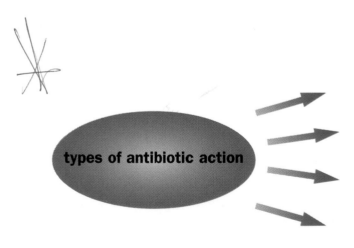

damages the bacterial cell wall
(e.g., penicillins and cephalosporins)

modifies protein synthesis
(e.g., erythromycin and tetracycline)

modifies energy metabolism.
(e.g., sulfonamides)

modifies DNA synthesis.
(e.g., ofloxacin and ciprofloxacin)

types of antibiotic action

ANTI-INFECTIVES

Antibiotic (Antimicrobial)

The terms antibiotic or antimicrobial refer to chemicals of bacterial microorganisms which suppress the growth of other microorganisms. Antimicrobials can be expanded to include both synthetic and naturally occurring antibiotics. Antimicrobials can be either **bacteriostatic** (inhibiting bacterial growth) or **bactericidal** (bacteria killing). These agents act by modifying protein synthesis, energy metabolism, DNA metabolism, and by damaging the bacteria's cell wall.

Antiviral

Antivirals inhibit the replication of viruses (**virustatic**). The viral microorganism will invade the host cell and proliferate using the cell's DNA and RNA. To effectively treat viral infections, the drug needs to stop the viral replication without destroying the patient's healthy cells. Mutations and resistance are common setbacks with this therapy. Antimicrobials are not effective with viral infections, but may be used in cases of accompanying secondary bacterial infection. **Protease inhibitors** (i.e. saquinavir, indinavir and nelfinavir) have been successful in blocking the enzyme responsible for viral replication. Other antiviral agents include: zidovudine and acyclovir.

Antifungal

Antifungals are used to treat fungal infections. Fungi are plant-like microorganisms commonly found in molds and yeast. The drugs chosen to treat these mycosis or mycotic infections are usually **fungicidal**. The fungal cell is destroyed as the drug prevents cell permeability and nutrition. Common fungal infections include: candidiasis (vaginal yeast infection), ringworm, and athlete's foot. Nystatin and fluconazole are popular antifungal drugs.

 antibiotic (antimicrobial) drug that destroys microorganisms.

antiviral drug that attacks a virus.

antifungal drug that destroys fungi or inhibits its growth.

antimycobacterial drug that attacks mycobacteria, the organisms that cause tuberculosis and leprosy.

antiprotozoal drug that destroys protozoa.

antihelminthic drug that destroys worms.

bactericidal bacteria killing.

bacteriostatic bacteria inhibiting.

virustatic drug that inhibits the growth of viruses.

ANTIBIOTICS

Ampicillin (Omnipen®, various)

Action and Indication

A penicillin-like bactericidal antibiotic that inhibits cell wall synthesis and offers both gram positive and gram negative coverage. Infections such as upper respiratory, urinary, GI, and meningitis can be successfully treated with this agent.

Dosage

250-1000 mg (1 g) every 4-6 hours, PO; 500-2000 mg (2 g) every 6 hours, IM or IV. Site, severity, and patient condition will dictate appropriate dosage.

Route

PO tablets, liquid suspension; IM, IV.

Side Effects

GI upset, allergic reaction.

gram positive/negative
a laboratory method for identifying microorganisms based on staining characteristics.

Warnings

Doses should be taken 30 minutes before or 2 hours after meals. Should not be used in patients with a history of penicillin or cephalosporin allergy. May reduce the effeciveness of oral contraceptives.

Special Patient Teaching Considerations

Note meal times to assure administration efficacy. Notify physician if any side effects or signs of allergies occur. Liquid medication should be stored in the refrigerator.

 The effectiveness of oral contraceptives may be reduced in antibiotic therapy and the risk of this is greater with broad spectrum antibiotics.

Ampicillin with Clavulanate Potassium (Augmentin®)

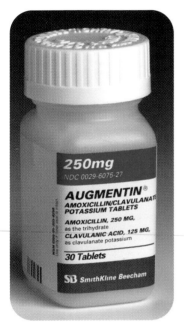

Augmentin®
(ampicillin with clavulanate potassium)
Courtesy of Smith, Kline, Beecham

Action and Indication

This semi-synthetic antibiotic inhibits bacterial cell wall synthesis. Clavulanate is a beta lactamase inhibitor and together, these agents provide gram positive coverage for organisms such as strep and most staph. Lower respiratory, urinary tract, sinus, and ear infections are often treated with this drug.

Dosage

Usual adult dosage is 250 mg every eight hours or 500 mg every 12 hours. This dosage may be increased in more severe cases. For children, the mg of the suspension and child's body weight in kilograms is essential to know. For example, if the suspension is 200-400 mg, 45 mg per kilo every 12 hours is recommended for a child over 3 months old. Some sources indicate the dosage may be less (40 mg per kilo) and given in 3 divided doses.

Route

PO tablets or liquid suspension.

Side Effects

Allergic reaction and GI upset such as diarrhea and vomiting. Also, possible elevated liver function studies.

Warnings

Should not be used in patients with a history of drug allergies (particularly to penicillins), liver or kidney dysfunction, or diabetes. May reduce the effeciveness of oral contraceptives.

Special Patient Teaching Considerations

The suspension is very sensitive to temperature and must be refrigerated. Notify a physician of the occurrence of diarrhea as it could indicate the start of serious bowel inflammation. This drug may be taken without regard to meals. Recognize that this agent contains a penicillin product and the patient's allergy history must be related to the physician.

ANTIBIOTICS

Cefuroxime Axetil (Ceftin®)

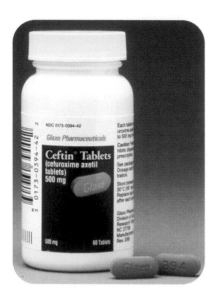

Ceftin®
(cefuroxime axetil)
Courtesy of Glaxo Wellcome Inc.

Action and Indication

This agent is a **second generation cephalosporin** which acts to inhibit bacterial cell wall synthesis. It is used to treat selected gram positive and gram negative microorganisms, including upper respiratory, urinary tract, and gonorrhea infections. Lyme disease may also be treated with this agent.

Dosage

Usual adult dosage is 125-500 mg 2 times a day for 10 days, depending on severity of the infection. Children's doses are calculated upon their weight and infection severity.

Route

PO tablets and suspension; IV. Note: IV dosage is 750-1500 mg every 8 hours.

Side Effects

Nausea/vomiting, diarrhea, and possible allergic response.

Warnings

There is a possibility of a secondary bacterial infection. Caution should be used in patients with a history of kidney dysfunction and/or penicillin allergy. Contraindicated for patients with previous cephalosporin allergy.

Special Patient Teaching Considerations

Notify the physician if the patient develops persistent diarrhea or allergy symptoms.

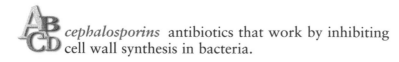

cephalosporins antibiotics that work by inhibiting cell wall synthesis in bacteria.

Cefprozil Monohydrate (Cefzil®)

Action and Indication

A **cephalosporin** antibiotic, this drug is indicated for cases of moderate to severe bacterial infections such as bronchitis, pneumonia, tonsillitis, and strep throat.

Dosage

Depending on site and severity of infection. For example, 250-500 mg 1-2 times a day for 10 days.

Route

PO, tablets and liquid.

Side Effects

GI upset such as nausea, abdominal pain, and diarrhea.

Warnings

Caution should be used in patients with a history of diuretic use and/or kidney dysfunction, diabetes, or colitis. Caution should be used in patients with a history of allergy to penicllins and it is contraindicated for patients with a known allergy to cephalosporins.

Special Patient Teaching Considerations

Oral contraceptives may not be as effective while taking this drug and glucose urine tests may be altered. For liquid suspensions, the bottle must be shaken before dispensing.

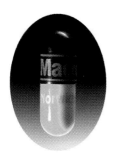

Macrobid®

Nitrofurantoin (Macrobid®) is an antibiotic used to treat acute cystitis caused by certain strains of Escherichia coli or Staphylococcus saprophyticus. It has a limited tissue distribution which results in lower rates of effectiveness but also lesser systemic toxicity than some other antibiotics.

Macrobid®
(nitrofurantoin)
Courtesy of Procter & Gamble

ANTIBIOTICS

Cefaclor (Ceclor®)

Action and Indication

This second generation **cephalosporin** inhibits synthesis in strep, most staph, E-coli, and Haemophilus influenzae infections.

Dosage

For adults: 250-500 mg PO every 8 hours. For children, 20 mg per 2.2 pounds (1kilogram) of body weight, per day and then divided into smaller doses and taken every eight hours.

Route

PO capsules or liquid suspension.

Side Effects

GI upset, especially diarrhea and allergic reactions including rash and itching.

Warnings

Caution should be used in patients with a history of GI disease or allergy to penicllins. This agent is contraindicated for patients with a known allergy to cephalosporins.

Special Patient Teaching Considerations

Although cefaclor works best on an empty stomach, it may cause GI upset, so check with your physician to determine the most appropriate dose time for you. Notify your physician of any known history of allergic response or signs of allergic response.

Cephalexin Hydrochloride (Keflex®)

Action and Indication

This **first generation cephalosporin** antibiotic works to inhibit bacterial cell wall synthesis of microorganisms such as E. Coli, proteus, staph, and selected strep.

Dosage

For adults: 250 – 500 mg every 6-12 hours, depending on infection severity. For children: 25-50 mg per kilogram of body weight, per day and given in divided doses.

Route

PO pulvules, liquid suspension.

Side Effects

GI upset such as nausea and diarrhea, possible allergic response.

Warnings

Caution should be used in patients with a history of diabetes, colitis, or allergy to penicllins. This agent may reduce the effeciveness of oral contraceptives. It is contraindicated for patients with a known allergy to cephalosporins.

Special Patient Teaching Considerations

Notify your physician of any developing allergic response and/or persistent diarrhea. Be aware of possible decrease in effectiveness of oral contraceptives while taking this medication.

ANTIBIOTICS

Levofloxacin (Levaquin®)

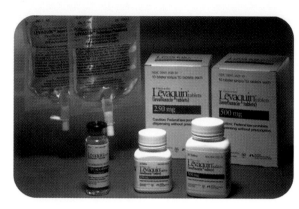

Levaquin®
(levofloxacin)
Courtesy of Ortho-McNeill
Pharmaceutical Company

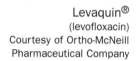

Action and Indication

A **quinolone** antibiotic that is often indicated in cases of pneumonia, bronchitis, sinus and urinary tract infections.

Dosage

250-500 mg once a day, dependent upon source and severity of infection. This medication is not recommended for use in children since it has been reported to cause potential developing bone and joint damage.

Route

PO tablets.

Side Effects

Headache, anxiety, dizziness, and GI effects such as abdominal pain, diarrhea, and gas.

Warnings

This drug may cause a serious allergic response. Patients should look for signs of rash, facial swelling, difficulty swallowing, difficulty breathing, and/or tachycardia. Nervous reactions from restlessness to convulsions have also been reported. Caution should be used in patients with a history of kidney dysfunction. Other drugs such as Ibuprofen and naproxen may increase nervous order reactions. Warfarin and theophylline may also cause a drug interaction.

Special Patient Teaching Considerations

Notify a physician immediately of any signs of adverse effects.

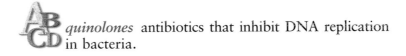

quinolones antibiotics that inhibit DNA replication in bacteria.

Ciprofloxacin (Cipro®)

Action and Indication

A synthetic broad spectrum **quinolone** antibiotic used to treat selected gram positive microorganisms such as staph and gram negative microorganisms such as pseudomonas that cause lower respiratory, urinary tract, and joint infections.

Dosage

Dependent on route chosen and infection severity. For example, 250-750 mg two times per day, PO; or 200-400 mg every 12 hours, IV. Note: this drug is not recommended for anyone under the age of 18.

Route

PO tablets; IV.

Side Effects

GI effects such as nausea, abdominal pain, and diarrhea; possible allergic response.

Warnings

Possible quinolone allergic reaction. Interaction with theophylline. A culture of the suspected microorganism should be done prior to selecting this agent. Ciprofloxacin may produce CNS effects such as confusion, tremor, or possibly seizure activity.

Special Patient Teaching Considerations

Can interact with zinc and calcium as found in antacids and multi-vitamins to reduce bioavailability. Avoid excessive sunlight, caffeine intake, theophylline, and operation of dangerous machinery.

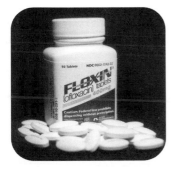

Floxin®

Oflaxacin (Floxin®) is another broad spectrum **quinolone** antibiotic for oral or intravenous administration. It is used to treat selected strains of microorganisms involved in lower respiratory, urinary tract, skin, prostate, and opthalmic infections.

Floxin®
(ofloxacin)
Courtesy of Ortho-McNeill
Pharmaceutical Company

ANTIBIOTICS

Azithromycin (Zithromax®)

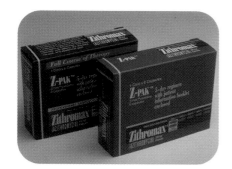

Zithromax®
(azithromycin)
Courtesy of Pfizer

Macrolide antibiotics are effective against a wide range of microorganisms and are primarily bacteriostatic.

Action and Indication

This **macrolide** antibiotic interferes with protein synthesis and is chemically related to erythromycin. It is indicated for infections of the upper and lower respiratory tract, skin, urinary tract, and selected sexually transmitted diseases. Zithromax offers good coverage of both gram positive and gram negative microorganisms.

Dosage

The suggested dosages are dependent upon the infecting organism and severity of infection. For example, in adults with certain respiratory conditions and skin infections, 500 mg on the first day followed by 250 mg each day for 3-5 days is recommended. In children with strep throat or ear infections, 10-12 mg per kilo of body weight once daily for 5 days is indicated.

Route

PO tablets, capsules or liquid suspension.

Side Effects

GI symptoms such as abdominal pain, diarrhea, nausea/vomiting.

Warnings

Use caution in patients with history of liver dysfunction or of drug allergy, especially regarding macrolide antibiotics. Agents containing aluminum or magnesium such as antacids could cause an unwanted drug interaction if taken concurrently with azithromycin.

Special Patient Teaching Considerations

Take this drug at least 1 hour before or two hours after eating. Complete the course of Zithromax, as directed. Report any allergy related symptom or persistent diarrhea to your physician.

Clarithromycin (Biaxin®)

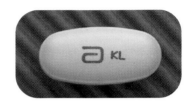

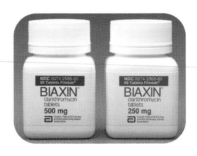

Biaxin® tablets
(clarithromycin)
Courtesy of Abbott Laboratories

Action and Indication

A **macrolide** antibiotic drug often prescribed in cases of respiratory infections such as sinusitis, bronchitis, and pneumonia. Tonsillitis and certain skin infections may also be treated with this agent.

Dosage

Dependent upon severity of condition. For example, 250-500 mg two times a day for 1-2 weeks.

Route

PO tablets.

Side Effects

GI such as diarrhea and nausea.

Warnings

This product is chemically similar to erythromycin and may result in reactions similar to that agent. For example, warfarin, digoxin, and triazolam may have drug interactions with clarithromycin. Use caution in patients with history of kidney dysfunction. Clarithromycin should not be taken by pregnant women. It is not recommended to take Propulsid while taking clarithromycin.

Special Patient Teaching Considerations

Notify your physician if you experienced a drug sensitivity to similar drugs such as azithromycin, troleandomycin, or erythromycin.

ANTIBIOTICS

Penicillin V Potassium (Veetids®, Beepen-VK®, various)

Action and Indication

This anti-infective antibiotic drug is used to treat infections such as middle ear, skin, upper and lower respiratory tract. The mechanism of this bactericidal agent is to inhibit bacterial wall synthesis.

Dosage

Dependent upon microorganism targeted, severity of the infection, and patient condition. For example, with mild to moderate strep infections, 125-250 mg every 6-8 hours for 10 days. For moderate to severe pneumococcal infections, 500 mg every 6 hours for 2 days until fever is gone.

Route

PO tablets and liquid suspension.

Side Effects

GI distress such as abdominal pain, nausea/vomiting, and diarrhea. Possible allergic reactions such as rash, itching or severe anaphyllactic reaction if the patient is sensitive to this form of drug.

Warnings

Possible allergic reaction. With females, oral contraceptives may be less effective while taking this agent. If possible, culture a specimen to conclusively determine infecting organism and appropriate drug choice.

Special Patient Teaching Considerations

Notify the physician of any penicillin or cephalosporin allergies. Patient should be alert to the possibility of a secondary infection and notify their doctor if this should occur. Complete the entire course of this drug, as directed.

Amoxicillin (Amoxil®, Trimox®)

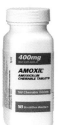
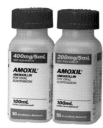

Amoxil®
(amoxicillin)
Courtesy of Smith, Kline, Beecham

Action and Indication

An antibiotic used to treat respiratory tract infections, urinary tract infections, skin infections, and venereal disease caused by specific organisms against which it is effective.

Dosage

For lower respiratory infections in adults: 500 mg three times a day, PO; and children: 40 mg/kg/day. All other in adults: 250 mg three times a day, PO; and children: 20 mg/kg/day.

Route

PO capsules, liquid.

Side Effects

GI upset, allergic response, including possible anaphylactic shock.

Warnings

Contraindicated for patients with history of hypersensitivity reactions to penicillins.

Special Patient Teaching Considerations

Be alert to signs of hypersensitivity reactions (e.g., skin rashes) and any signs of secondary infections resistant to amoxicillin. Discontinue use and notify physician immediately if hypersensitive reactions occur.

ANTIBIOTICS

Sulfisoxazole (Gantrisin®)

Gantrisin®
(sulfisoxazole)
Courtesy of Roche

Action and Indication

Used mostly to treat children in cases of acute, recurring, or chronic urinary tract infections. May also be used in cases of conjunctivitis, bacterial meningitis, and in combination with penicillin or erythromycin for treatment of ear infections.

Dosage

To start, one-half of the regular dose or 75 mg per 2.2 pounds of body weight (1 kilogram) over a 24 hour period and divided into 4-6 doses. This is followed by maintenance dosing with 150 mg/kg per 24 hrs. The dose should not exceed 6 grams over a 24 hour period.

Route

PO tablets and liquid suspension; ophthalmic solution.

Side Effects

GI upset, blood disorders, allergic reaction including cyanosis of skin and chills.

Warnings

Possible sulfa drug allergic reaction. Note: The combination sulfa agents Bactrim and Septra are widely used today, replacing Gantrisin as the drug of choice for the general population older than infancy. These drugs contain trimethoprim and are available in injection form for use in severe cases such as HIV.

Special Patient Teaching Considerations

Gantrisin is a **sulfa drug** and the physician should be notified if any side effects or allergic responses occur. Children should also have frequent complete blood counts if taking this drug for a prolonged period. Patients should maintain an adequate fluid intake to prevent crystalluria and stone formation. Gantrisin is not recommended for use in infants less than 2 months of age except in the treatment of congenital taxoplasmosis as adjunctive therapy with pyrimethamine.

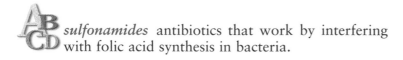

sulfonamides antibiotics that work by interfering with folic acid synthesis in bacteria.

Trimethoprim + Sulfamethoxazole (Bactrim®, Septra®)

Action and Indication

A **sulfa antibiotic** that blocks folic acid synthesis. It is used in the treatment of urinary tract infections, bronchitis and middle ear infections. Effective use of this agent is subject to culture and sensitivity reports.

Dosage

Dependent upon infection location, severity and patient age. For example, UTI treated outpatient, 1 double strength tablet, 2 times a day for 3 days. UTI treated in-patient, 5 mg/kg/day of trimethoprim and 25 mg/kg/day of sulfamethoxazole, given IV in 2-3 divided doses.

Route

PO tablets or oral suspension, IV.

Side Effects

GI effects such as nausea, vomiting, and possible pancreatitis. Allergic reactions such as skin rash, depression, and seizures are also possible.

Warnings

Use caution in patients with history of asthma, liver or kidney dysfunction, chronic alcoholism, malabsorption syndrome, or folic acid deficiency. This drug is contraindicated in cases of sulfa allergy, for pregnant patients at term or during the nursing period, and for infants less than two months of age. Complete blood counts (CBC) and creatinine levels should be monitored frequently. Culture and sensitivity tests should be performed prior to selecting this drug for treatment.

Special Patient Teaching Considerations

Notify the physician of any sign of allergic response and if pregnancy occurs during the course of this treatment. Also, severe intestinal inflammation may occur, and bouts of diarrhea should be reported. Avoid alcohol while taking this medication.

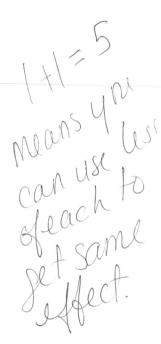

1+1 = 5
means you
can use less
of each to
get same
effect.

ANTIBIOTIC

Tetracycline Hydrochloride (Achromycin®)

Action and Indication

This is a broad spectrum bacteriostatic antibiotic used to treat mycoplasma, rickettsia, chlamydia, and borrelia burgdorferi microorganisms. Inhibiting bacterial protein synthesis, this agent is prescribed in cases of Lyme Disease, Rocky Mountain Spotted Fever, Typhus, upper respiratory, and urinary tract infections. It is often indicated for the treatment of facial acne.

Dosage

250-500 mg four times a day PO and 500-1000 mg every 12 hours. IV for more severe cases.

Route

PO liquid or capsules, IV

Side Effects

Blood disorder, headache, GI upset, allergic response

Warnings

Tetracycline is contraindicated in pregnant patients due to problems in fetal bone and tooth development (may discolor teeth). Also, children under the age of eight could experience similar symptoms. In addition, photosensitivity and kidney toxicity may also develop.

Special Patient Teaching Considerations

Do not take if pregnant. Take precautions regarding exposure to sunlight to avoid sunburn or skin irritations.

Metronidazole (Flagyl®)

Action and Indication

This antibacterial and antiprotozoal agent is often prescribed for vaginal, urinary tract, and amebic infections such as dysentery. Flagyl has an excellent abscess penetration ability.

Dosage

Dependent on the infecting organism and the severity of the infection. Could range from 250 mg-750 mg PO, three times a day. If the infectious process is serious, IV Flagyl could be given at 500 mg every 6-8 hours. One day treatment regimes have been ordered at 2 grams PO taken as a single or divided dose.

Route

PO tablets or IV.

Side Effects

GI upset, tiredness, weakness, and possible blood disorders.

Warnings

Patients receiving lithium may have their serum lithium levels raised if also taking this drug. Concurrent use of alcohol could cause an Antabuse-like reaction consisting of abdominal cramps, nausea/vomiting, headaches and flushing. Prolonged use of this drug (perhaps for treatment of Crohn's Disease) could lead to peripheral neuropathy.

Special Patient Teaching Considerations

If a female is being treated for vaginal trichomonas, any and all sexual partners need to receive identical therapy to prevent reinfection. Note: Most males are asymptomatic (do not show symptoms) for trichomonas. Alcohol should not be consumed while taking this medication as serious complications could arise. The patient should notify her physician if she becomes pregnant.

*Do not drink alcohol with this

ANTIVIRALS

Zidovudine (AZT®, Retrovir®, ZDV®)

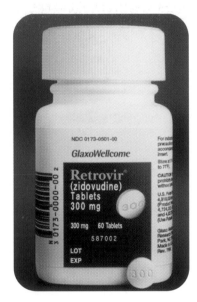

Retrovir®
(ziduvodine)
Courtesy of Glaxo Wellcome Inc.

Action and Indication

This agent is used to treat HIV by inhibiting protease and preventing the replication of the virus in the host's RNA and DNA.

Dosage

200 mg three times a day for prophylaxis and treatment of active disease. Post exposure to disease, prophylaxis should begin as soon as possible and continue for 4 weeks. For children 3 months to 12 years of age, 2 mg/per kilogram of body weight every 6 hours for 6 weeks beginning as soon as possible after exposure. The actual dosage is determined according to patient size and illness severity.

Route

PO capsules or syrup.

Side Effects

The side effects may be worse in patients whose illness and symptoms of the illness are greater. Change in taste, GI upset, difficult breathing, insomnia, and malaise may occur.

Warnings

Blood diseases, including severe anemia, may develop. Long-term effects of this drug are not yet known. Liver function studies should be conducted while using this agent.

Special Patient Teaching Considerations

Notify the physician of any changes in general health and condition. Frequent blood counts or blood transfusions may be necessary. Note: taking this drug does not reduce the risk of transmission of HIV.

Acyclovir (Zovirax®)

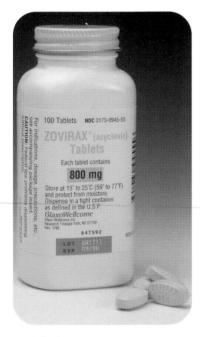

Zovirax®
(acyclovir)
Courtesy of Glaxo Wellcome Inc.

Action and Indication

This antiviral drug is used to treat varicella-zoster (chickenpox), herpes zoster (shingles), and herpes simplex 1 and 2. The goals of this therapy are to shorten the clinical course of the infection and prevent recurrences by inhibiting DNA synthesis and replication of the virus.

Dosage

Dosage depends on the disease and severity of the disease being treated. For example, genital herpes may require 200-400 mg PO four to five times daily while varicella-zoster may require 800 mg PO every 4-6 hours.

Route

PO capsules, tablets, or liquid; topical ointment; and IV for severe genital herpes or herpes simplex encephalitis.

Side Effects

If taken PO, GI upset, including nausea and vomiting, may occur. IV administration may cause rash or phlebitis.

Warnings

Good hydration is important to avoid renal complications while taking this drug.

Special Patient Teaching Considerations

This medication can be taken without regard for meals. Maintain good hydration. Report any side effects to the physician.

ANTIFUNGALS

Nystatin (Mycostatin® Cream or Ointment, Mycolog-II®)

Action and Indication

This agent acts as both a **fungicidal** and **fungistatic** agent. It is often prescribed in the treatment of candidasis or yeast-like fungal infection. In cases of oral candidasis, a Nystatin suspension may be ordered to "swish and swallow". Note: Mycolog II® is a combination product containing the topical steroid triamcinolone.

Dosage

Topical: Apply to skin twice a day. Oral suspension may range from 0.5 million units four times a day to 1.5 million units six times a day.

Route

Topical or oral suspension for "swish and swallow."

Side Effects

Local skin irritations, inflammation around the mouth and rare excessive growth of hair on face.

Warnings

This drug is occasionally though rarely capable of producing steroid-like reactions.

Special Patient Teaching Considerations

Store this product away from heat and light.

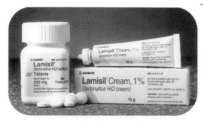

Lamisil®
(terbinafine hydrochloride)
Courtesy of Novartis
Pharmaceutical Corporation

Lamisil® (terbinafine hydrochloride)

Terbinafine hydrochloride tablets are indicated for the treatment of onychomycosis, a fungal infection of the toenails or fingernails.

6 weeks for an effective response

Fluconazole (Diflucan®)

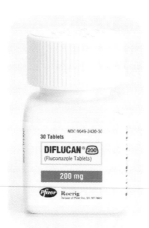

Diflucan®
(fluconazole)
Courtesy of Pfizer

Action and Indication

An antifungal used to treat candidiasis and crytoccocal meningitis.

Dosage

Varies according to the location and severity of the infection. For example: 150 mg in a single dose for vaginal infections and 400 mg first day, followed by 200 mg once a day until spinal fluid is negative, when treating meningitis.

Route

PO tablets, liquid suspension or IV.

Side Effects

Abdominal pain, nausea, headache, and dizziness

Warnings

Caution should be used in patients with a history of liver dysfunction. Allergic reaction possible.

Special Patient Teaching Considerations

The patient should notify her physician if she becomes pregnant. This medication may be taken with or without meals. Report side effects or signs of allergic response to the physician.

DRUG CHART

GENERIC NAME	TRADE NAME	ROUTE	GENERIC NAME	TRADE NAME	ROUTE
ANTIBIOTICS			Ceftriaxone	Rocephin	Inj.
AMINOGLYCOSIDES			Cefepime	Maxipime	Inj.
Amikacin	Amikin	Inj.	**GLYCOPEPTIDES**		
	Various	Inj.	Vancomycin	Vancocin	PO, Inj.
Gentamicin	Garamycin	Inj., Eye, Top.		Various	Inj.
	Various	Inj., Eye, Top.	**MACROLIDES**		
Neomycin	Mycifradin	PO, Eye, Top.	Azithromycin	Zithromax	PO
	Various	PO, Eye, Top	Clarithromycin	Biaxin	PO
Spectinomycin	Trobicin	Inj.	Dirithromycin	Dynabac	PO
Streptomycin	Streptomycin	Inj.	Erythromycin	Emycin	PO
Tobramycin	Nebcin	Injectable		E.E.S.	PO
	Tobrex	Eye		Eryc	PO
	Various	Injectable		Various	PO, Inj., Eye, Top.
ANTIMYCOBACTERIALS			Erythromycin / Sulfisoxazole	Pediazole	PO
Clofazimine	Lamprene	PO		Eryzole	PO
Cycloserine	Seromycin	PO	**MONOBACTAMS**		
Ethambutol	Myambutol	PO	Aztreonam	Azactam	Inj.
Isoniazid	INH	PO, Inj.	**PENICILLINS**		
	Various	PO	Penicillin G	Bicillin	Inj.
Pyrazinamide	PZA	PO		Wycillin	Inj.
Rifabutin	Mycobutin	PO		Various	Inj.
Rifampin	Rifadin	PO, Inj.	Penicillin V	Pen Vee K	PO
	Various	PO, Inj.		V Cillin K	PO
Rifapentine	Priftin	PO		Various	PO
CABEPENEMS			Amoxicillin	Amoxil	PO
Imipenem / Cilastatin	Primaxin	Inj.		Trimox	PO
Meropenem	Merrem	Inj.		Various	PO
CEPHALOSPORINS			Ampicillin	Omnipen	PO, Inj.
Cefadroxil	Duricef	PO		Polycillin	PO, Inj.
	Ultracef	PO		Various	PO, Inj.
Cefazolin	Ancef	Inj.	Amoxicillin / Clavulanic Acid	Augmentin	PO
	Kefzol	Inj.	Ampicillin / Sulbactam	Unasyn	Inj.
Cephalexin	Keflex	PO	Carbenicillin	Geocillin	PO
	Various	PO	Mezlocillin	Mezlin	Inj.
Cephradine	Velosef	PO	Piperacillin	Pipracil	Inj.
	Anspor	PO	Piperacillin / Tazobactam	Zosyn	Inj.
Cefaclor	Ceclor	PO	Ticarcillin	Ticar	Inj.
	Various	PO	Ticarcillin / Clavulanic Acid	Timentin	Inj.
Cefdinir	Omnicef	PO	Dicloxacillin	Dynapen	PO
Cefotetan	Cefotan	Inj.		Various	PO
Cefoxitin	Mefoxin	Inj.	Nafcillin	Unipen	Inj.
Cefprozil	Cefzil	PO	Oxacillin	Prostaphlin	PO, Inj.
Cefuroxime	Ceftin	PO		Various	PO, Inj.
	Zinacef	PO	**QUINOLONES**		
	Kefurox	PO	Ciprofloxacin	Cipro	PO, Eye
Cefixime	Suprax	PO	Levofloxacin	Levaquin	PO
Cefoperazone	Cefobid	Inj.	Lomefloxacin	Maxaquin	PO
Cefotaxime	Claforan	Inj.	Norfloxacin	Noroxin	PO
Cefpodoxime	Vantin	PO		Chibroxin	Eye
Ceftazidime	Fortaz	Inj.	Ofloxacin	Floxin	PO, Inj., Ear
	Various	Inj.		Ocuflox	Eye
Ceftibuten	Cedax	PO	Sparfloxacin	Zagam	PO
Ceftizoxime	Cefizox	Inj.	Trovafloxacin	Trovan	PO

GENERIC NAME	TRADE NAME	ROUTE
TETRACYCLINES		
Demeclocycline	Declomycin	PO
Doxycycline	Vibramycin	PO, Inj.
	Various	PO, Inj.
Minocycline	Minocin	PO
	Various	PO
Tetracycline	Sumycin	PO
	Various	PO, Inj., Eye
URINARY ANTI-INFECTIVES		
Fosfomycin	Monurol	PO
Methanimine	Hiprex	PO
	Various	PO
Nitrofurantoin	Macrobid	PO
	Various	PO
Trimethoprim	Trimpex	PO
	Various	PO
ANTIVIRALS		
Acyclovir	Zovirax	PO, Inj.
Amantadine	Symmetrel	PO
	Various	PO
Cidofovir	Forvade	Inj.
Famciclovir	Famvir	PO
Fomivirsen	Vitravene	Inj.
Foscarnet	Foscavir	Inj.
Ganciclovir	Cytovene	PO, Inj., Eye implant
Penciclovir	Denavir	Top.
Ribavirin	Virazole	Inj.
Rimantadine	Flumadine	PO
Valacyclovir	Valtrex	PO
Vidarabine	Vira-A	Eye
ANTIRETROVIRALS		
PROTEASE INHIBITORS		
Amprenavir	Agenerase	PO
Indinavir	Crixivan	PO
Nelfinavir	Viracept	PO
Ritonavir	Norvir	PO
Saquinavir	Invirase	PO
	Fortovase	PO
REVERSE TRANSCRIPTASE INHIBITORS		
Abacavir	Ziagen	PO
Delavirdine	Rescriptor	PO
Didanosine, DDI	Videx	PO
Efavirenz	Sustiva	PO
Lamivudine, 3TC	Epivir	PO
Lamivudine/Zidovudine	Combivir	PO
Nevirapine	Viramune	PO
Stavudine, d4T	Zerit	PO
Zalcitabine	Hivid	PO
Zidovudine, ZDV	Retrovir	PO, Inj.

GENERIC NAME	TRADE NAME	ROUTE
ANTIFUNGALS		
Flucytosine	Ancobon	PO
Griseofulvin	Fulvicin PG	PO
	Various	PO
Terbinafine	Lamisil	PO, Top.
Clotrimazole	Lotrimin	Top., Vag.
	Mycelex	PO, Top., Vag.
	Various	Top., Vag.
Fluconazole	Diflucan	PO
Itraconazole	Sporanox	PO
Ketoconazole	Nizoral	PO, Top.
Miconazole	Monistat	Top., Vag.
Terconazole	Terazol	Vag.
Tioconazole	Vagistat	Vag.
Amphotericin B	Fungizone	PO, Inj., Top.
	Various	PO, Inj., Top.
Nystatin	Mycostatin	PO, Top.
	Various	PO, Top.
OTHER ANTI-INFECTIVES		
Bacitracin	Bacitracin	PO, Inj., Top.
Chloramphenicol	Chloromycetin	PO
Clindamycin	Cleocin	PO, Inj., Top.
Loracarbef	Lorabid	PO
Metronidazole	Flagyl	PO, Inj., Top.
	Various	PO, Inj., Top.
Polymyxin B	Aerosporin	Top., Eye
Neomycin / Polymyxin B/ Bacitracin	Neosporin	Top.
	Various	Top.
Polymyxin B / Bacitracin	Polysporin	Top.
	Various	Top.
ANTIMALARIALS		
Chloroquine	Aralen	PO, Inj.
Hydroxychloroquine	Plaquenil	PO
Primaquine	Primaquine	PO
Pyrimethamine	Daraprim	PO
Quinine	Quinine	PO
ANTIPROTOZOALS		
Atovaquone	Mepron	PO
Dapsone	Dapsone	PO
Pentamidine	Pentam	Inj.
	Various	Inj.
Trimetrexate	Neutrexin	Inj.

REVIEW

KEY CONCEPTS

✔ Anti-infectives treat disease produced by microorganisms such as bacteria, viruses, fungi, protozoa and parasitic worms.

✔ The terms antibiotic or antimicrobial refer to chemicals of bacterial microorganisms which suppress the growth of other microorganisms.

✔ Antimicrobials can be either bacteriostatic (inhibiting bacterial growth) or bactericidal (bacteria killing).

✔ Antimicrobials act by modifying protein synthesis, energy metabolism, DNA metabolism, or by damaging the bacteria's cell wall.

✔ Antivirals inhibit the replication of viruses (virustatic).

✔ Mutations and resistance are common setbacks with antiviral therapy.

✔ Antimicrobials are not effective with viral infections, but may be used in cases of accompanying secondary bacterial infection.

✔ Fungi are plant-like microorganisms commonly found in molds and yeast.

✔ Antifungals used to treat these mycosis or mycotic infections are usually fungicidal. The fungal cell is destroyed as the drug prevents cell permeability and nutrition.

✔ Gram stain identification (positive/negative) is a laboratory method for identifying microorganisms based on staining characteristics.

✔ The effectiveness of oral contraceptives may be reduced in antibiotic therapy and the risk of this is greater with broad spectrum antibiotics.

✔ Many patients have allergies to entire classes of antibiotics (e.g., penicillins, cephalosporins, etc.) and other antibiotics of the same class should generally not be used with those patients.

✔ Macrolide antibiotics are effective against a wide range of microorganisms and are primarily bacteriostatic.

✔ Antimycobacterials are agents that treat tuberculosis, leprosy and the MAC complex in AIDS.

✔ Antiprotozoals are agents that treat malaria, vaginitis and sleeping sickness.

✔ Antihelminthics are agents that treat parasitic worms in the GI tract.

SELF TEST

MATCH THE GENERIC AND TRADE NAMES.   *answers are in the back of the book*

1. Acyclovir   _____   Amoxil

2. Amoxicillin   _____   Augmentin

3. Amoxicillin/Clavulanic Acid   _____   Biaxin

4. Cefprozil   _____   Ceftin

5. Cefuroxime   _____   Cefzil

6. Cephalexin   _____   Garamycin

7. Clarithromycin   _____   Keflex

8. Doxycycline   _____   Levaquin

9. Gentamicin   _____   Macrobid

10. Levofloxacin   _____   Retrovir

11. Nitrofurantoin   _____   Vibramycin

12. Zidovudine   _____   Zovirax

CHOOSE THE BEST ANSWER.   *answers are in the back of the book*

1. Of the following anti-infective agents, which one would be used to treat Tuberculosis or Leprosy?
   a. antibiotics
   b. antimycobacterials
   c. antiprotozoals
   d. antihelminthics

2. Which of the following is an antifungal agent?
   a. acyclovir
   b. fluconazole
   c. cefaclor
   d. metronidazole

3. Which of the following is an antiviral agent?
   a. acyclovir
   b. fluconazole
   c. cefaclor
   d. metronidazole

4. An individual who is allergic to penicillin may have a "cross-sensitivity" or allergic reaction to which of the following drugs?
   a. acylcovir
   b. fluconazole
   c. cefaclor
   d. metronidazole

ANTINEOPLASTICS

Antineoplastics inhibit the new growth of cancer cells or *neoplasms*.

Typically, cancer cells are abnormal in structure and growth rate. They offer no useful function, have unusual genetic content, and often reproduce quickly and uncontrollably. Antineoplastics present a **chemotherapeutic** approach to the treatment of cancer and together with surgery, radiation and perhaps alternative medicine, comprise an often hopeful and successful treatment protocol.

The term *malignancy* is used to denote the presence of a life-threatening cancerous group of cells or tumor.

If this original (primary) cell group spreads to other areas, often via the lymphatic or circulatory systems, it is said to have **metastasized**. Treatment to **remission** (state of cancer inactivity) or cure is more successful if little or no metastasis has occurred. However, current chemotherapeutic research and development is offering encouragement for cancers in later stages of growth.

The side effects caused by many of these drugs are often uncomfortable and serious.

They include immunosuppression (compromising one's immune system), anemia (decreased count of red blood cells), alopecia (hair loss), GI ulceration, and dehydration/weight loss caused by nausea and vomiting.

normal cell mitosis

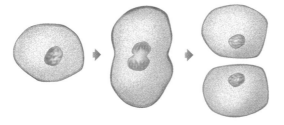

lymphocyte a type of white blood cell that releases antibodies that destroy disease cells.

metastasis when cancer cells spread beyond their original site.

neoplasm a new and abnormal tissue growth, often referring to cancer cells.

remission a state in which cancer cells are inactive.

The Lymphatic System

The lymphatic system is the center of the body's **immune system**. It collects plasma water from the blood vessels, filters it for impurities through the **lymph nodes**, and returns the **lymph** fluid back to the general circulation. Carried in the lymph are **lymphocytes**, a type of white blood cell that releases **antibodies** that attack and destroy **antigens** like bacteria and disease cells (including cancer). This is the body's **immune response** to antigens. **T-cells** and **B-cells** are the primary lymphocytes. Maintenance of the body's lymphocyte supply is largely performed by the bone marrow.

Antineoplastic drugs are targeted at cells with fast growth rates, which not only includes cancer cells but bone marrow as well. As a result, a serious side effect of antineoplastics is that they depress the immune system (**immunosuppression)**, leaving chemotherapy patients prone to infections.

Controlling Cell Growth

Normal cell growth (shown at left) is highly structured and steady, but cancer cells often reproduce quickly and uncontrollably. Antineoplastic drugs act on various stages of the cell replication process to stop the growth of cancerous cells.

Since cancer cells can mutate in many ways, different chemicals are used to stop their growth. This results in the "cocktail" approach to chemotherapy, in which a number of drugs are administered to a patient. Of course, these cocktails also affect normal cells, so they are administered in cycles that allow patients to recover from their adverse effects before the next round of administration.

Antimetabolites

Classified in accordance with the substances they interfere with, these antineoplastic drugs inhibit cell growth and replication by mimicking natural metabolites and taking their place within the cells. These fake metabolites inhibit the synthesis of important cellular enzymes, including DNA.

Alkyating Agents

These drugs interfere with mitosis or cell division by binding with DNA and preventing cellular replication. The early alkylating drugs were developed in World War I to introduce chemical warfare. Known as nitrogen mustard gases, these chemicals possessed properties which inhibited cellular growth and sperm counts while depressing bone marrow and damaging intestinal mucosa. Although these agents will adversely affect all cells, those that are growing at a more rapid rate (presumably cancerous) will be more affected. Nitrosureas, a more recent type of alkyating agent, are lipid soluble and pass easily into the brain where they are effective in treating brain cancers.

The rosy periwinkle of Madagascar is the source of the antineoplastic vincristine.

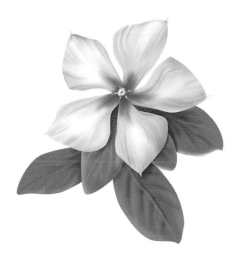

Due to the toxicity of many antineoplastics, normal healthy cells are destroyed along with the cancerous cells.

Rapidly replicating cells such as those of the GI tract, bone marrow, and hair follicles are most often affected by selected antineoplastics, causing nausea/vomiting, bone marrow suppression, and hair loss.

Current widely used antineoplastic drugs include *alkylating agents* (nitrogen mustards), *antimetabolites,* and *plant alkaloids.*

They are usually given in cycles (e.g., 3-4 weeks between treatments), allowing rest and recovery periods for the patient. In theory, during the healthy cells recovery, neoplastic cells are entering a rapid division phase and are destroyed in greater numbers when chemotherapy is again begun. Drug resistance to a particular antineoplastic agent may occur, however, so a combination of these drugs may be given at one time to assure effectiveness. This "cocktail," as it is sometimes called, offers drugs of different actions and structure to address whatever type of cancerous cell group is suspected to be present.

Hormones, antibiotics, and radioactive isotopes are also classified as antineoplastic agents, generally for specific site treatment.

For example, if a tumor is found to be hormone dependent, surgical removal of the affected organ is often indicated (e.g., prostate, breast, or uterus), thus eliminating the chance for hormonal support. In addition, the synthetic antiestrogen agent, tamoxifen, is often used for the treatment of breast cancer in post-menopausal women. Certain antibiotics such as bleomycin and doxorubicin will be ordered to treat skin cancers, lymphomas, and leukemias. The radioactive isotopes, such as gold (AU198) and iodine (I131), are also generally organ specific, but are radioactive and special caution is needed during their use.

Plant Alkaloids

Derived from natural products or semisynthetically produced using natural products, some of these drugs inhibit the enzyme topoisomerase.

Topoisomerase is required for molecular cell growth or mitosis and therefore certain plant alkaloids interfere with cellular DNA replication. Other mechanisms of growth inhibition are not clearly understood.

ALKYLATING AGENTS

Cyclophosphamide (Cytoxan®)

Action and Indication

Interferes with the cell's (DNA) ability to replicate. This drug may be used alone or in combination with other drugs and can be prescribed for breast cancer, leukemias, ovarian cancer, Hodgkin's Lymphoma, and others.

Dosage

PO dose may range from 1-5 mg per 2.2 pounds (1kilo) of body weight per day. The actual dose is dependent upon the tumor.

Route

PO or IV (usually in combination when given IV).

Side Effects

Immunosuppression, development of a secondary cancer (up to several years after the drug is given), hemorrhagic cystitis, hair loss, anorexia, and nausea/vomiting.

Warnings

Patients should drink large amounts of water to reduce chance of cystitis and other urinary complications, such as urolithiasis (renal stones). Dosing needs to be adjusted in cases of liver and kidney failure as well as white cell count fluctuations.

Special Patient Teaching Considerations

Drink large amounts of water. Keep appointments for blood work. Take this drug on an empty stomach unless GI upset occurs. Store liquid cyclophosphamide in the refrigerator.

Cisplatin (Cis-P®, Platinol®)

Action and Indication

This agent may be used for multiple malignancies, especially those found in the ovary and the lung. Cisplatin is included in many published studies and recommended regimes for these cancers. As long as the patient demonstrates progress, this therapy should continue.

Dosage

Often dosed in combination with other antineoplastics. For example: 40 mg-100 mg/m^2, IV, day 1 and/or day 29, repeating every 4-6 weeks. The actual selected dosage is tumor dependent.

Route

IV.

Side Effects

Kidney toxicity, neuropathy, hearing complications, electrolyte depletion due in part to severe nausea/vomiting.

Warnings

IV hydration may be necessary to avoid renal toxicity. Frequent electrolyte blood levels, hearing tests and kidney function blood tests should be conducted. Contraindicated for pregnant women.

Special Patient Teaching Considerations

Drink fluids often. Follow through with the recommended blood tests. The patient should notify her physician if she becomes pregnant as fetal harm could occur.

Body Surface Area

Chemotherapy dosages are generally based on body surface area (BSA), which is always given in meters squared (m^2). See the discussion on BSA in Chapter 6.

Blood Counts

Blood counts are monitored for a variety of conditions and treatments. Since antineoplastics have a direct effect on all cells, monitoring blood counts for various factors (red blood cells, white blood cells, platelets, or other indices) is important.

ALKYLATING AGENTS

Busulfan (Myleran®)

Action and Indication

Used to treat progressive bone marrow and spinal cord related cancers, but non-specific for phase of cell division.

Dosage

To begin, 4-8 mg daily, followed by a maintenance dose of 1-3 mg daily.

Route

PO.

Side Effects

Skin pigmentation, suppression of bone marrow and spinal cord cell components (myelosuppression), and possible lung complications. Prolonged use could lead to ovarian or testiscular depression.

Warnings

Adrenal studies need to be conducted while patient is taking this drug due to possibility of developing adrenal insufficiency. Frequent complete blood counts (CBCs) should be performed and WBC and platelet changes monitored.

Special Patient Teaching Considerations

Lung complications (fibrosis) could occur long after treatment has ended. Report any unusual respiratory symptoms to the physician. Keep appointments for blood level monitoring.

Methotrexate (Rheumatrex®)

Action and Indication

Interferes with cell replication by inhibiting an essential enzyme. This agent may be used to treat lymphomas, certain leukemias, and some forms of breast, uterine, and lung cancer. May also be used in severe cases of rheumatoid arthritis.

Dosage

Individual and tumor dependent. An example could be 20-25 mg IV per week or 40 mg/m^2 IV on days 1 and/or 8. Smaller oral doses are used for non-neoplastic disease.

Route

PO, IV, or intrathecally (spinal cord).

Side Effects

Bone marrow depression, nausea/vomiting, and other GI upset, liver toxicity and dizziness.

Warnings

The patient should be monitored for symptoms of respiratory distress, confusion, and decrease in fertility.

Special Patient Teaching Considerations

Take this medication only as prescribed. Report any symptoms of tingling or numbness in hands and feet, seizure, dry cough, fever or difficulty breathing (dyspnea) to the physician.

ANTIMETABOLITES

5-Fluorouracil (5-FU®, 5% Efudex® Cream)

Action and Indication

The most active and common antineoplastic agent used for the treatment of colorectal cancer. It inhibits the cell replication process by impairing protein synthesis of RNA. May be used in combination with other antineoplastics such as levamisole, leucovorin, and interferon.

Dosage

The dosage is tumor and severity dependent. It is often given bolus (at once) via IV, but has proven to be very effective clinically when given in a continuous infusion over the period of perhaps 5 days. An example may be 450 mg/m^2, bolus daily for five days, followed by the same amount given weekly for 1 year. This regime would typically allow for a 3-4 week rest period.

Route

IV (bolus or continuous infusion), 2%, 5% topical agent.

Side Effects

GI upset (including inflammation), WBC deficiency, and dermatitis.

Warnings

Patients who already are immunocompromised with poor nutritional status should not receive this drug. Continous infusion has been found to be less disruptive to the blood forming organs than bolus treatment.

Special Patient Treatment Considerations

Notify the physician in the event of severe nausea/ vomiting or GI related bleeding. Keep appointments for regular blood count checks. Avoid prolonged sun exposure and wear sunglasses if eyes are sensitive to sunlight.

Mercaptopurine (6-MP®, Purinethol®)

Action and Indication

Inhibits RNA synthesis and cell replication. May be indicated as maintenance in cases of acute leukemia. Often used in combination with methotrexate. The goal of maintenance therapy is to prolong remission by assuring inability of cancer cell growth. This drug is also indicated in cases of ulcerative colitis.

Dosage

Dependent on severity of condition. For example, 60 mg/m^2 for 28 days monthly.

Route

PO scored tablets.

Side Effects

Myelosuppression and liver toxicity

Warnings

Drug interactions are possible with Bactrim, Septra, and allopurinol. The dosage should be reduced if given with allopurinol or patient has a compromised liver and/or kidney condition.

Special Patient Teaching Considerations

Report symptoms of side effects to the physician. Keep blood count appointments.

PLANT ALKALOIDS

Vincristine (Oncovin®)

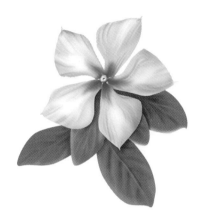

the rosy periwinkle

Action and Indication

A derivative of the periwinkle plant, this natural antineoplastic agent inhibits cell mitosis and tumor growth. Vincristine is often indicated in cases of leukemias and solid tumors.

Dosage

Site and severity dependent. For example, when used in combination with other antineoplastics, doses may range from 1.5 mg/m^2 IV days 1 and 7 and repeat every 3 weeks for lung cancer, to 1 mg IV per week for breast cancer.

Route

IV.

Side effects

Shortness of breath, renal toxicity, immunosuppression, and possible tissue irritation/necrosis due to IV infiltration.

Warnings

Patient should be monitored for signs of neuromuscular effects, bone marrow depression, and severe constipation. Caution is needed when administrating this drug via IV. Avoid skin contact and infiltration.

Special Patient Teaching Considerations

Notify the physician in the event of severe side effect symptoms. Keep appointments for blood level testing. If constipated, contact the physician before taking a laxative. Drink several glasses of water daily.

Paclitaxel (Taxol®)

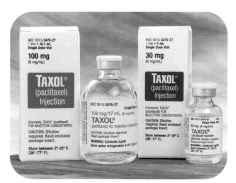

Taxol®
(paclitaxel)
Courtesy of Bristol, Myers, Squibb

Action and Indication

Derivative of the yew tree, this plant alkaloid interferes with mitosis by stabilizing essential elements (cellular proteins -Tubulin) which are needed to promote cellular replication. Cellular reorganization and growth process is thus inhibited. Indications include: head (brain), neck, lung, and malignant melanoma cancers. This agent is extremely toxic and usually used as a second line if more conventional protocols fail.

Dosage

Dependent on severity of condition. For example: 135-175 mg/m^2, over 3 hours, every 3 weeks.

Route

IV.

Side Effects

Allergic reaction, nausea/vomiting, hypotension.

Warnings

This drug needs to be preceded by an antihistamine, steroid or Benadryl to prophylactically treat any hypersensitivity reactions that may occur. Vital sign monitoring, particularly blood pressure, needs to be done frequently during administration.

Special Patient Teaching Considerations

Notify the physician in the event of any allergic reaction.

PLANT ALKALOIDS

Etoposide (VePesid®, VP-16®)

Action and Indication

A semisynthetic derivative of the mayapple plant, this antineoplastic agent inhibits the cellular agent topoisomerase and prevents cellular replication.

Dosage

Will vary in accordance with the cancer site, severity and patient condition. An example may be 35-100mg/m^2/day for 5 consecutive days.

Route

PO capsules or IV.

Side effects

Allergic response, blood forming organ depression, nausea, vomiting.

Warnings

Administer slowly to avoid hypotension. Complete blood counts should be performed.

Special Patient Teaching Considerations

Notify the physician in the event of any allergic reaction. Keep appointments for blood tests.

Tamoxifen Citrate (Nolvadex®)

Action and Indication

An anticancer agent with antiestrogen properties. Tamoxifen is often used in cases of breast cancer due to its ability to bind estrogen receptors and compete with estradiol for estrogen receptor protein.

Dosage

10-20 mg two times a day.

Route

PO tablets.

Side Effects

Menstrual dysfunction, vision changes, hot flashes, and GI effects such as nausea/vomiting.

Warnings

Blood results should be monitored for prothrombin levels of patients taking warfarin and those with a decrease in WBC's and platelets. CBC's and calcium levels should be assessed on a regular basis. At the start of this therapy, bone and/or tumor pain may actually increase, indicating the drug is being effective.

Special Patient Teaching Considerations

Do not take this medication if you are or become pregnant. Notify the physician in the event of abnormal vaginal bleeding and cramping or vision difficulties.

DRUG CHART

Generic Name	Trade Name	Route	Generic Name	Trade Name	Route
Alkylating Agents			**Interleukens**		
Altretamine	Hexalen	PO	Aldesleukin, IL-2	Proleukin	Inj.
Busulfan	Myleran	PO			
Dacarbazine	DTIC-Dome	Inj.	**Monoclonal Antibodies**		
Procarbazine	Matulane	PO	Rituxamab	Rituxan	Inj.
Thiotepa	Thioplex	Inj.	Trastuzumab	Herceptin	Inj.
Chlorambucil	Leukeran	PO			
Cyclophosphamide	Cytoxan	PO, Inj.	**Natural Antineoplastics**		
	Various	Inj.	Asparaginase	Elspar	Inj.
Ifosfamide	Ifex	Inj.		Oncaspar	Inj.
Mechlorethamine	Mustargen	Inj.	Daunorubicin	Cerubidine	Inj.
Melphalan	Alkeran	PO	Doxorubicin	Adriamycin	Inj.
Carmustine, BCNU	BiCNU	Inj.		Various	Inj.
	Gliadel	Implant	Idarubicin	Idamycin	Inj.
Lomustine, CCNU	CeeNU	PO	Valrubicin	Valstar	Intravesicle
Streptozocin	Zanosar	Inj.	Bleomycin	Blenoxane	Inj.
Carboplatin	Paraplatin	Inj.	Dactinomycin	Cosmegen	Inj.
Cisplatin	Platinol	Inj.	Mitomycin	Mutamycin	Inj.
			Plicamycin	Mithracin	Inj.
Anthracendiones			Irinotecan	Camptosar	Inj.
Mitoxantrone	Novantrone	Inj.	Topotecan	Hycamtin	Inj.
			Etoposide, VP-16	VePesid	Inj.
Antimetabolites				Various	Inj.
Hydroxyurea	Hydrea	PO	Teniposide	Vumon	Inj.
	Droxia	PO	Docetaxel	Taxotere	Inj.
Methotrexate, MTX	Methotrexate	PO, Inj.	Paclitaxel	Taxol	Inj.
	Various	PO, Inj.		Paxene	Inj.
Cladribine	Leustatin	Inj.	Vinblastine	Velban	Inj.
Fludarabine	Fludara	Inj.		Various	Inj.
Mercaptopurine, 6-MP	Purinethol	PO	Vincristine	Oncovin	Inj.
Pentostatin	Nipent	Inj.	Vinorelbine	Navelbine	Inj.
Thioguanine, 6-TG	Thioguanine	PO			
Capecitabine	Xeloda	PO	**Hormones**		
Cytarabine, ARA-C	Cytosar-U	Inj.	**Anti-Estrogens**		
	DepoCyt	Inj.	Raloxifene	Evista	PO
Floxuridine	FUDR	Inj.	Tamoxifen	Nolvadex	PO
Fluorouracil, 5-FU	Adrucil	Inj.	Toremifene	Fareston	PO
	Efudex	Topical	**Anti-Androgens**		
	Various	Inj., Topical	Bicalutamide	Casodex	PO
Gemcitabine	Gemzar	Inj.	Flutamide	Eulexin	PO
			Nilutamide	Nilandron	PO

KEY CONCEPTS

✔ Cancer cells (neoplasms) are abnormal in structure and growth rate. The term malignancy is used to denote the presence of a life-threatening cancerous group of cells or tumor.

✔ If the original cancer cell group spreads to other areas it is said to have metastasized. Treatment to remission or cure is more successful if little or no metastasis has occurred.

✔ The side effects caused by many antineoplastics include immunosuppression (compromising one's immune system), anemia (decreased count of red blood cells), alopecia (hair loss), GI ulceration, and dehydration/weight loss caused by nausea and vomiting.

✔ Lymphocytes are a type of white blood cell that releases antibodies that attack and destroy antigens like bacteria and disease cells (including cancer). T-cells and B-Cells are the primary lymphocytes. Maintenance of the body's lymphocyte supply is largely performed by the bone marrow.

✔ Antineoplastic drugs are targeted at cells with fast growth rates, which includes cancer cells and bone marrow, with the result that they also tend to depress the immune system.

✔ Current widely used antineoplastic drugs include alkylating agents (nitrogen mustards), antimetabolites, and plant alkaloids. Hormones, antibiotics, and radioactive isotopes are also classified as antineoplastic agents, generally for specific site treatment.

✔ Antimetabolites inhibit the synthesis of DNA (and thertefore cell growth and replication) by mimicking natural metabolites and taking their place within cells. Alkyating agents (nitrogen mustards) interfere with mitosis or cell division by binding with DNA to prevent cell replication.

✔ Antineoplastics are usually given in cycles (e.g., 3-4 weeks between treatments), allowing rest and recovery periods for the patient.

CHOOSE THE BEST ANSWER.

answers are in the back of the book

1) The drug tamoxifen (Nolvadex®) is used specifically
   a. for individuals with certain types of prostatic cancers.
   b. for individuals with certain types of breast cancers.
   c. as an alkylating agent.
   d. as an antimetabolite.

2) Which of the following could be a potential side effect of chemo drugs?
   a. alopecia and anemia
   b. immunosuppression
   c. GI disturbances and dehydration/weight loss
   d. All of the above

3) Of the following statements, which one is false?
   a. The lymphatic system is the center of the body's immune system.
   b. Metastasis occurs when cancer cells spread beyond their original site.
   c. The use of more than one drug is recommended in chemotherapy over the use of just one drug.
   d. The difficulty in treating cancer is that typically, cancer cells are normal in structure and growth rate as normal cells.

4) Which of the following drugs is considered an alkylating agent?
   a. cyclophosphamide
   b. methotrexate
   c. 5-FU
   d. paclitaxel

CARDIOVASCULAR AGENTS

Some of the most widely used medications available are used to treat diseases and conditions of the cardiovascular system.

Cardiovascular agents include **antianginals, antiarrhythmics, antihypertensives, vasopressors, antihyperlipidemics, thrombolytics** and **anticoagulants**. They are used in treating myocardial infarction (heart attack), angina, cerebral vascular accident (CVA) or stroke, hyper/hypotension (high/low blood pressure), congestive heart failure (CHF), coronary artery disease (CAD), arrhythmias, high cholesterol, unwanted blood clots, and arteriosclerosis.

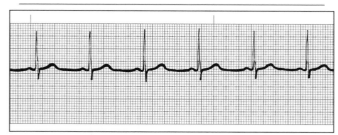

An EKG strip for a normal heart rhythm — variations from this pattern indicate an arrhythmia. The type of arrhythmia can be determined by the nature of the variation.

Arrhythmias

Normally, the electrical system of the heart causes it to contract (or beat) in a regular and organized rhythm that can be graphed by an **electrocardiogram** (**EKG** or **ECG**). An arrhythmia is an abnormal heart rhythm that can interfere with the heart's ability to pump in an effective, organized manner. Arrhythmias range from minor to life-threatening. They are classified by degree of seriousness, site of origin (where the electrical impulse causing the rhythm came from), and rate or speed. Familiar arrhythmias include:

➡ tachycardia;
➡ bradycardia;
➡ premature or ectopic beats;
➡ flutter and fibrillation.

THE HEART

Conduction

The heart is a pump that uses complex chemical and electrical processes to function. Chemically charged particles (ions) stimulate heart muscle to contract and relax systematically, pumping blood through the cardiovascular system. This contraction and relaxation is referred to as the **cardiac cycle**.

The **SA node** is the fastest generating electrical impulse area of the heart and it sets the pace. The atria and ventricles follow the conduction signal while the **AV node** together with the fine fibers (**Purkinje Fibers**) at the base of the heart transmit the impulse.

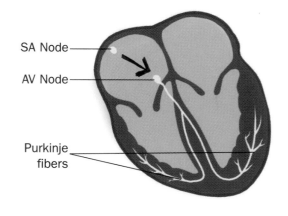

SA Node
AV Node
Purkinje fibers

---

arrhythmia an abnormal heart rhythm.
cardiac cycle the contraction and relaxation of the heart that pumps blood through the cardiovascular system.
diastolic pressure the minimum blood pressure when the heart relaxes; the second number in a blood pressure reading.
electrocardiogram (EKG or ECG) a graph of the heart's rhythms.

embolism, embolus a clot that has traveled in the bloodstream to a point where it obstructs flow.
myocardium heart muscle.
systolic pressure the maximum blood pressure when the heart contracts; the first number in a blood pressure reading.
thrombus a blood clot.

The Heart and Circulation

The heart is a muscular organ which powers blood circulation for the entire body. Divided into four chambers, the right and left **atria** (top chambers) and the right and left **ventricles** (bottom chambers), the heart receives deoxygenated blood into the right side (referred to as **pulmonary circulation**) and oxygenated blood into the left side (referred to as **systemic circulation**).

The right ventricle pumps blood to the lungs where it will mix with oxygen. The left ventricle pumps oxygenated blood to the body. The **myocardium** (heart muscle) is supplied fresh oxygen-rich blood by the **coronary arteries**, which branch from the **aorta** and circle back to the heart.

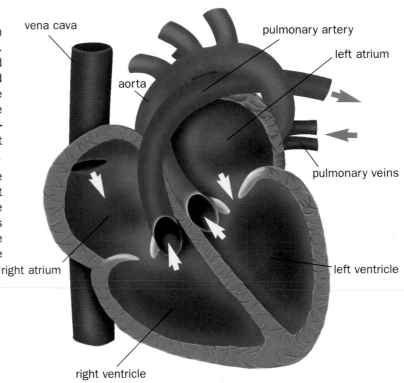

vena cava

aorta

right atrium

pulmonary artery

left atrium

pulmonary veins

left ventricle

right ventricle

Blood Clotting

Clotting is an essential function of blood that prevents excessive blood loss from injuries. Though **clotting factors** are the primary influence on clotting (see Chapter 18), adequate **platelets** and healthy blood vessel walls are also important. Too much clotting can be dangerous, however. If a clot (**thrombus**) is formed in the bloodstream, it can be carried to a location where it blocks a blood vessel and blood flow. Such blockages are called **embolisms**, and they can cause strokes and death.

Blood Pressure

Blood pressure is the outward pressure of the blood against the arteries as it is pumped through the body by the heart. Current literature recommends a blood pressure no higher than 135/85 for 40% of a normal healthy adult's day. The first number is the **systolic** value that represents the maximum pressure as the heart contracts to pump blood out. The second number is the **diastolic** value that represents the minimum pressure in the artery as the heart relaxes.

CARDIOVASCULAR AGENTS

CLASSES

Antianginals

[handwritten: Angina is when coronary arteries are becoming blocked = pain in the chest]

[handwritten: narrowing of arteries]

[handwritten: nitroglycerin - patients should sit down cause they could get dizzy.]

Antianginals are used to treat cardiac related chest pain (angina) resulting from ischemic heart disease.

Patients with this condition suffer a lack of oxygen and blood flow to the myocardium. Nitrates, beta-blockers, and calcium channel blockers are examples of antianginals.

Antiarrhythmics

[handwritten: Propranolol (Inderal)]

Antiarrhythmics are used to treat irregular heart rhythms.

They regulate the conduction activity of the heart by inhibiting abnormal pacemaker cells or recurring abnormal impulses and restoring a normal rhythm. Antiarrhythmics include beta blockers and drugs that block sodium channels, potassium ion channels, and calcium channels.

Antihypertensives

Antihypertensives are used to reduce a sustained elevation in blood pressure.

Factors affecting blood pressure include stress, blood volume, arterial narrowing, age, gender and general condition of health. Common antihypertensives include beta-blockers to reduce cardiac output, diuretics to decrease fluid volume, ACE inhibitors to reduce salt and water retention and inhibit vascular constriction, and calcium channel blockers to relax blood vessels.

Vasopressors

Vasopressors act to increase blood pressure.

If a patient is in a state of shock due to decreased blood volume, inadequate cardiac output or severe infection, fluids may be introduced to provide adequate blood volume. In addition to fluid replacement, vasopressors may be used to help supply blood to the brain and kidney.

Antihyperlipidemics

Antihyperlipidemics are used to lower high levels of cholesterol that can lead to blocked blood vessels.

Cholesterol is a **lipid** normally present in the body that is essential for healthy cell function. Proteins and carbohydrates, as well as fat are responsible for natural cholesterol production. Cholesterol levels are measured as **total cholesterol, LDL (low-density lipoprotein)**, and **HDL (high-density lipoprotein)**. Excess amounts of LDL can lead to blocked blood vessels and cardiovascular problems. HMG-CoA Reductase inhibitors are used to treat high LDL levels.

Thrombolytics / Anticoagulants

↳ destroy clot

Thromb = destroys

anti = prevents

Thrombolytics are used to dissolve blood clots and anticoagulants are used to prevent their formation.

Thrombolytics can be dangerous since blood clotting can be disturbed, resulting in profuse bleeding and even bleeding to death. However, in cases of impending myocardial infarction or stroke, a travelling blood clot (**embolus**) can be dissolved and the stroke prevented. There has been much success with this group of drugs in recent years. A common thrombolytic agent is alteplase. Common anticoagulants include warfarin and heparin.

TYPES OF ACTION

Beta blockers	Drugs that reduce the oxygen demands of the heart muscle.
Calcium channel blockers	Drugs that relax the heart by reducing heart conduction.
Diuretics	Drugs that decrease blood pressure by decreasing blood volume. They decrease volume by increasing the elimination of salts and water through urination.
ACE inhibitors	The "-pril" drugs, they relax the blood vessels. Note: the "-sartan" drugs are considered a subgroup of ACE inhibitors.
Vasodilators	Drugs that relax and expand the blood vessels.

ANTIANGINALS

[handwritten: Patch   Patch   Sublingual   Patch]

Nitroglycerin (Nitro-Bid®, Nitro-Dur®, Nitrostat®, and Transderm-Nitro®)

Action and Indication

Nitroglycerin acts to dilate the coronary artery walls, thus increasing the flow of blood and oxygen. This will ease the chest pain (angina pectoris) caused by the coronary artery constriction.

Dosage

Varies as to severity of chest pain and route of administration chosen. For example, at onset of chest pain, take 1 sublingual tablet. This may be repeated every five minutes until pain subsides. If pain continues after 15 minutes and 3 tablets, the physician should be notified immediately. A skin patch may be applied every 12 to 24 hours to prevent angina attacks.

Route

Sublingual tablets, nasal spray, topical patch, ointment, IV.

Side Effects

Headache, dizziness, hypotension, lightheadedness, nausea/vomiting.

Warnings

[handwritten: 1 month use →]

Headache pain can be severe and tolerance can be quickly reached. Sublingual tablets may loose their effectiveness after a few months. The patient's supply should be fresh. APAP (liquid low-dose acetaminophen) may be used for headache pain.

Special Patient Teaching Considerations

Alcohol and aspirin should be avoided when taking this drug. Also, lightheadedness, dizziness, and severe headache may occur. Do not change dose to avoid the headache. Operate machinery with caution. If wearing a patch, clean old administration area well before applying to new site. Dispose of patches carefully, as the residue could be harmful to children or pets. Ensure nitroglycerin tablets are fresh (within a few months) for optimal effectiveness and do not transfer pills from original container. This will preserve their potency.

Nifedipine (Procardia®, Adalat®)

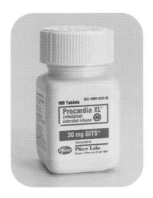

Procardia® XL
(nifedipine)
Courtesy of Pfizer

Action and Indication

This **calcium channel blocker** is indicated in cases of angina and may also be used to treat hypertension. The mechanism of this agent is to relax arterial walls leading to easing blood flow and lowering of blood pressure.

Dosage

To start, 10 mg taken three times a day. This may increase to 30 mg 3-4 times a day, with a maximum of 120 mg daily. Some sources state an allowed maximum of 180 mg daily. Note: Regular and long-acting forms of Procardia are available and will vary in their recommended dosages.

Route

PO, capsules.

Side Effects

Hypotension, fluid retention, decreased urine output, flushing and tachycardia.

Warnings

It is recommended to lower the dosage for elderly and patients with a history of liver dysfunction. Procardia has been reported to increase digoxin levels in blood. Monitor the patient's blood pressure for occurrence of hypotension and be aware of other drug therapy such as beta blockers which may cause hypotension with concurrent use. Note: Procardia is used for cases of angina while Procardia XL is indicated for hypertension. *Neither of these drugs should be prescribed immediately following a heart attack and are not recommended for use in children.*

Special Patient Teaching Considerations

Report symptoms of hypotension, angina, and/or edema to the physician. Avoid use of alcohol to reduce risk of drowsiness.

Do Not Take alcohol with this drug

ANTIANGINALS

Verapamil Hydrochloride (Calan®, Isoptin®)

Action and Indication

A **calcium channel blocker** causing decreased cardiac conduction. Used to treat supraventricular arrhythmias, angina, and hypertension.

Dosage

Depending on indication and on choice of regular or sustained release. For example, 40-120 mg PO three times a day.

Route

PO, IV.

Side Effects

Hypotension, dizziness, bradycardia, shortness of breath, congestive heart failure, constipation.

Warnings

Contraindicated in patients with a low blood pressure, atrial fibrillation or flutter, and heart block.

Special Patient Teaching Considerations

Notify the physician of other medical conditions and drugs being taken (e.g., beta blockers). Verapamil may be contraindicated. Notify the physician of any signs of adverse effects.

Isosorbide Mononitrate (Imdur®, Ismo®, Monoket®)

Action and Indication
A vasodilator which is used to treat coronary artery disease. This drug may also help prevent angina attacks from occurring.

Dosage
30-60 mg to start, once a day. This dosage may be increased to a maximum of 120 mg daily.

Route
PO, tablets (regular and extended release are available).

Side Effects
Headache, hypotension, and dizziness.

Warnings
Caution should be used in patients with a history of hypotension or nitrate allergies, or who are taking other drug therapies such as diltiazem hydrochloride, verapamil hydrochloride, and/or nifedipine.

Special Patient Teaching Considerations
Do not abruptly stop taking this medication. Due to possible dizziness and lightheadedness, do not operate dangerous machinery and avoid alcohol while taking isosobide mononitrate. This medication has been known to cause false low serum cholesterol readings.

ANTIARRHYTHMICS

Bretylium Tosylate (Bretylol®)

Action and Indication

Class III antiarrhythmic used to treat serious life-threatening ventricular arrhythmias, such as ventricular tachycardia.

Dosage

Dependent upon patient weight, severity of ventricular arrhythmia, and current American Heart Association guidelines. For example, initially 5 mg/kg given IV push, followed in 1-2 minutes with defibrillation. If successful, a maintenance infusion of 1-2 mg/min is started.

Route

IV, IVP (IV push). only

Side Effects

Nausea, vomiting, hypotension, initial rises in norepinephrine that may lead to a rise in blood pressure and heart rate. Other arrhythmias may occur.

Warnings

Monitor patient for signs of vomiting and prevent aspiration. This is a very serious drug and this intensive care or emergency room patient should be cardiac monitored and observed at all times. The drug lidocaine is often tried first before employing this agent.

Special Patient Teaching Considerations

Report any sign of nausea or other feelings of discomfort.

only to treat severe arrhythmias
- given in a hospital setting

Lidocaine Hydrochloride (Xylocaine®)

Action and Indication

A **class I sodium channel blocker** antiarrhythmic used to treat severe arrhythmias, generally ventricular in nature.

Dosage

Dependent on patient weight, severity of arrhythmia, and current American Heart Association treatment protocol. For example, 1 mg to 1.5 mg/kg IV bolus initially. If patient converts to normal sinus rhythm, follow up with a maintenance dose of 1-4 mg/min. The elderly and those with liver disease or congestive heart failure (CHF) may receive a lesser dose. All patients usually receive up to a 50% reduction in the dosage past the first 24 hours.

Route

IV.

Side Effects

Sedation, seizures, irritability, hypotension.

Warnings

The decision to initiate this therapy is a professional one rendered by the physician in charge. Once the therapy is initiated and the patient converts to a normal rhythm and/or ventricular ectopy slows or ceases, maintenance must be continued to assure optimal benefit.

Special Patient Teaching Considerations

This is a very serious drug to receive. Often the intensive care or emergency room patient is not aware of its delivery. If they are awake and alert, it is important to present a calming and reassuring attitude and ask them to notify you if they experience any unusual discomfort.

only to treat severe arrhythmias
-given in a hospital setting

ANTIHYPERTENSIVES

Diltiazem Hydrochloride (Cardizem®, Tiazac®)

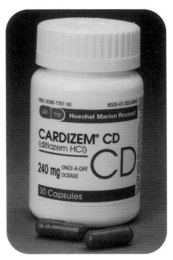

Cardizem® CD
(diltiazem hydrochloride)
Courtesy of Hoechst Marion
Roussel

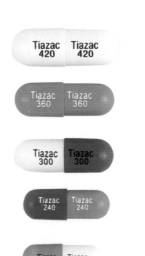

Action and Indication

This agent is a **calcium channel blocker** that acts to dilate blood vessels and reduce blood pressure and anginal pain. It is also known to control ventricular rate during atrial fibrillation or flutter.

Dosage

Dependent upon severity of the condition and preparation. For example, to treat angina or hypertension: 30-90 mg of regular tablets, 3-4 times a day; or 60-180 mg of sustained release tablets, two times a day. For more severe arrhythmia conditions: IV at 0.25 mg/kg of body weight to be given over 2 min.

Route

PO, tablets and capsules. Also available as IV infusion.

Side Effects

Hypotension, flushing, nausea, bradycardia, and possible heart block could occur.

Warnings

Caution should be used in patients with history of congestive heart failure, or if the patient is taking certain beta blockers (atenolol, propanolol), cimetidine, or digoxin.

Special Patient Teaching Considerations

Check pulse regularly to determine if its rate is slow. Notify physician of a rate below 50 beats per minute. *Do not abruptly stop this medication as anginal attacks could occur.*

Tiazac®
(diltiazem hydrochloride)
Courtesy of Forest Pharmaceuticals

Doxazosin Mesylate (Cardura®)

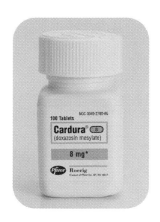

Cardura®
(doxazosin mesylate)
Courtesy of mfr

Action and Indication
Due to its peripheral vascular dilatation effects, this **alpha receptor blocker** is used to treat varied conditions such as hypertension, congestive heart failure, and benign prostatic hypertrophy.

Dosage
Most sources agree that the usual dosage is 1 mg daily. This amount may be increased by 2 mg up to a maximum of 16 mg especially in cases of hypertension.

Route
PO, tablets.

Side Effects
Dizziness, hypotension, and fatigue. Fainting could also occur.

Warnings
It is important to monitor the patient's blood pressure following the initial dose of this medication and the complete blood count (CBC) while taking this drug.

Special Patient Teaching Considerations
It may take several weeks to realize an optimal therapeutic effect of Cardura. The patient's condition could become worse if he or she does not take this agent regularly. Due to the drowsy effect this medication may have, do not operate dangerous machinery.

ANTIHYPERTENSIVES

Losartan Potassium (Cozaar®)

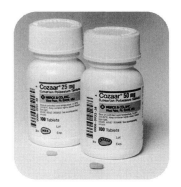

Cozaar®
(losartan potassium)
Courtesy of Merck Archives

Action and Indication

Cozaar is an antihypertensive drug that blocks angiotensin II receptors and prevents the hormone angiotensin II from constricting blood vessels and raising blood pressure.

Dosage

50 mg to a maximum of 100 mg daily, with reduced dosage for patients with liver dysfunction.

Route

PO, tablets.

Side Effects

Possible hypotension, particularly if taking concurrently with a diuretic. Lightheadedness or even fainting could occur. Other side effects may include upper respiratory infection with cough.

Warnings

This drug should not be used by pregnant or lactating women.

Special Patient Teaching Considerations

Do not take this drug if you are pregnant. Fetal death could occur, especially during the second or third trimester. Cozaar should be taken regularly and at the same time daily to realize its optimal effect. Also notify the physician in the event of GI symptoms that cause dehydration. Fluid depletion could cause serious hypotension while taking this medication.

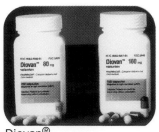

Diovan®
(valsartan)
Courtesy of Novartis Pharmaceutical
Corporation

Valsartan (Diovan®)

Valsartan is an **ACE inhibitor** used for the treatment of hypertension. It may be used alone or with other agents. *Like other ACE inhibitors, it is contraindicated for pregnant women, since fetal death can result.*

Losartan Potassium + Hydrochlorothiazide (Hyzaar®)

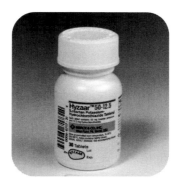

Hyzaar
(losartan potassium/
hydrochlorothiazide)
Courtesy of Merck Archives

Action and Indication

This antihypertensive agent works in combination by supplying losartan to prevent angiotensin II from constricting blood vessels and hydrochlorothiazide to increase urine output and decrease vascular fluid volume. Both actions contribute to the lowering of blood pressure.

Dosage

One tablet (losartan 50 mg and hydrochlorothiazide 12.5 mg) once a day. It is possible to increase the dosage, if needed, to a maximum of two tablets per day. A decreased dose may be indicated for patients with liver dysfunction.

Route

PO, tablets.

Side Effects

Potential allergic reactions. Low potassium, hypotension, dizziness, and possible respiratory infection.

Warnings

This drug should not be used by pregnant or lactating women. Use with other diuretic or antihypertensive therapy may result in adverse effects. Caution should be used in patients with a history of lupus, diabetes, asthma, gout, or kidney disease.

Special Patient Teaching Considerations

Do not take this drug if you are pregnant. Fetal death could occur, especially during the second or third trimester. Avoid alcohol while taking Hyzaar and notify a physician if you also take drugs such as prednisone, insulin, narcotic painkillers, sulfa drugs, troleandomycin, or lithium. Hyzaar can be taken without regard to meals.

ANTIHYPERTENSIVES

Amlodipine Besylate (Norvasc®)

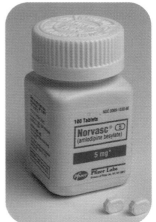

Norvasc®
(amlodipine besylate)
Courtesy of Pfizer

Action and Indication

This antihypertensive **calcium channel blocker** is used to treat both hypertension and angina. The action of Norvasc includes dilating blood vessels and slowing heart rate.

Dosage

Initially 5mg daily to a suggested maximum of 10 mg daily. The elderly, those with liver dysfunction, or otherwise compromised patients, would receive a decreased dose.

Route

PO, tablets.

Side Effects

Hypotension, dizziness, fluid retention, heart palpitations.

Warnings

This drug should be reduced gradually. Use caution in patients with a history of liver disease and heart failure.

Special Patient Teaching Considerations

Norvasc may be taken without regard to meals. Notify the physician if there are not positive results in 24-48 hours.

Felodipine (Plendil®)

Action and Indication

This antihypertensive is a **calcium channel blocker** that acts as a peripheral vessel dilator to lower blood pressure. Plendil also acts to reduce cardiac muscle contraction and improve the flow of oxygen to the myocardium and prevent angina.

Dosage

Suggested initial dose is 5 mg daily with a maintenance dose of 5-20 mg daily. Usually the dose is adjusted in 2 week intervals. This medication dosage is normally reduced for the elderly and those with liver dysfunction.

Route

PO, tablets.

Side Effects

Headache, lower extremity edema, hypotension, and flushing of the skin.

Warnings

Some sources indicate that this drug may increase digoxin levels in the blood. As with other calcium channel blockers such as verapamil and nifedipine, allergic reaction is possible in some patients. Selected beta blockers may also cause an unwanted drug interaction.

Special Patient Teaching Considerations

Notify a physician if lower extremity edema or signs of hypotension (dizziness, lightheadedness, tachycardia) occur. Take this medication whole. Note that it may take several weeks to feel the optimal effects of this drug. Patients should notify their dentist when taking this medication as they may experience dental discomfort such as swollen gums and sore mouth.

ANTIHYPERTENSIVES

Metoprolol Tartrate (Lopressor®)

Action and Indication

This **beta blocker** is indicated for the treatment of hypertension, angina, and status post myocardial infactions. The demand for oxygen by the myocardium is decreased due to the beta blocking action of Lopressor. The rate and force of the heart contractions are reduced, lowering blood pressure and allowing the heart's muscle to decrease its work load.

Dosage

For both angina and hypertension, the recommended dosage is 100 mg daily taken in two divided doses. This dosage may be increased to a maximum of 400 mg per day.

Route

PO tablets and long acting tablets.

Side Effects

Hypotension, bradycardia, rash, itching, possible depression, and disorientation.

Warnings

Use caution in patients with history of bradycardia and heart block, asthma, or liver dysfunction. The antihypertensive drug reserpine could cause an undesired drug interaction.

Special Patient Teaching Considerations

Take this medication with meals. Check pulse regularly. If heart rate drops below 50 beats per minute, notify a physician. Some sources claim that Lopressor may cause drowsiness. Avoid use of dangerous machinery while taking this medication.

Furosemide (Lasix®)

Action and Indication

A *loop diuretic*, this drug acts to increase renal blood flow and promote urination. Loop diuretics will generally maintain their effectiveness even in cases of impaired renal function. This agent is often prescribed for cases of congestive heart failure (CHF), edema (tissue water retention), and hypertension. However, it is ineffective in cases of total renal failure as a functioning kidney is a prerequisite for its use.

Dosage

20-120 mg two times a day in divided doses, with the second dose given 6-8 hours after the first dose. Usually no more than 400 mg are given at one time and the total daily dose should not exceed 600 mg. The patient condition and disease severity will dictate the dosage.

Route

PO tablets, and solution IM, IV.

Side Effects

Hypotension, reduced electrolytes such as potassium and sodium, anemia, blurred vision, and hearing loss.

Warnings

Caution patient regarding signs and symptoms of hypokalemia (decreased potassium levels), photosensitivity, and previous allergic response to sulfa drugs.

Special Patient Teaching Considerations

Furosemide does not "cure" blood pressure but may help control it. Watch for signs of muscle weakness or rapid/ irregular heart beat. These symptoms may mean a depletion of potassium and the physician may suggest eating supplements (bananas, raisins, orange juice, and tomato juice).

ANTIHYPERTENSIVES

Benazepril Hydrochloride (Lotensin®)

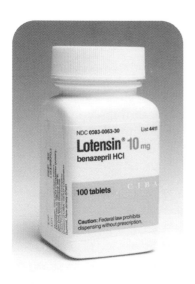

Lotensin®
(benazepril hydrochloride)
Courtesy of Novartis Pharmaceutical
Corporation

Action and Indication

The mechanism of this **ACE inhibitor** is to prevent angiotensin from increasing salt and water retention. It may be used alone or in combination with thiazide diuretics – as in **Lotensin HCT®** which combines **hydrochlorothiazide** and benazepril in the formulation.

Dosage

Without the concurrent use of another diuretic, the suggested dosage is 10 mg daily to start, with an increase to 20-40 mg daily. The maximum recommended dose is 80 mg per day. The larger amounts would be administered in divided doses 2 times per day. If the patient is also receiving another diuretic or has a kidney dysfunction, the suggested dose would be less.

Route

PO tablets.

Side Effects

Headache, dizziness, angioedema (swelling in the face or tongue, difficulty breathing), symptoms of hyerkalemia such as dry mouth, irregular heart beat, muscle pain, and possible nausea.

Warnings

Should not be used if pregnant. Use caution in patients with history of renal disease, diuretic therapy, and congestive heart failure.

Special Patient Teaching Considerations

Do not use if pregnant. Do not abruptly stop taking this medication. Desired results may not occur for 2-3 weeks. Notify physician immediately of side effects. Refrain from taking salt substitutes or potassium supplements while on Lotensin.

Bisoprolol Fumarate + Hydrochlorothiazide (Ziac®)

Action and Indication

An antihypertensive drug that combines properties of a synthetic **beta-blocker** (bisoprolol) and a **thiazide diuretic** (hydrochlorothiazide). Both reduce blood pressure and their effects together are additive.

Dosage

This drug is available in various strengths. An initial dose would be 2.5 mg bisprolol and 6.5 mg of hydrochlorothiazide taken daily. This dosage may be increased every 2 weeks to a maximum of 20 mg of bisoprolol with 12.5mg of hydrochlorothiazide daily. The dosages depend upon the patient and condition.

Route

PO tablets.

Side Effects

Hypotension, vertigo, sleep disturbances, possible palpitations, and rare bronchospasm.

Warnings

Contraindicated for patients with a history of overt cardiac failure, cardiogenic shock, second or third degree AV block, marked sinus bradycardia, and anuria. Caution should also be used if the patient has a history of diabetes, peripheral vascular disease, or liver/kidney dysfunction. Beta blockers are generally contraindicated if patients have a history of bronchospasm (i.e., asthma). Ziac should also not be combined with the use of other beta blockers as their effect could be increased.

Special Patient Teaching Considerations

Do not abruptly stop taking this medication. Notify a physician if any side effects occur, especially if cardiac or respiratory related. Diabetics note: hypoglycemic symptoms, especially tachycardia, may be masked when taking beta blockers.

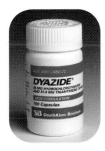

Dyazide®

Dyazide® combines the diuretic drugs hydrochlorathiazide and triamterene. Triamterene helps minimize the potassium loss caused by hydrochlorathiazide.

Dyazide®
(triamterene and hydrochlorothiazide)
Courtesy of Smith, Kline, Beecham

ANTIHYPERTENSIVES

Atenolol (Tenormin®)

Action and Indication

This **beta blocker** is often prescribed in cases of hypertension, angina, and cardiac arrhythmias such as SVT (supra ventricular tachycardia). Since beta blockers decrease the force and rate of contractions, this drug may also be indicated in treatment of myocardial infarctions. Some sources indicate usage in cases of migraine headache, alcohol withdrawal, and anxiety.

Dosage

50-100 mg per day in a single dose. For less severe cases, as little as 25 mg per day may be indicated, and for more severe cases such as heart attack, the dosage will be 5 mg IV over 5 minutes with possible repeat in 10 minutes.

Route

PO tablets or IV infusion.

Side Effects

Bradycardia, nausea, tiredness, and possible dizziness.

Warnings

Caution should be used in patients with history of coronary artery disease, congestive heart failure, asthma, kidney disease, or diabetes.

Special Patient Teaching Considerations

This medication should not be stopped abruptly as angina or infarction could occur. Take pulse regularly and notify a physician if it is below 50.

Terazosin Hydrochloride (Hytrin®)

Action and Indication

This antihypertensive **alpha receptor blocker** causes peripheral dilatation and is indicated in cases of high blood pressure and benign prostatic hypertrophy. It may be prescribed for use as sole therapy or used in combination with other antihypertensives or beta blockers.

Dosage

Initally, 1 mg daily at bedtime is recommended. Tolerance is assessed and possible increase is indicated. 1-5 mg daily with a maximum of 20 mg daily is suggested. For BPH, this drug may be prescribed for a 4-6 week interval.

Route

PO tablet.

Side Effects

Possible hypotension, especially in the first several doses; syncope and nasal congestion.

Warnings

Patients should be monitored initially to assess for orthostatic hypotension or other signs of intolerance.

Special Patient Teaching Considerations

Take the initial dose at bedtime in case of hypotension symptoms which may occur. Report any hypotensive signs to a physician. With each new dosage change or at the start of this therapy, avoid tasks which involve potentially perilous activity (e.g., driving, operating machinery, climbing). Also report any signs of painful erection to the physician as this could lead to impotence.

ANTIHYPERTENSIVES

Lisinopril (Prinivil®, Zestril®)

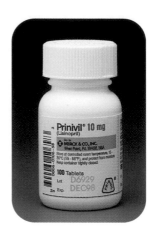

Prinivil®
(lisinopril)
Courtesy of Merck Archives

Action and Indication

An **ACE inhibitor** that acts to dilate both arterial and venous blood vessels to lower blood pressure. Improvement in exercise tolerance, left ventricular size, and mortality rate have been documented.

Dosage

10 mg PO once a day. Once blood pressure is adjusted, the dosage may increase to 20-40 mg per day. Dosage may be lower if patient is also taking diuretics.

Route

PO tablets.

Side Effects

Hypotension, dizziness, high potassium (hyperkalemia, especially if renal function is impaired), irritating cough, decreased urine output, and chest pain.

Warnings

ACE inhibitors should not be taken with potassium supplements. *This drug is also contraindicated for patients who are pregnant.*

Special Patient Teaching Considerations

This drug should not be used by pregnant women. Continue taking this drug as prescribed, even though you may feel better. Lisinopril may take several weeks to deliver the optimum effect. Do not take potassium supplements at the same time you are taking this drug.

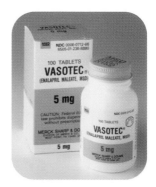

Vasotec®
(enalapril maleate)
Courtesy of Merck Archives

Enalapril Maleate (Vasotec®)

Enalapril is a popular **ACE inhibitor** antihypertensive with similar effects to others in its class. It is used alone or in combination with other antihypertensive agents, particularly thiazide diuretics. Allergic reaction is possible and it is contraindicated for patients with hypersensitivity to ACE inhibitors. *Note: ACE inhibitors should not be used by pregnant women.*

Hydrochlorothiazide (Esidrix®, hydroDIURIL®, various)

Action and Indication

A **diuretic** used to treat hypertension, edema, congestive heart failure, cirrhosis of the liver, and kidney dysfunction. This diuretic promotes elimination of urine and excess body fluid.

Dosage

Dependent on condition to be treated. For example, for hypertension the suggested doasge is 12.5-50 mg given as one single or two divided doses. For cases of edema, the dosage may be 25-100 mg in a single, divided, or alternate day dose. Children's doses would calculated according to their body weight.

Route

PO tablets

Side Effects

Hypotension, dizziness, low serum electrolytes such as potassium which could lead to cardiac irregularities and muscle cramps, and GI symptoms such as abdominal cramps and diarrhea.

Warnings

Use with caution in patients with history of renal disease, sulfa drug allergy, bronchial asthma, gout, elevated serum creatinine, or glucose intolerance. Monitor regularly for electrolyte imbalance, particularly regarding potassium.

Special Patient Teaching Considerations

Watch for signs of low blood pressure (dizziness, lightheadedness upon rising, headache) and for signs of low potassium (rapid or irregular heart beat, muscle weakness). Be cautious with exercise as too much activity may cause a depletion of fluid, low blood pressure, or low potassium level.

VASOPRESSORS

Dobutamine Hydrochloride (Dobutrex®)

Action and Indication

May be indicated if patient is more stable, but still at risk for shock. A second line vasopressor used after blood pressure is above 100 systolic.

Dosage

Dependent on severity and patient condition. For example, 2-20 micrograms/kg/min.

Route

IV.

Side Effects

Hypertension, increased heart rate, and chest pain.

Warnings

This drug is very serious and should be administered only in a monitored situation. It may increase insulin requirements and not be effective if the patient is also taking beta blockers. Note: the peak effect may not occur until 10 minutes after administration.

Special Patient Teaching Considerations

Physician should be notified of other drug therapy the patient is receiving and any complaints of side effects (rapid heart rate).

Dopamine Hydrochloride (Intropin®)

Action and Indication

Increases renal blood flow, fluid volume, and vascular resistance contributing to increased blood pressure. May be used in combination with norepinephrine in critical life-threatening situations.

Dosage

Dependent on severity of shock, patient condition, and weight. For example, to increase fluid volume via urine output, 2 micrograms/kg/min. Severe hypotension may require higher doses such as 5 micrograms/kg/min.

Route

IV, often using a central line.

Side Effects

Chest pain, rapid heart rate with increased arrhythmias such as premature ventricular contractions (PVCs).

Warnings

This is a serious drug usually seen only in emergency/intensive care situations where the patient is experiencing shock or CPR is being employed. Severe heart failure in an ER/CCU controlled situation may be an indication however. The patient needs to be monitored throughout this drug's administration and afterward. If the patient also has peripheral vascular disease, their legs may become oxygen deprived due to the vascular constricting properties of this agent. Observation is recommended.

Special Patient Teaching Considerations

If the patient is alert, it is important to ask them for their medical history, including the names of medications they regularly take. Psychotropic drugs could cause a decrease in dopamine's effectiveness.

ANTIHYPERLIPIDEMIC

Lovastatin (Mevacor®)

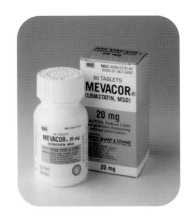

Mevacor®
(lovastatin)
Courtesy of Merck Archives

Action and Indication

A cholesterol lowering medication which is generally indicated when diet and exercise programs fail. Patients with **hypercholesterolemia** are prone to arteriosclerosis and will benefit from the action of this drug.

Dosage

The suggested starting dose is 20 mg per day, with a maximum dose of 80 mg per day. The larger amounts may be administered in divided doses.

Route

PO tablets.

Side Effects

Elevated liver function studies, GI symptoms such as abdominal pain and cramps, nausea and diarrhea.

Warnings

Liver function tests every 6-12 weeks initially and 6 months thereafter are suggested while the patient is taking this drug. Use caution in patients with history of diabetes, liver or kidney disease, hypothyroidism, or excess serum protein. This drug is contraindicated for patients who are also taking cyclosporine, nicotinic acid, or gemfibrozil. Patients should be monitored for signs or symptoms of kidney damage.

Special Patient Teaching Considerations

Do not use alcohol while taking this drug. Remember, Mevacor is not a replacement for a healthy diet and/or good exercise program. It is adjunct therapy. Mevacor is not recommended for use in children or pregnant women.

 hypercholesterolemia excessive amount of cholesterol in the blood.

Atorvastatin Calcium (Lipitor®)

Action and Indication

This drug is indicated in cases of high cholesterol as it works to clear LDL (low density lipoprotein) from blood and inhibit the synthesis of new LDL.

Dosage

To start, 10 mg once a day is recommended with a suggested maximum of 80 mg daily.

Route

PO tablets.

Side Effects

Flu-like symptoms, eyesight changes, back pain, and GI effects such as abdominal pain, indigestion , and constipation.

Warnings

Other cholesterol lowering drugs may be taken at the same time, to enhance the effects of Lipitor. Liver function tests are suggested following 6-12 weeks of use. Should not be used if pregnant.

Special Patient Teaching Considerations

Do not take this drug if pregnant. Tagamet, Lanoxin, erythromycin, oral contraceptives, and Diflucan are examples of drugs that may cause an interaction with Lipitor. Take this drug at the same time each day and be aware that it may take up to two weeks to show results. Report any muscle pain or damage to your physician and remember this drug is an adjunct therapy. It should not replace a healthy diet or exercise program.

ANTIHYPERLIPIDEMIC

Simvastatin (Zocor®)

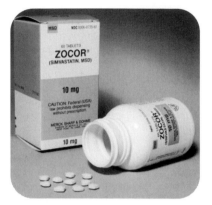

Zocor® 10 mg tablets

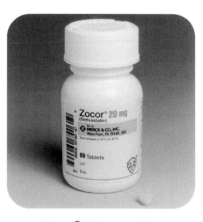

Zocor® 20 mg tablets

Zocor®
(simvastatin)
Courtesy of Merck Archives

Action and Indication

An **HMG-CoA Reductase inhibitor**, one of the "statin" drugs, Zocor lowers total cholesterol, LDL cholesterol, and triglyceride levels while increasing HDL cholesterol levels.

Dosage

5-10 mg taken once a day, usually at bedtime. This dose may be increased or decreased every 4 weeks. The suggested maximum dose is 40 mg daily. Patients with severe kidney dysfunction would receive a lower dosage.

Route

PO tablets.

Side Effects

Headache, elevated liver function tests, abdominal pain, and possible elevated CPK levels.

Warnings

Zocor is contraindicated in patients with liver disease, who have an allergy history to Zocor, or who are pregnant. Caution your patients regarding feelings of muscle weakness or pain. Monitor liver function and CPK (muscle tissue damage indicator) levels.

Special Patient Teaching Considerations

Remember that Zocor is not a replacement for a therapeutic diet and exercise regime. These measures should be continued, as ordered, while taking this medication.

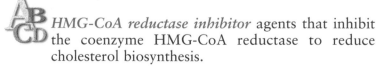

HMG-CoA reductase inhibitor agents that inhibit the coenzyme HMG-CoA reductase to reduce cholesterol biosynthesis.

Fluvastatin sodium (Lescol®)

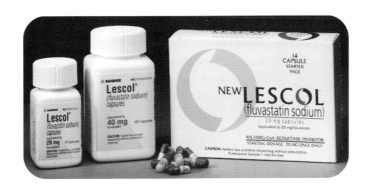

Lescol®
(fluvastatin sodium)
Courtesy of Novartis
Pharmaceutical Corporation

Action and Indication

This **HMG-CoA Reductase inhibitor** acts to lower total cholesterol, LDL cholesterol and triglyceride levels while increasing HDL cholesterol levels.

Dosage

20 mg daily initially to 80 mg daily maximum. It is recommended that the higher dose be split into two doses per day.

Route

PO capsules.

Side Effects

Flu-like symptoms, back pain and GI effects such as nausea, diarrhea, abdominal pain.

Warnings

Serum liver enzyme studies should be conducted prior to starting this therapy and at 6-12 week intervals. *Should not be used if pregnant.* Use caution in patients with history of kidney dysfunction or complaints of muscle weakness and/or pain.

Special Patient Teaching Considerations

Notify your physician of side effects occurring, particularly muscle pain and weakness. It is important to remember that Lescol is adjunct therapy to a low fat, low cholesterol diet. Exercise and ideal body weight should be maintained.

ANTIHYPERLIPIDEMIC

Pravastatin Sodium (Pravachol®)

Action and Indication

An **HMG-CoA Reductase inhibitor,** Pravachol reduces total cholesterol and the synthesis of LDL. Also lowers triglyceride levels and increases HDL levels.

Dosage

Initially, 10-20 mg daily with a possible increase to 40 mg daily.

Route

PO tablets.

Side Effects

Elevated liver function studies, weakness, and possible headache.

Warnings

Caution is advised for patients with a history of alcoholism or liver dysfunction. *Pregnant women should not take this drug.* Liver function studies should be performed at regular intervals.

Special Patient Teaching Considerations

Do not drink alcohol while taking this medication. Notify your physician should you become pregnant and give your doctor an accurate drug therapy history. Agents such as erythromycin, warfarin, cimetidine, niacin, and gemfibrozil may cause an unwanted drug interaction.

Alteplase (Activase®)

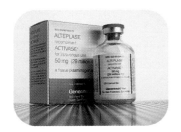

Activase®
(alteplase)
Courtesy of Genentech, Inc.

Alteplase is known as a ***tissue plasminogen activator***, or ***tPA***.

Action and Indication

Works to cause **lysis** (breakdown) of formed clot (thrombus) by assisting fibrin breakdown. Blood flow and oxygenation is thus restored to the ischemic myocardium. This drug is indicated in cases of life threatening pulmonary embolus and myocardial infarctions.

Dosage

Dependent on condition and severity. (For example, if considering the patient's weight in an MI, 15 mg given IV bolus (at one time) and followed by 0.75 mg/kg over 30 min (not to exceed 50 mg). This may also be followed with 0.50 mg/kg over 1 hour (not to exceed 35 mg).

Route

IV.

Side Effects

May cause intracranial bleeding and arrhythmias

Warnings

There are many risks associated with this serious drug. New guidelines are still becoming available. Each situation must be professionally judged independently as to whether the benefits would outweigh the risks. Contraindications may include: pregnancy, prolonged CPR, history of stroke and intracranial bleed, recent brain or major surgery, and active or recent internal bleeding.

Special Patient Teaching Considerations

Accuracy of health history is very important. Notify the physician of any signs of adverse effects.

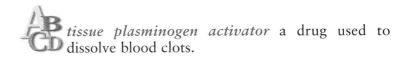

ABCD ***tissue plasminogen activator*** a drug used to dissolve blood clots.

ANTICOAGULANTS

Warfarin Sodium (Coumadin®)

Action and Indication

This agent inhibits blood clot formation by interfering with Vitamin K coagulation factors. It is often prescribed in cases of suspected and unwanted blood clot formation (i.e., atrial fibrillation, thrombophlebitis or occasion of recurring heart attack or stroke) or when the clotting time is too low and platelet counts are too high. Known as a "blood thinner."

Dosage

2-5 mg per day to start, depending on patient's condition and monitored clotting times (PT's, PTT's). A maintenance dose of up to 10 mg per day may be indicated.

Route

PO

Side Effects

Bleeding, difficulty breathing, dizziness, low blood pressure.

Warnings

The patient's clotting times must be continually monitored while receiving this therapy and afterward as it takes several days to return to normal clotting once the drug is discontinued. There could be potency issues if brands of this agent are changed. Contraindicated in pregnancy.

Special Patient Teaching Considerations

This medication may make clotting more difficult in the event of injury. Seek immediate attention should this occasion arise. Notify all medical personnel if seeking treatment (including dentists). Avoid the use of alcohol while taking this drug. Do not take OTC medications (including aspirin) without consulting with a physician. *Many drugs will interact with warfarin and it is essential that the physician be notified of all other drug therapy.*

Clotting Times

Prothrombin Time Testing (PTT) is used to assess a patient's clotting time. It measures the plasma's ***prothrombin*** or ***natural clotting factor.*** Slowing the patient's clotting time to about two to two and a half times the normal rate lessens the likelihood of dangerous thrombosis, but will not cause excessive bleeding. PTTs are conducted frequently on patients receiving anticoagulant therapy to make sure clotting times are appropriate.

Heparin

Action and Indication

This anticoagulation agent acts to inhibit clot formation by potentiating the anticoagulant action of antithrombin III. It may also allow the natural thrombolytic system to eradicate the existing clot. Commercially, this drug is obtained from hog intestines or beef lungs. It is often indicated in severe cases of arterial and venous thrombosis, including DVT (deep vein thrombosis) and as adjunctive therapy for myocardial infarctions.

Dosage

Dependent upon event targeted and patient condition. For example, for DVT prevention (prophylaxis) 5000 units SQ (subcutaneous), every 12 hours.

Route

SQ, IV. Caution: when administering SQ heparin. Site of choice is abdominal. Do not rub the area post injection as local bleeding or bruising could occur.

Side Effects

Bleeding, bloodshot eyes, mild decrease of platelets, hypersensitivity, and possible hair loss (alopecia).

Warnings

Patient coagulation studies need to be consistantly monitored and dosage chosen accordingly. Note: methods for adjusting IV heparin levels to PTT's vary widely. Contraindicated in patients with active bleeding, recent surgery or severe hypertension.

Special Patient Teaching Considerations

Medical history needs to be accurate. Notify the physician of any signs of bleeding or side effects.

DRUG CHART

Generic Name	Trade Name	Route
BETA BLOCKERS		
Acebutolol	Sectral	PO
Atenolol	Tenormin	PO, Inj.
	Various	PO, Inj.
Betaxolol	Kerlone	PO
Bisoprodol	Zebeta	PO
Carvedilol	Coreg	PO
Esmolol	Brevibloc	Inj.
Labetalol	Normodyne	PO, Inj.
	Trandate	PO, Inj.
Levobunolol	Betagan	Eye
Metoprolol	Lopressor	PO, Inj.
	Various	PO, Inj.
Nadolol	Corgard	PO
Pindolol	Visken	PO
	Various	PO
Propranolol	Inderal	PO, Inj.
	Betachron	PO
	Various	PO, Inj.
Sotalol	Betapace	PO
Timolol	Blocadren	PO
CALCIUM CHANNEL BLOCKERS		
Amlodipine	Norvasc	PO
Bepridil	Vascor	PO
Diltiazem	Cardizem	PO, Inj.
Felodipine	Plendil	PO
Isradipine	DynaCirc	PO
Nicardipine	Cardene	PO, Inj.
Nifedipine	Procardia	PO
	Adalat CC	PO
	Various	PO
Nisoldipine	Sular	PO
Verapamil	Calan	PO
	Isoptin	PO, Inj.
	Various	PO, Inj.
NITRATES		
Isosorbide Dinitrate	Isordil	PO
	Various	PO
Isosorbide Mononitrate	Imdur	PO
	Ismo	PO
	Monoket	PO
Nitroglycerin	Nitro-Bid	PO, Inj.
	Various	PO, Inj., Transdermal

Generic Name	Trade Name	Route
CARDIAC GLYCOSIDES		
Digitoxin	Crystodigin	PO
Digoxin	Lanoxin	PO, Inj.
ANTIARRHYTHMICS		
CLASS I		
Disopyramide	Norpace	PO
Encainide	Enkaid	PO
Flecainide	Tambocor	PO
Lidocaine	Xylocaine	Inj.
Mexiletine	Mexitil	PO
Moricizine	Ethmozine	PO
Phenytoin	Dilantin	PO, Inj.
Procainamide	Pronestyl	PO, Inj.
	Various	PO, Inj.
Propafenone	Rythmol	PO
Quinidine	Cardioquin	PO
	Quinaglute	PO
	Various	PO, Inj.
Tocainide	Tonocard	PO
CLASS III		
Amiodarone	Cordarone	PO, Inj.
	Pacerone	PO
Bretylium	Bretylol	Inj.
Ibutilide	Corvert	Inj.
ANGIOTENSIN II RECEPTOR ANTAGONISTS		
Candesartan	Atacand	PO
Eprosartan	Teveten	PO
HCTZ / Losartan	Hyzaar	PO
HCTZ / Valsartan	Diovan HCT	PO
Irbesartan	Avapro	PO
Losartan	Cozaar	PO
Telmisartan	Micardis	PO
Valsartan	Diovan	PO
(note: HCTZ stands for hydrochlorothiazide)		
ACE INHIBITORS		
Benazepril	Lotensin	PO
Benazepril / HCTZ	Lotensin HCT	PO
Captopril	Capoten	PO
Enalapril	Vasotec	PO, Inj.
Enalapril / HCTZ	Vaseretic	PO
Fosinopril	Monopril	PO
HCTZ / Lisinopril	Prinizide	PO
	Zestoretic	PO

GENERIC NAME	TRADE NAME	ROUTE	GENERIC NAME	TRADE NAME	ROUTE
Lisinopril	Prinivil	PO	**ADRENERGIC AGONISTS**		
	Zestril	PO	Dopamine	Intropin	Inj.
Moexipril	Univasc	PO		Dopastat	Inj.
Quinapril	Accupril	PO	Dobutamine	Dobutrex	Inj.
Ramipril	Altace	PO	Epinephrine	Adrenalin	Inj.
Spirapril	Renormax	PO		Various	Inj.
Trandolapril	Mavik	PO	Isoproterenol	Isuprel	Inj.
ALPHA-BLOCKERS			**ANTICOAGULANTS**		
Doxazosin	Cardura	PO	Antithrombin III	Thrombate III	Inj.
Phenoxybenzamine	Dibenzyline	PO	Ardeparin	Normiflo	Inj.
Phentolamine	Regitine	Inj.	Dalteparin	Fragmin	Inj.
	Vasomax	Inj.	Danaparoid	Orgaran	Inj.
Prazosin	Minipress	PO	Enoxaparin	Lovenox	Inj.
	Various	PO	Heparin	Heparin	Inj.
Tamsulosin	Flomax	PO		Various	Inj.
Terazosin	Hytrin	PO	Lepirudin	Refludan	Inj.
Yohimbine	Yocon	PO	Pentosan	Elmiron	PO
	Various	PO	Warfarin	Coumadin	PO
CENTRAL ACTING ADRENERGIC AGENTS			**THROMBOLYTIC AGENTS**		
Clonidine	Catapres	PO	Alteplase, TPA	Activase	Inj.
	Various	PO	Anistreplase	Eminase	Inj.
Guanabenz	Wytensin	PO	Reteplase, r-PA	Retavase	Inj.
Guanfacine	Tenex	PO	Streptokinase	Streptase	Inj.
Methyldopa	Aldomet	PO, Inj.		Kabikinase	Inj.
	Various	PO, Inj.	Urokinase	Abbokinase	Inj.
DIURETICS					
Amiloride	Midamor	PO			
Bumetanide	Bumex	PO, Inj.			
	Various	PO, Inj.			
Chlorthalidone	Hygroton	PO			
	Various	PO			
Ethacrynic Acid	Edecrin	PO, Inj.			
Furosemide	Lasix	PO, Inj.			
Hydrochlorothiazide (HCTZ)	Esidrix	PO			
	Hydrodiuril	PO			
	Various	PO			
Indapamide	Lozol	PO			
Metolazone	Zaroxyolyn	PO			
	Mykrox	PO			
Spironolactone	Aldactone	PO			
	Various	PO			
Torsemide	Demadex	PO, Inj.			
Triamterene	Dyrenium	PO			

REVIEW

KEY CONCEPTS

✔ The heart is a pump that uses complex chemical and electrical processes to function. Chemically charged particles (ions) stimulate heart muscle to contract and relax systematically, pumping blood through the cardiovascular system.

✔ The heart is divided into four chambers, the right and left atria (top chambers) and the right and left ventricles (bottom chambers). The heart receives deoxygenated blood into the right side (referred to as pulmonary circulation) and oxygenated blood into the left side (referred to as systemic circulation). The right ventricle pumps blood to the lungs where it will mix with oxygen. The left ventricle pumps oxygenated blood to the body.

✔ Normally, the electrical system of the heart causes it to contract (or beat) in a regular and organized rhythm that can be graphed by an electrocardiogram (EKG or ECG). An arrhythmia is an abnormal heart rhythm that can interfere with the heart's ability to pump in an effective, organized manner. They range from minor to life-threatening.

✔ Blood pressure is the outward pressure of the blood against the arteries as it is pumped through the body by the heart. It is measured as systolic pressure/diastolic pressure (e.g., 110/70). The systolic value represents the maximum pressure as the heart contracts. The diastolic value represents the minimum pressure in the artery as the heart relaxes.

✔ Antianginals are used to treat cardiac related chest pain (angina) resulting from ischemic heart disease. Patients with angina suffer a lack of oxygen and blood flow to the myocardium.

✔ Antiarrhythmics are used to treat irregular heart rhythms. They regulate the conduction activity of the heart by inhibiting abnormal pacemaker cells or recurring abnormal impulses and restoring a normal rhythm.

✔ Antihypertensives are used to reduce a sustained elevation in blood pressure.

✔ Factors affecting blood pressure include stress, blood volume, arterial narrowing, age, gender and general condition of health.

✔ Vasopressors act to increase blood pressure.

✔ Antihyperlipidemics are used to lower high levels of cholesterol, which is measured as total cholesterol, LDL (low-density lipoprotein), and HDL (high-density lipoprotein). Excess amounts of LDL can lead to blocked blood vessels and cardiovascular problems.

✔ Thrombolytics are used to dissolve blood clots and anticoagulants are used to prevent their formation.

✔ Beta blockers are agents that reduce the oxygen demands of the heart muscle.

✔ Calcium channel blockers are agents that relax the heart by reducing heart conduction.

✔ Diuretics are agents that decrease blood pressure by decreasing blood volume. They decrease volume by increasing the elimination of salts and water through urination.

✔ ACE inhibitors relax the blood vessels.

✔ Vasodilators are agents that relax and expand the blood vessels.

SELF TEST

MATCH THE GENERIC AND TRADE NAMES.   *answers are in the back of the book*

1. Benazepril	_____	Calan
2. Digoxin	_____	Cardizem
3. Diltiazem	_____	Cardura
4. Doxazosin	_____	Coumadin
5. Felodipine	_____	Dilantin
6. Furosemide	_____	Lanoxin
7. Lisinopril	_____	Lasix
8. Metoprolol	_____	Lopressor
9. Nifedipine	_____	Lotensin
10. Phenytoin	_____	Plendil
11. Verapamil	_____	Prinivil
12. Warfarin	_____	Procardia

CHOOSE THE BEST ANSWER.   *answers are in the back of the book*

1. Which of the following is an ACE Inhibitor?

    a. alteplase
    b. furosemide
    c. lisinopril
    d. nitroglycerin

2. Of the following statements, which one is false?

    a. Vasopressors act to decrease blood pressure
    b. Antiarrhythmics are used to treat irregular heart rhythms
    c. Antianginals are used to treat cardiac related chest pain

3. What specific classes of drugs are used to inhibit the potential for clot formation?

    a. antianginals
    b. antihyperglycemics
    c. antilipidemics
    d. anticoagulants

4. This drug is specifically used to dilate the coronary artery walls, thus increasing the flow of blood and oxygen to the heart.

    a. alteplase
    b. furosemide
    c. lisinopril
    d. nitroglycerin

DERMATOLOGICALS

The skin is the body's protective barrier.

It is the largest of the body's organs and protects the other organs against microorganisms, trauma, extreme temperature and other harmful elements. It is comprised of several layers: the epidermis (top layer), dermis (middle layer), and subcutaneous tissue (bottom layer). Within these layers, structures such as hair follicles and shafts, sebaceous and sweat glands, veins, arteries, and sensory nerves are found.

Dermatological refers to a drug used to treat a condition or disease related to the skin.

Pathological medical conditions and diseases which occur on or in the skin can be caused by inflammation, infection, growth rate changes, trauma, or structural dysfunction. Examples of skin conditions are: burns, cuts, rashes, dandruff, eczema, and skin cancer.

THE SKIN

The skin, also called the **Integumentary System,** is generally 3-5 millimeters thick, though it is thicker in the palms of the hands and soles of the feet and thinner in the eyelids and genitals. The outer layer of the epidermis (called the **stratum corneum**) is constantly replenished with new cells from underneath. The turnover time from cell development to shedding (**sloughing**) is about 21 days.

Skin Conditions

The following are examples of skin reactions that selected dermatologicals address:

➡ trauma (burns, cuts, abrasions, bruises).

➡ fluid accumulation (edema, cellulitis, blisters).

➡ discoloration and pigmentation, rashes, freckles, drug or allergy related photosensitivity,

➡ hyper or hypo melanin (skin pigment).

➡ dry skin or scaling (dandruff).

➡ cancers (basal cell, squamous cell or melanoma).

➡ non-malignant growths (keratoses).

In addition, the following common skin diseases are often treated with both prescription and non-prescription medications:

➡ eczema.

➡ psoriasis.

➡ acne.

➡ fungal infections (athlete's foot, ringworm).

➡ viral infections (herpes simplex).

➡ general dermatitis, hives or other allergic reactions caused by food, plants, insects, or sunburn.

dermatological a product used to treat a skin condition.

integumentary system the skin.

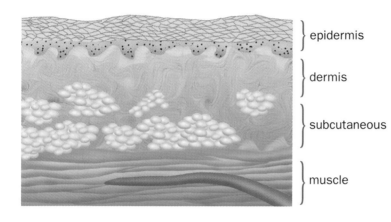

epidermis

dermis

subcutaneous

muscle

Other Structures

Contained within the skin are accessory structures: hair follicles, sweat glands, sebaceous glands, and nails.

Note also that the subcutaneous layer is not always considered a part of the skin but simply loose connective tissue that separates the skin from the underlying organs. It is, however, so closely interconnected that it is generally described with the integumentary system.

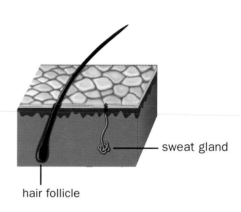

sweat gland

hair follicle

Dermatological Agents

Steroids, antihistamines, and inti-infectives are commonly used to treat skin disorders. Examples of commonly prescribed dermatological agents include:

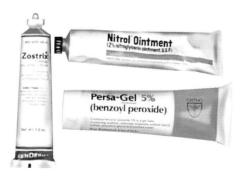

- ➥ hydrocortisone cream
- ➥ diphenhydramine
- ➥ silver sulfadiazine cream
- ➥ doxycycline hyclate
- ➥ ofloxacin

Note: The drying agent zinc oxide is often seen in a combination product with the local anesthetic camphor, moisture absorbing agent kaolin, and an anti-infective such as triclosan when treating diaper rash.

DERMATOLOGICALS

Hydrocortisone Cream (Anusol-HC®, Hytone®, etc.)

Action and Indication

This is a **steroidal** cream used to treat inflammation, itching of the skin, and other dermatological problems. It acts to inhibit the production of epidermal DNA and reduce chemical factors, such as prostaglandins, that contribute to skin inflammation.

Dosage

Depending on the commercial product, hydrocortisone is available in 0.25%–1% tubes OTC and at higher concentrations by prescription. A typical application would be a light layer 2 to 4 times daily.

Route

Topical.

Side Effects

Burning, local irritation, dryness, acne-like eruptions.

Warnings

If too much of this drug is absorbed through the skin, it can have a systemic effect and produce steroid-like reactions (excessive hair growth, moon face). Avoid close contact with the eyes.

Special Patient Teaching Considerations

Notify the physician if the original skin problem has not cleared or if a secondary one occurs. Avoid prolonged and heavy use.

Diphenhydramine Hydrochloride (Benadryl®)

Action and Indication

This is an **antihistamine** with anticholinergic properties used to treat allergic inflammation and swelling responses. Note: This agent may also be indicated in cases of insomnia, motion sickness, and parkinsonian episodes seen in drug reactions.

Dosage

Patient condition dependent. For example, 25-50 mg PO, 3-4 times a day. Lower PO dosages are available in OTC products.

Route

PO chewable tablets, capsules, liquid. For more severe cases, diphenhydramine may be given IM or IV.

Side Effects

Drowsiness, GI upset, upper respiratory congestion, and possible sedation.

Warnings

Contraindicated for newborns, infants, or nursing mothers. Caution should be used in patients with a history of narrow-angle glaucoma, hyperthyroidism, and bronchial asthma.

Special Patient Teaching Considerations

This drug may cause drowsiness. Caution should be used in daily activities, especially for those that require alertness, e.g., operating machinery.

DERMATOLOGICALS

Silver Sulfadiazine (Silvadene® Cream 1%)

Action and Indication

This **sulfa antibiotic** agent is used to treat burn cases. It may be used in combination with other drugs for more severe 2nd or 3rd degree events and contains anti-inflammatory as well as antibacterial properties.

Dosage

Application of a single thin layer over the affected area 1-2 times a day.

Route

Topical.

Side Effects

Allergic or sensitivity response and possible skin discoloration.

Warnings

Should not be used by patients with known sulfa drug allergy. Caution should be used in patients with a history of drug allergy or liver or kidney disorder.

Special Patient Teaching Considerations

Use this product sparingly and avoid prolonged use. If the affected area is not healing, notify the physician.

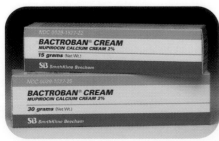

Bactroban®

Mupirocin (Bactroban®) is an antibiotic ointment indicated for treatment of impetigo due to certain staph and strep infections.

Bactroban®
(mupirocin)
Courtesy of Smith, Kline, Beecham

Doxycycline Hyclate (Doryx®, Vibramycin®)

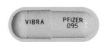

100 mg capsule

50 mg capsule

Vibramycin®
(doxycycline hyclate)
Courtesy of Pfizer

Action and Indication

A broad-spectrum **tetracycline group antibiotic** that is used for acne and a variety of bacterial infections such as urinary tract infections, Rocky Mountain Spotted Fever, and amoebic dysentery.

Dosage

Dependent upon disease treated and severity. For example: 100 mg, two times a day PO on the first day, followed by 100 mg 1-2 times a day for the next 6 days.

Route

PO capsules, tablets or liquid (for dermatological considerations).

Side Effects

As with tetracycline, developmental tooth discoloration may occur in fetuses or children under the age of 8. Hypersensitivity, photosensitivity and allergic response may also occur, e.g., angioedema (chest pain, swelling of face, throat and extremities), and dysphagia (difficulty swallowing).

Warnings

May cause tooth discoloration during tooth development. Secondary infections and allergic reactions are possible. Drugs such as antacids and iron supplements may decrease the absorption of this agent.

Special Patient Teaching Considerations

Be aware of possible photosensitive reactions and avoid prolonged exposure to the sun or tanning booths. Notify a physician of any side effects. Although this medication may be taken without regard to meals, it may be taken with milk to avoid possible gastric upset. These tablets or capsules should be swallowed whole.

DERMATOLOGICALS

Clotrimazole and Betamethasone Dipropionate (Lotrisone®)

Action and Indication

This product is a topical antifungal (clotrimazole) and steroid (betamethasone) combination medication used to treat cases of athlete's foot, ringworm, and jock itch. The antifungal element will control yeast growth while the steroid component will address associated inflammation and itching.

Dosage

This product is available in tubes of 15 and 45 grams. Apply lightly and gently to the affected areas two times a day. *This product is not recommended for use on children or pregnant women.*

Route

Topical cream.

Side Effects

Local irritation, blisters, hives, rash, and possible signs of steroidal use such as edema and Cushing's syndrome (bruises, hypertension, mood swings, edema and weight gain).

Warnings

Allergic reaction possible. Should not be used by pregnant women. Monitor the patient for signs or symptoms of Cushing's syndrome.

Special Patient Teaching Considerations

Use only as directed and apply this medication sparingly and gently. Notify the physician of any signs of adverse effects or if there is no improvement in condition after about two weeks of treatment.

Ofloxacin (Floxin®)

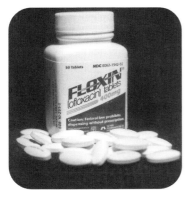

Floxin®
(ofloxacin)
Courtesy of Ortho-McNeill
Pharmaceutical Company

Action and Indication

This gram positive and gram negative broad-spectrum antibiotic is used to treat dermatological infections as well as staph aureus, MRSA, and chlamydia.

Dosage

Dependent upon site and severity of infection. For example: for mild to moderate skin infections, 400 mg PO, every 12 hours to total 800 mg daily for 10-14 days.

Route

PO tablets for mild cases; IV for more severe cases.

Side Effects

GI upset, headache, insomnia, dizziness, or light headedness.

Warnings

Although rare, allergic responses to this drug could be very severe. Should not be used by patients with known quinolone allergies. Caution should be used in patients with a history of seizures or kidney disease.

Special Patient Teaching Considerations

Notify the physician immediately of any signs of adverse effects. Avoid excessive sun exposure and drink plenty of fluids when taking this drug. This drug may be taken without regard to meals.

DRUG CHART

Generic Name	Trade Name	Route	Generic Name	Trade Name	Route
ANTIHISTAMINES			TOPICAL ANTIFUNGALS		
Diphenhydramine	Benadryl	PO, Inj., Top.	Econazole	Spectazole	Top.
	Various	PO, Inj., Top.	Clotrimazole	Lotrimin	Top.
Hydroxyzine	Atarax	PO, Inj.	Ketoconazole	Nizoral	Top.
	Vistaril	PO, Inj.	Clotrimazole / Betamethasone	Lotrisone	Top.
	Various	PO, Inj.			
			TOPICAL ANTINEOPLASTICS		
TOPICAL ANALGESICS			Fluorouracil, 5-FU	Efudex	Top.
Benzocaine	Americaine	Top.			
Capsaicin	Zostrix	Top.	TOPICAL VITAMIN ANALOGS		
	Various	Top.	Alitretinoin	Panretin	Top.
			Tretinoin	Renova	Top.
ANTIPSORIATIC AGENTS				Retin-A	Top.
Methotrexate	Various	PO, Inj.		Various	Top.
Acitretin	Soriatane	PO			
Calcipotriene	Dovonex	Top.	TOPICAL CORTICOSTEROIDS		
Coal Tar	Various	Top.	Betamethasone	Valisone	Top.
Methoxsalen	Oxsoralen	PO, Top.		Various	Top.
Tazarotene	Tazorac	Top.	Clobetasol	Temovate	Top.
				Cormax	Top.
TOPICAL SUNSCREENS			Desonide	Desowen	Top.
Padimate O	Chap Stick	Top.		Tridesilon	Top.
	Various	Top.	Fluocinolone	Synalar	Top.
Para-Aminobenzoic Acid (PABA)	Various	Top.		Various	Top.
			Fluocinonide	Lidex	Top.
TOPICAL ANTI-INFECTIVES			Fluticasone	Cutivate	Top.
Chlorhexidine	Hibiclens	Top.	Hydrocortisone	Cortaid	Top.
	Various	Top.		Various	Top.
Mupirocin	Bactroban	Top.	Mometasone	Elocon	Top.
Silver Sulfadiazine	Silvadene	Top.	Triamcinolone	Aristocort	Top.
	SSD	Top.		Kenalog	Top.

KEY CONCEPTS

✔ The skin is the largest of the body's organs and protects the other organs against microorganisms, trauma, extreme temperature and other harmful elements.

✔ The skin is also called the Integumentary System. It is generally 3-5 millimeters thick, though it is thicker in the palms of the hands and soles of the feet and thinner in the eyelids and genitals.

✔ The skin is comprised of several layers: the epidermis (top layer), dermis (middle layer) and subcutaneous tissue (bottom layer). Within these layers, structures such as hair follicles and shafts, sebaceous and sweat glands, veins, arteries and sensory nerves are found.

✔ The subcutaneous layer is not always considered a part of the skin but simply loose connective tissue that separates the skin from the underlying organs. It is, however, so closely interconnected that it is generally described with the integumentary system.

✔ The outer layer of the epidermis (called the stratum corneum) is constantly replenished with new cells from underneath. The turnover time from cell development to shedding (sloughing) is about 21 days.

✔ Pathological medical conditions and diseases which occur on or in the skin can be caused by inflammation, infection, growth rate changes, trauma, or structural dysfunction. Examples of skin conditions are: burns, cuts, rashes, dandruff, eczema, and skin cancer.

✔ Steroids, antihistamines, and inti-infectives are commonly used to treat skin disorders.

CHOOSE THE BEST ANSWER.   *answers are in the back of the book*

1. The drying agent zinc oxide (ZnO_2) is often seen in a combination product with a local anesthetic, moisture absorbing agent and antibiotic. Which of the following ingredients would be considered as the local anesthetic?
   a. camphor
   b. kaolin
   c. triclosan
   d. diphenhydramine

2. What medication below would be used as a topical antibiotic specifically for burns?
   a. hydrocortisone
   b. silver sulfadiazine
   c. diphenhydramine
   d. ofloxacin

3. The outer layer of the epidermis is constantly replenished with new cells from underneath. The turnover time from cell development to shedding of the epidermis is about
   a. 11 hours
   b. 11 days
   c. 21 hours
   d. 21 days

4. Which of the following medications below would be considered a corticosteroid?
   a. hydrocortisone
   b. silver sulfadiazine
   c. diphenhydramine
   d. ofloxacin

ELECTROLYTIC AGENTS

Maintaining the proper balance of body fluids is essential to health and body function.

Water is the primary element in the body, accounting for more than half of body weight. It is found inside cells (**intracellular fluid**) and outside them (**extracellular fluid**) in plasma and tissue (**interstitial**) fluid.

Electrolytes **are water soluble minerals that are contained in our body fluids as salts.**

They form electrically charged particles called **ions**, which attract water. They have both positive and negative charges and are responsible for fluid movement into and out of cells. Changes in the body's normal electrolyte count affect fluid movement and balance and consequently various body functions.

Examples of common electrolytes include sodium (Na^+), potassium (K^+), calcium (Ca^{++}), chloride (Cl^-) and magnesium (Mg^{++}).

The plus and minus signs indicate their electrical charges. Functions these electrolytes affect include blood pressure, blood coagulation, muscle contractions, myocardial conduction, energy levels and enzyme production. In the following pages, electrolyte disorders and suggested therapies for restoring normal sodium, potassium, calcium and magnesium balance will be identified and explored.

anions a negatively charged ion.

cations a positively charged ion.

dissociation when a compound breaks down and separates into smaller components.

electrolytes a substance that in solution forms ions that conduct an electrical current.

extracellular fluids the fluid outside the body's individual cells found in plasma and tissue fluid.

intracellular fluids cell fluid.

interstitial fluid tissue fluid.

ions electrically charged particles.

Opposites Attract

Water molecules (H_2O) are **polarized**. That is, they have positively and negatively charged sides. For this reason, many compounds **dissociate** (come apart) in water to form ions and the ions in turn **associate** with the water molecules.

The dissociation of sodium chloride (NaCl) into Na^+ and Cl^- ions followed by their association with water molecules is depicted at right. H_2O is attracted at its negative pole to the positive sodium ion and at its positive pole to the negative chloride ion.

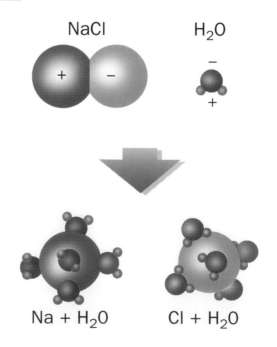

NaCl   H₂O

Na + H₂O   Cl + H₂O

Hypernatremia (high serum sodium concentration)

Sodium is a major cation and profoundly effects the fluid movement in and out of the body's cells. Hypernatremia is the condition of having too much sodium. It results from excessive water deficit, water loss exceeding sodium loss, or in cases of fluid overload where sodium gain is greater than the water gain. Patients at risk include infants, elderly, those with conditions such as diabetes insipidus, severe debilitation, or an illness that would produce profuse sweating, fever and/or protracted vomiting and diarrhea. In addition, those receiving IV sodium, diuretics, mannitol, and strong laxatives are also capable of becoming hypernatremic.

Patients with hypernatremia may experience spastic and hypertonic muscular responses, restlessness, thirst, and ataxia (abnormal lack of coordination). In severe cases, seizures, coma, or even death could occur.

Therapy

Along with treating the underlying medical disorder which may have lead to this condition, a 5% dextrose IV solution would be indicated to replace the water deficit or 0.45%-0.9% NaCl to replace intravascular volume. Caution: serum sodium levels must be decreased slowly to avoid risk of cerebral edema, neurological damage, seizures or even death. Drugs such as vasopressors and antidiuretics may be prescribed as adjunctive treatment.

Hyponatremia (low serum sodium concentration)

Hyponatremia is a sodium deficit that causes fluid to move out of the cells in an effort to increase blood volume and make up for the extracellular loss. Its symptoms include tachycardia, poor skin turgor, decreased urination, muscle cramps, nausea/vomiting and hypotension. If the decrease of sodium is rapid, more severe symptoms such as seizure, disorientation, and coma could occur.

Therapy

Since the etiology of hyponatremia is often dehydration, GI illness (vomiting/diarrhea), or excessive use of diuretics, therapy usually involves fluid and sodium replacement (i.e. 0.9% NaCl to infuse over a period of 6-12 hours). In certain circumstances, where water levels are at a significantly higher percentage than sodium, causing fluid volume to be high, loop diuretics may be necessary to encourage the loss of water. Both water and salt (sodium) may also be restricted in this case.

ELECTROLYTIC AGENTS

Hyperkalemia (high potassium levels)

Hyperkalemia is a condition of high potassium levels manifested by muscle weakness, possible paralysis and loss of feeling in the legs, traveling up to the arms. Muscle twitching and cramping can also occur as the potassium level rises. Excessive potassium levels can lead to cardiac arrhythmias, including heart block.

Therapy

The patient receiving potassium therapy needs to be frequently assessed regarding their ECG results. There will be definitive changes noted should this condition be present. Calcium may be administered to correct arrhythmias, although it does not actually lower potassium levels. IV glucose, insulin, or sodium bicarbonate will promote movement of the potassium out of the cells. If a patient already has ECG changes, the resin sodium polystyrene sulfonate would not be indicated, but it does effectively rid the body of potassium. Hemodialysis may be employed should this condition continue.

Hypokalemia (low potassium levels)

Hypokalemia is a condition of low potassium levels that is often attributed to dehydration and fluid loss due to GI illness (vomiting/diarrhea), fever, diuretics, surgery or medical condition necessitating the use of naso-gastric drainage. Signs and symptoms of hypokalemia include: cardiac arrhythmias with marked ECG changes, glucose intolerance, muscle weakness, cramping, and possible paralysis.

Therapy

Potassium replacement therapy is often indicated and may be administered PO or IV (for severe cases). Sustained-release oral products are found to be more easily tolerated as they are not as upsetting to the GI tract. Chloride and non-chloride salts as well as potassium sparing diuretics may also be prescribed in some cases.

Hypercalemia (high calcium levels)

Hypercalemia is a condition of high calcium levels often caused by hyperparathyroidism, due to benign parathyroid tumor growth. Certain malignancies such as of the breast, skin and bladder may also lead to this condition. While there are definitive ECG changes associated with hypercalemia, it often is asymptomatic except in cases associated with cancers where nausea/vomiting, anorexia, frequent urination, and thirst may be present.

Therapy

Normal Saline

A solution of 0.9% sodium chloride and distilled water. It has an ion concentration similar to blood serum.

IV normal saline may be ordered for hydration and diuretics may follow to increase urine output. Drugs such as furosemide, prednisone, gallium nitrate, and mithramycin may be indicated while calcitonin IV is used in emergency situations.

Hypocalemia (low calcium levels)

Hypocalemia, or low calcium levels, may be related to hypoparathyroidism, vitamin D deficiency, GI diseases, or surgery. Tetany, hyperexcitability of nerve and muscle fibers, is a major symptom of hypocalemia. A decrease in myocardial contractility and muscle spasms and cramps may also occur.

Therapy

IV administration of soluble calcium salts (e.g., carbonate, chloride, gluconate) is a common form of treatment while certain cases may require oral calcium supplements, magnesium and vitamin D.

ELECTROLYTIC AGENTS

Hypermagnesemia (high magnesium levels)

Hypermagnesemia often occurs in cases of kidney filtration rate dysfunction. Patients who are receiving magnesium products (i.e., antacids) to treat ulcers, early labor, or eclampsia (a pregnancy based condition causing high blood pressure and fluid retention) are at a higher risk to develop high serum magnesium levels. Muscle weakness and diminished reflexes may occur in cases of mild hypermagnesemia, while paralysis, respiratory distress, heart block, and sedation leading to coma or death can occur with higher concentrations.

Therapy

IV calcium will address both the cardiovascular and the neuromuscular effects of hypermagnesemia. IV furosemide and saline will promote the excretion of magnesium. Vasopressors, ventilation, and pacemakers may be necessary until the magnesium levels are lowered.

Hypomagnesemia (low magnesium levels)

Hypomagnesemia may be due to malabsorption disorders, loss of GI fluids, excessive diuretic usage, or deprivation diets. Hyperreflex, muscle twitching, depression, confusion, delirium, and ventricular arrhythmias are common signs and symptoms of this condition. If the case is mild, and the patient is not symptomatic, oral magnesium supplements may be indicated.

Therapy

IV magnesium supplements would be ordered as the severity increased.

Note: IV magnesium is diluted to about 20% to avoid pain and venous damage during administration. Magnesium is also infused slowly and may need to be repeated due to a large percentage of excretion.

Potassium Chloride (K-Dur®, Micro-K®, Slow-K®, and Kaon-Cl®)

Action and Indication

This product is used in the prevention and treatment of hypokalemia (low potassium levels). This condition may occur while taking diuretics, digitalis, or during certain disease states.

Dosage

4-10 tablets or capsules of potassium chloride daily is recommended in the treatment of low potassium levels. For hypokalemia prevention, 2-3 tablets or capsules is suggested. The amount of potassium equals 20-100 mEq daily with no more than 40 mEq given in a single dose.

Route

PO tablets or capsules.

Side Effects

Hyperkalemia and GI effects such as diarrhea, abdominal pain, blockage, and possible bleeding.

Warning

Use caution in patients with history of liver or kidney disease, heart disease, diabetes, dehydration, severe burns, and ulcers. Use caution in patients taking ACE inhibitors. Ventricular ectopy and arrhythmias may be reduced with serum potassium levels of 4.0 mEq/L or greater.

Special Patient Teaching Considerations

Notify physician of black or tarry stools and do not change brands of potassium chloride.

Used for hypokalemia

DRUG CHART

Generic Name	Trade Name	Route
ACIDIFYING AGENTS		
Ammonium Chloride (NH_4Cl)	Various	Injectable
ALKALINIZING AGENTS		
Sodium Bicarbonate ($NaHCO_3$)	Various	Inj.
Sodium Lactate ($C_3H_5NaO_3$)	Various	Inj.
ELECTROLYTE REPLACEMENTS		
Potassium Chloride (KCl)	Various	PO, Inj.
Calcium Chloride ($CaCl_2$)	Various	Inj.
Calcium Gluconate	Various	Inj.
Sodium Chloride ($NaCl$)	Various	Inj.
Magnesium Sulfate ($MgSO_4$)	Various	Inj.
DIURETICS		
Amiloride	Midamor	PO
Bumetanide	Bumex	PO, Inj.
	Various	PO, Inj.
Chlorthalidone	Hygroton	PO
	Various	PO
Ethacrynic Acid	Edecrin	PO, Inj.
Furosemide	Lasix	PO, Inj.
	Various	PO, Inj.
Hydrochlorothiazide, HCTZ	Various	PO
Indapamide	Lozol	PO
	Various	PO
Metolazone	Zaroxolyn	PO
	Mykrox	PO
Spironolactone	Aldactone	PO
	Various	PO
Torsemide	Demadex	PO, Inj.
Triamterene	Dyrenium	PO
Triamterene / Hydrochlorothiazide	Dyazide	PO
OVER THE COUNTER ELECTROLYTE REPLACEMENTS		
	Gatorade	PO
	Pedialyte	PO

KEY CONCEPTS

✔ Proper fluid balance is essential to health and body function. Water is the primary element in the body, accounting for more than half of body weight. It is found inside cells (intracellular fluid) and outside them (extracellular fluid) in plasma and tissue (interstitial) fluid.

✔ Water molecules (H_2O) are polarized. That is, they have positively and negatively charged sides. For this reason, many compounds dissociate in water to form ions and the ions in turn associate with the water molecules. Anions are negatively charged ions. Cations are positively charged.

✔ Electrolytes are water soluble minerals contained in body fluids as salts. They form ions that attract water. They have both positive and negative charges and are responsible for fluid movement into and out of cells. Examples of common electrolytes include sodium (Na^+), potassium (K^+), calcium (Ca^{++}), chloride (Cl^-) and magnesium (Mg^{++}).

✔ Hypernatremia is the condition of having too much sodium. It can result from excessive water deficit, water loss exceeding sodium loss, or where sodium gain is greater than the water gain.

✔ Hyponatremia is a sodium deficit that causes fluid to move out of the cells in an effort to increase blood volume and make up for the extracellular loss.

✔ Hyperkalemia is a condition of high potassium levels manifested by muscle weakness, possible paralysis and loss of feeling in the legs, traveling up to the arms.

✔ Hypokalemia is a condition of low potassium levels often attributed to dehydration and fluid loss.

✔ Hypercalemia is a condition of high calcium levels often caused by hyperparathyroidism.

✔ Hypocalemia, or low calcium levels, may be related to hypoparathyroidism, vitamin D deficiency, GI diseases, or surgery.

✔ Hypermagnesemia a condition of high magnesium levels with symptoms ranging from mild to severe, including fatal. Hypomagnesemia a condition of low magnesium levels.

CHOOSE THE BEST ANSWER. *answers are in the back of the book*

1. Hyperparathyroidism is often associated with:
   a. hyperkalemia
   b. hpercalcemia
   c. hypermagnesemia
   d. none of the above

2. Of the following electrolytes, which one has a negative (-) charge?
   a. sodium (Na)
   b. potassium (K)
   c. calcium (Ca)
   d. chloride (Cl)

3. Which of the following electrolytes is associated with hypokalemia?
   a. sodium (Na)
   b. potassium (K)
   c. calcium (Ca)
   d. chloride (Cl)

4. Which electrolyte is considered the major cation that profoundly effects the fluid movement in and out of the body's cells?
   a. sodium (Na)
   b. potassium (K)
   c. calcium (Ca)
   d. chloride (Cl)

GASTROINTESTINAL AGENTS

Gastrointestinal agents are used to treat disorders of the stomach and/or the intestines.

The drugs that address and treat various stomach and intestinal disorders include enzymes, antidiarrheals, antiemetics (anti-vomiting), antiulcer agents, laxatives, and stool softeners.

The GI organs are intimately related to the digestive system as a whole.

The other alimentary tract organs (mouth and esophagus), the accessory organs of digestion (salivary, gastric, and intestinal glands, liver, gall bladder, and pancreas), and the organs of elimination (rectum and anus) are often affected by direct GI disorders. For example, it is not uncommon for a colon cancer to metastasize not only to the stomach, but to the pancreas, liver, and rectum as well. As a result, although specific site antineoplastic drugs and treatments are available, agents may be used that treat more than one site and cell type at a time. **Gastric reflux** is another example. Gastric hyperacidity will often travel toward the chest and throat area via the esophagus. Antacid drugs that inhibit acidity of the stomach will provide for rest and healing of the esophagus when this happens.

THE DIGESTIVE SYSTEM

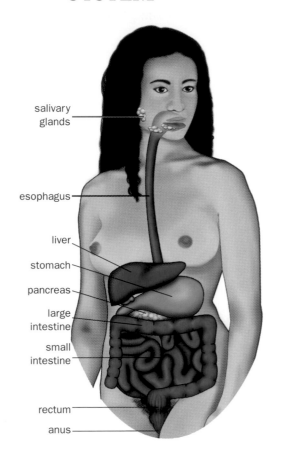

The stomach lies in the upper left quadrant of the abdomen between the lower end of the esophagus and the beginning of the small intestine (duodenum). This organ serves to store and chemically break down food using hydrochloric acid and pepsinogen. **Chyme** is the semi-liquid form of food as it enters the duodenum. **Peristalsis** is the wave-like motion which moves the food products along the intestinal tract.

Together, the small intestine and the large intestine make up about 28 feet of bowel (intestine). Most food absorption takes place in the small intestine. The large intestine absorbs water and connects to the rectum and anus for stool evacuation.

The GI organs are large in mass compared to other systems' organs and play a major role in normal body function. As a result, dysfunction, abnormality or other pathologic medical conditions of the GI tract may require serious and immediate drug therapy as well as other forms of medical or surgical intervention. Similar to other organ systems, preventive care and early detection of pathology is suggested and encouraged.

chyme the semi-liquid form of food as it enters the intestinal tract.

peristalsis the wave like motion of the intestines that moves food through them.

GASTROINTESTINAL AGENTS

Enzymes

Pepsin is a normally present gastric enzyme that breaks down proteins. However, in the absence of pepsin, it is still possible for the digestive system to break down protein molecules into amino acids using **proteolytic enzymes** from the pancreas that are found in the small intestine. These enzymes are capable of attacking starches and fats. If a patient's condition warrants treatment using **enzyme therapy** (as with cystic fibrosis and chronic pancreatitis), products that contain pancreatin, an agent prepared from hog pancreas, or pancrelipase may be indicated. **Malabsorption** conditions such as **steatorrhea**, where fat is inadequately digested and is excreted in large amounts in feces, may be treated with pancrelipase.

Antidiarrheals

Diarrhea is a condition of frequent watery stools which results from microorganism invasion, drug or stress reaction, and/or other circumstances causing a decrease in intestinal absorption of water, an increased secretion of electrolytes into the intestines or an excessive amount of mucus production. **Antiperistalsis drugs** slow the movement of the intestinal contents to allow for greater water and electrolyte absorption. Loperamide is a common antiperistalsis agent and diphenoxylate plus atropine is another popular antidiarrheal agent. Bismuth subsalicylate (Pepto-Bismol) is a **secretion inhibitor** that acts to prevent organisms from attaching to the intestinal mucosa and may deactivate certain toxins as well. In cases of infectious diarrhea, antibiotics such as metronidazole and vancomycin may also be indicated and ordered in conjunction with other therapies. Note: Some antibiotics can kill normal bacterial flora or facilitate regrowth of resistant microorganisms, and so lead to diarrhea.

Antiemetics

This class of drugs treats the condition of nausea and vomiting. There are many causes for this condition which is usually a symptom or side effect as opposed to being the actual condition itself: food or drug reaction or allergy, pregnancy, anxiety, exhaustion, dehydration, and a large number of diseases or illnesses such as cancer, or a microorganism related infectious process such as a middle ear infection. Often, antiemetics are ordered concurrently with other drug therapies used to treat the underlying condition. Vomiting is a reflex that occurs from a variety of stimuli. The treatment is to reduce the hyperactivity of stimuli receptors and lower the impulse rate. Also, decreasing the sensitivity to emetic chemicals found in the blood will inhibit the vomiting reflex. Dehydration and electrolyte imbalance are of major concern with prolonged vomiting.

GASTROINTESTINAL AGENTS

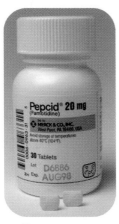

Pepcid® (famotidine) is used for short-term treatment of acid reflux and stomach ulcers.

Courtesy of Merck Archives

Gastric Reflux

Gastric Reflux is a more serious gastric acid condition that is often treated with a strong antacid.

Enemas

Enemas may be placed into this category since they are indicated in cases of constipation, pre-medical treatment, and to ease the stress of bowel movements. Fleets, sodium biphosphate and sodium phosphate, is a popular saline enema.

Antacid/Antiulcer Agents

Antacids, generally composed of inorganic salts such as calcium carbonate, aluminum hydroxide, and magnesium hydroxide are popular antiulcer agents that act to neutralize existing acid, as opposed to inhibiting its production. Antacids are most indicated at the onset of hypergastric activity, are pain relieving yet short acting, and not strong enough for a diagnosed ulcer condition. Caution should be exercised to not rely on anatacids alone or for a prolonged time. If ulcer symptoms persist, the physician should be notified. Maalox is an example of a common antacid.

Cimetidine is a **histamine receptor antagonist.** It inhibits the secretion of gastric acid by blocking the effects of histamine. This type of agent was first approved for use in 1977 and revolutionized standard antacid therapy. Cimetidine has a history of drug interactions, however, and improved histamine antagonists (ranitidine, famotidine, and nizatidine) have since been developed.

Peptic ulcer is caused by hypergastric acidity that erodes tissue in localized areas of the stomach and intestines. While these lesions are normally benign, they may produce symptoms that are mild and of minor discomfort or they may be more serious and extend to underlying layers of connective tissue and smooth muscle. In these cases, blood vessels can be affected and bleeding can occur. A special dietary regime (i.e., frequent, small, bland, non-acid containing meals) together with selected drug therapy is commonly recommended for treatment of this condition.

Laxatives and Stool Softeners

These agents are commonly prescribed to treat **constipation,** the condition of dehydrated stool in which bowel movements are infrequent, hard, and often painful and difficult. Aside from changing a patient's diet, fluid intake and activity level, drug therapy may be suggested. Laxatives promote defecation without stress or pain and are often suggested for use prior to certain medical procedures related to the bowel (e.g., colonoscopy, barium enema), for constipation, and for patients who have hemorrhoids, recent hernia surgery, or a heart attack.

There are several types of laxatives available: **bulk forming,** that swell as they mix with intestinal contents; **stimulant,** that irritate the lining and nerves of the intestine; **saline,** that rapidly promote watery stool by drawing water into the intestine; and **osmotic,** that increase the stool's water content using osmosis. The osmotic laxative is often used as a **retention enema,** although it can be powerful and cause cramping. Lactulose (Chronulac® Syrup) is an example of a commonly prescribed saline laxative.

Docusate sodium (Colace®) is a commonly ordered **stool softener,** or emollient laxative. It promotes the mixing of fatty and watery intestinal substances to soften the stool's contents and ease the evacuation of feces.

Pancrelipase (Pancrease®, Creon®, Viokase®, Ultrase®, Cotazym®)

Action and Indication

This pancreatic enzyme is given to patients with pancreatic enzyme deficiencies due to blockage of pancreas or common bile duct, cystic fibrosis, or chronic pancreatitis. These capsules contain lipase, protease, and amylase and aid in the digestion of fats, proteins, and starches.

Dosage

Dosage will vary with severity of deficiency and patient condition. May range from 1-3 capsules or tablets with meals and 1 with snacks, ranging from 4,000-20,000 units with each meal.

Route

PO capsules or tablets.

Side Effects

GI upset. Allergic reaction is rare but possible.

Warnings

Contraindicated for patients with acute pancreatitis or allergic response to pork protein. Possible drug interactions with antiulcer or antacid agents. It may be necessary to give a histamine blocker at the same time to avoid gastric acid destruction of the enzyme.

Special Patient Teaching Considerations

Do not take antacids without a doctor's permission and notify the physician if an allergic response occurs. Do not change brands as that could effect the drug's efficacy. Also, note that keeping this agent in the mouth can cause mouth sores.

ANTIDIARRHEALS

Loperamide Hydrochloride (Imodium®, Imodium AD®)

Action and Indication

This agent inhibits peristalsis of the GI tract and halts diarrhea. Often prescribed for cases of "Traveler's Diarrhea" and to reduce stool volume from a colonostomy.

Dosage

To start, 2 capsules, caplets, or teaspoons (4 mg) followed by one capsule, caplet, or teaspoon (2 mg) after each loose stool. Daily dosage should not exceed 8 capsules (16 mg).

Route

PO capsules, caplets, or cherry-flavored liquid.

Side Effects

GI distress, possible allergic reaction including rash, drowsiness, dry mouth.

Warnings

This medication is not indicated for cases of acute diarrhea or diarrhea caused by bacteria (i.e., food poisoning). Caution should be used in children under the age of two or for the elderly, as these patients are in greater danger of developing dehydration. Patient's medical history is important, especially if the patient has had liver disease since extreme nervousness and/or seizures could develop.

Special Patient Teaching Considerations

Notify the physician if any signs of abdominal distention or constipation occur. Drink plenty of fluids and perhaps suck on hard candy to avoid dry mouth discomfort. Since drowsiness could occur, caution with daily activities should be exercised. If symptoms of diarrhea persist or become worse (severe cramping, blood in stools, fever), notify the physician immediately.

Diphenoxylate Hydrochloride and Atropine Sulfate (Lomotil®)

Action and Indication

A narcotic-like antidiarrheal that slows GI movement. Note: Atropine is added to reduce the narcotic potential of this medication.

Dosage

2 tablets or teaspoons 3-4 times a day, until diarrhea is controlled. A follow-up dosage of 2 tablets or teaspoons per day may be indicated.

Route

PO tablets, liquid.

Side Effects

Due to the **atropine effect** (drying of secretions), dry mouth, tachycardia and urinary retention could occur. Serious conditions such as paralytic ileus (stopping of peristalsis) and toxic megacolon (swelling of intestine with unabsorbed fluid) are possible.

Warnings

Patients must be monitored for signs of ileus (intestinal blockage) or a dilated colon. Patient history is important, especially if there have been incidences of obstructive jaundice, ulcerative colitis, liver or kidney disease. This product can become addictive. Certain antibiotics (i.e. Ceclor, Achromycin) may cause diarrhea.

Special Patient Teaching Considerations

Notify the physician if this condition does not improve in two days or if signs of abdominal distention, fluid retention, difficulty urinating, dizziness, or fever should occur. Drink plenty of fluids and eat bland foods. Avoid the concurrent use of alcohol.

ANTIEMETICS

Trimethobenzamide Hydrochloride (Tigan®)

Action and Indication

This agent acts to reduce nausea and vomiting, primarily in adults (caution should be used with children), by effecting the parasympathetic nervous system receptors in an anticholinergic response.

Dosage

250 mg PO 3-4 times a day. 200 mg PR (suppository) and IM 3-4 times a day.

Route

PO tablets; IM and PR.

Side Effects

Allergic skin reactions, drowsiness, blurred vision, depression, and possible parkinsonian-like symptoms.

Warnings

Allergic reaction possible. Caution should be exercised if treating children since there have been cases of Reye's Syndrome associated with Tigan use. Other conditions (e.g., appendicitis) may be masked while using this agent.

Special Patient Teaching Considerations

Do not give this product to children without a physician's consent. Report severe side effects and continuation of nausea/vomiting to your doctor. Watch for signs of drowsiness and take appropriate action (avoidance of activities that involve mental alertness).

Prochlorperazine Maleate (Compazine®)

Action and Indication
Treats nausea and vomiting by inhibiting the chemo-receptors and slowing response of the stimuli causing the nausea. This agent is indicated in cases of severe nausea.

Dosage
5-10 mg tablet PO three to four times per day; 10-15 mg PO long-acting spansule twice daily in divided doses; 25 mg PR (rectally via suppository), 2 times a day; 5-10 mg IM four to six times a day (not to exceed 40 mg in a 24 hour period).

Route
PO tablet, long-acting spansule, syrup; IM and PR.

Side Effects
Hypotension, drowsiness, muscle rigidity and abnormalities of movement, blurred vision, and agitation.

Warnings
This patient can experience an increased risk of seizure activity and tardive dyskinesia (twitching and muscle spasms). Elderly women are at a higher risk for this event. Allergic reaction possible.

Special Patient Teaching Considerations
Avoid usage of alcohol and barbiturates when taking this drug. Also avoid prolonged exposure to sunlight and heat. Do not abruptly discontinue this drug as dizziness, appetite changes, and tremors could occur.

ANTACID / ANTIULCER

Magnesium Hydroxide and Aluminum Hydroxide (Maalox®)

Action and Indication

A popular OTC antacid used to treat heartburn, acid indigestion, and forms of mild gastric discomfort such as gas and overeating. This agent acts to neutralize the acids, not inhibit their production.

Dosage

1-2 chewable tablets 1 hour after meals and bedtime or 2-4 teaspoons 1 hour after meals and at bedtime.

Route

PO chewable tablets or liquid suspension.

Side Effects

Cramps, constipation, increased thirst.

Warnings

Caution should be used in patients with history of Alzheimer's, kidney dysfunction, or sodium restrictions. Patients should take this agent two hours from taking other medications such as antibitotics, digoxin, lithium products, phenytoin, and iron salts. Absorption may be reduced.

Special Patient Teaching Considerations

Notify a physician if hyperacidity discomfort continues or black tarry stools occur. This agent is meant for short term symptom relief. If problems persist, a serious medical problem could be involved. Drink plenty of water with this product.

Cimetidine (Tagamet®)

Action and Indication

This antiulcer **histamine blocking agent** is commonly prescribed in cases of gastric reflux, intestinal and gastric ulcers, and ulcer prevention. Cimetidine acts to inhibit the secretion of gastric acid.

Dosage

Dependent upon indication and patient condition. For example, 800 mg PO every bedtime; 300 mg PO, 4 times a day with meals and at bedtime.

Route

PO tablets and liquid; IV.

Side Effects

Headache, agitation, confusion (esp. in the elderly), breast development in men.

Warnings

This agent will affect the blood levels of several common drugs (e.g., phenytoin, lidocaine, propranolol, and aminophylline). If the patient is also taking antacids, space them at least two hours apart. Caution should be used in patients with a history of liver and/or kidney dysfunction.

Special Patient Teaching Considerations

Take antacids two hours apart from cimetidine and avoid excessive amounts of caffeine or any alcohol while taking this drug. Notify a physician should black tarry stools appear as a bleeding ulcer could be present.

Famotidine (Pepcid®)

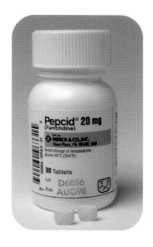

Pepcid®
(famotidine)
Courtesy of Merck Archives

Action and Indication

Pepcid is a **histamine blocker** that helps prevent excess acid release and selected medical conditions hyperacidity causes (e.g., duodenal and gastric ulcers, or acid refux from the stomach to the esophagus). This drug is also available in an over-the-counter preparation and indicated for treatment of heartburn and acid indigestion.

Dosage

To start, the recommended dose ranges from 20-40 mg once daily, depending upon the severity and type of condition to be treated. A maintenance dose may be suggested (e.g., 20 mg daily) after 4-8 weeks of acute treatment. This medication is also available in IV form for severe cases.

Route

Generally PO tablets or oral suspension. Also available for IV therapy.

Side Effects

Headache, abdominal discomfort, and possible hair loss.

Warnings

Possible allergic reaction. Use caution in patients with history of renal dysfunction. Patients should be assessed for signs or symptoms of GI cancer before prescribing this drug. Patients should avoid aspirin and use ibuprofen instead to avoid increased risk of GI bleeding.

Special Patient Teaching Considerations

Report chronic abdominal pain or difficulty swallowing to your physician. Do not continue taking over-the-counter Pepcid for a period of over two weeks, without notifying a physician.

Lansoprazole (Prevacid®)

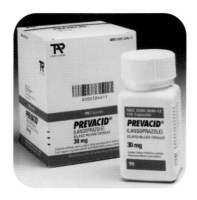

Prevacid®
(lanzoprazole)
Courtesy of Tap
Pharmaceuticals, Inc.

Action and Indication

This agent inhibits gastric acid secretion and is indicated in cases of duodenal ulcers, esophageal reflux, hyeracid diseases such as Zollinger-Ellison syndrome, and for bacterial events such as H. Pylori (Helicobacter pylori). It is used mostly for short treatment protocols and a reduction in dosage is recommended for patients with liver dysfunction.

Dosage

15-30 mg every day, before a meal, for 4-8 weeks, depending on the disease and it's severity.

Route

PO capsules and delayed release capsules.

Side Effects

GI effects such as diarrhea, nausea, and possible abdominal pain.

Warnings

Allergic reaction possible. For treatment of H. Pylori, antibiotics should be taken at the same time. Blood levels of gastrin should be monitored and prescription of a histamine blocking agent considered should the levels significantly increase.

Special Patient Teaching Considerations

Take this drug before a meal. Notify the physician regarding other concurrent drug therapy such as ampicillin and iron as these agents may interfere with the effectiveness of lanzoprazole.

ANTACID / ANTIULCER

Nizatidine (Axid®)

Action and Indication

Nizatidine is a **histamine blocker** prescribed in cases of duodenal and peptic ulcer disease. It is also used for heartburn and esophageal inflammation.

Dosage

300 mg daily at bedtime or 150 mg twice daily.

Route

PO, pulvules.

Side Effects

GI symptoms such as nausea, abdominal pain, and diarrhea. Possibly headache and weakness could also occur.

Warnings

Allergic reaction possible. Use caution in patients with kidney dysfunction.

Special Patient Teaching Considerations

Notify the physician if ulcer discomfort continues after 4-8 weeks of therapy. Further medical tests may be indicated. Note that taking aspirin at the same time could cause increased discomfort.

Ranitidine Hydrochloride (Zantac®)

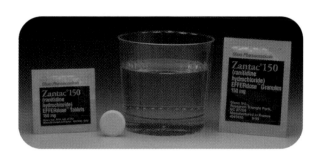

Zantac®
(ranitidine hydrochloride)
Courtesy of Glaxo Wellcome

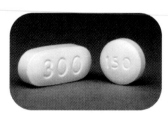

ranitidine hydrochloride
300mg and 150 mg tablets
Courtesy of Novopharm USA

Action and Indication

This anti-ulcer medication acts as a **histamine blocker** inhibiting acid production. It is indicated in cases of peptic ulcer disease, esophageal reflux, and Zollinger-Ellison syndrome.

Dosage

150 mg two times a day to start. A total of 300 mg may be prescribed to be taken once a day after dinner or at bedtime. Note: the above dosage regimes are meant for PO use. IV Zantac is also available for more serious cases.

Route

PO tablets or liquid; IV.

Side Effects

Possible severe headache, confusion, agitation, elevated liver function tests, and rare cardiac rhythm irregularities.

Warnings

Zantac may result in a false positive urine protein reading. Patients should not use selected antacids such as Maalox and Mylanta concurrently. Dosage may be decreased for patient's with kidney/liver dysfunction. Patient should be assessed for possibility of gastric carcinoma.

Special Patient Teaching Considerations

If GI distress symptoms persist while taking this drug, notify the physician.

ANTACID / ANTIULCER

Cisapride (Propulsid®)

Action and Indication

This agent acts to increase the release of acetylcholine which speeds gastric emptying and reduces esophageal sphincter pressure. Propulsid is indicated in cases of heartburn and esophageal reflux.

Dosage

10-20 mg taken 4 times a day, at least 15 minutes before meals and again at bedtime.

Route

PO tablets.

Side Effects

GI effects such as abdominal pain, nausea, bloating, and diarrhea.

Warnings

Contraindicated for use with ketoconazole, itraconazole, miconazole, fluconazole, erythromycin, clarithromycin, and troleandomycin. Should not be used in patients with gastrointestinal hemorrhage, obstruction, or perforation. Caution should be used in patients with history of cardiac disease as it may cause serious arrhythmia.

Special Patient Teaching Considerations

This drug is especially indicated for treatment of night time heartburn and should not be used for cases of day time heartburn. Avoid alcohol while taking this drug.

Omeprazole (Prilosec®)

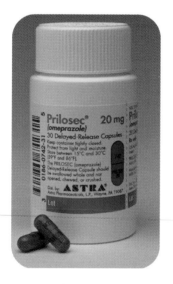

Prilosec®
(omeprazole)
Courtesy of AstraZeneca LP

Prilosec® (omeprazole) is an **acid pump inhibitor** (also called **proton pump inhibitor**) that decreases acid production.

Action and Indication

This drug is indicated in cases of peptic ulcer and esophageal reflux due to it's reduction of gastric acid synthesis. In conjunction with the antibiotic, Biaxin, this drug can also be used in cases of H. Pylori.

Dosage

20-40 mg daily for 4-8 weeks, depending on disease and disease severity. Severe hyperacidity may require higher doses such as 60 mg daily.

Route

PO capsules.

Side Effects

Headache and GI effects such as abdominal pain, nausea/vomiting, and diarrhea.

Warnings

Antibiotics for the treatment of H. Pylori must be started at the same time for best results. Blood levels of gastrin should be monitiored if the patient is receiving Prilosec on a long term basis. A histamine blocking agent may be indicated in cases of significantly increased gastrin levels. Patient should be assessed for gastric carcinoma as this drug can mask the symptoms.

Special Patient Teaching Considerations

Take this drug before a meal. The capsule should be swallowed whole. Avoid caffeine. It may take several days to feel positive effects of omeprazole. Take as directed and notify the physician if relief of symptoms has not occurred after one week.

LAXATIVES & STOOL SOFTENERS

Lactulose (Chronulac® Syrup, Duphalac®)

Action and Indication

Indicated in cases of constipation, this agent raises the osmotic pressure in the colon to increase the frequency and number of bowel movements.

Dosage

1-2 tablespoons daily to equal 15-30 mls initially. There is the possibility of an increase to a total of 60 mls daily.

Route

PO syrup.

Side Effects

Gas, diarrhea, cramps, possible nausea/vomiting.

Warnings

Neomycin can reduce the efficacy of this drug. Use caution in patients with history of diabetes since this product contains sugar.

Special Patient Teaching Considerations

Before taking this drug, notify the physician of any diabetic history or plans to breastfeed. After taking the drug, notify the physician if diarrhea occurs.

Docusate Sodium (Colace®)

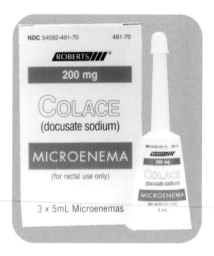

Colace®
(docusate sodium)
Courtesy of Roberts
Pharmaceutical Corporation

Action and Indication

This stool softener promotes easy bowel movements by mixing fat and water in the intestine, thus providing lubrication and softer fecal material. This drug is often used in cases where bowel movement straining could be detrimental to the patient (e.g., following childbirth or a heart attack, and in cases of hernias or high blood pressure).

Dosage

50-100 mg 1-2 times a day.

Route

PO tablets, capsules, oral solution, and syrup; PR rectal solution.

Side Effects

Rare, but allergic rash or bitter taste and nausea may occur.

Warnings

Should not be used concurrently with mineral oil.

Special Patient Teaching Considerations

Colace is indicated for short-term use, for minor constipation or hard stools. Notify the physician if abdominal pain, nausea, vomiting, or rectal pain or bleeding occur.

DRUG CHART

Generic Name	Trade Name	Route	Generic Name	Trade Name	Route
Antidiarrheals			**Antacids**		
Bismuth Subsalicylate	Pepto-Bismol	PO	Aluminum Hydroxide	Amphogel	PO
	Various	PO		Alu-Cap	PO
Diphenoxylate / Atropine	Lomotil	PO	Calcium Carbonate	Alka-Seltzer	PO
	Various	PO		Titralac	PO
Loperamide	Imodium	PO		Tums	PO
	Various	PO		Various	PO
Octreotide	Sandostatin	Inj.	Magnesium Aluminum Hydroxide	Maalox	PO
Kaolin / Pectin	Kaopectate	PO			
				Various	PO
Antiemetics					
Promethazine	Phenergan	PO, PR, Inj.	**Antiulcer**		
	Various	PO, PR, Inj.	proton pump inhibitors		
Prochlorperazine	Compazine	PO, PR, Inj.	Lansoprazole	Prevacid	PO
	Various	PO, PR, Inj.	Omeprazole	Prilosec	PO
Thiethylperazine	Torecan	PO, PR, Inj.	**Gastric Mucosal Agent**		
Trimethobenzamide	Tigan	PO, PR, Inj.	Misoprostol	Cytotec	PO
	Various	PO, PR, Inj.	Sucralfate	Carafate	PO
Dolasetron	Anzemet	PO, Inj.	**Histamine-2 Blockers**		
Granisetron	Kytril	Inj.	Cimetidine	Tagamet	PO, Inj.
Odansetron	Zofran	PO, Inj.		Various	PO, Inj.
			Famotidine	Pepcid	PO, Inj.
Anticholinergics				Mylanta-AR	PO
Dicyclomine	Bentyl	PO, Inj.		Various	PO, Inj.
	Antispas	PO, Inj.	Nizatidine	Axid	PO
	Various	PO, Inj.	Ranitidine	Zantac	PO, Inj.
Glycopyrrolate	Robinul	PO, Inj.		Various	PO, Inj.
	Various	PO, Inj.	Ranitidine Bismuth Citrate	Tritec	PO
Hyoscyamine	Cystospaz	PO			
	Levsin	PO			
	Various	PO			

GENERIC NAME	TRADE NAME	ROUTE
EMETICS		
Ipecac	Ipecac	PO
GASTROINTESTINAL ENZYMES		
Pancreatin	Donnazyme	PO
Pancrelipase	Ku-Zyme	PO
	Cotazym	PO
	Various	PO
Sacrosidase	Sucraid	PO
LAXATIVES / STOOL SOFTENERS		
Bisacodyl	Dulcolax	PO, PR
	Feen-A-Mint	PO
	Various	PO, PR
Lactulose	Cephulac	PO
	Various	PO
Methylcellulose	Citrucel	PO
Psyllium	Metamucil	PO
	Konsyl	PO
Senna	Senokot	PO
Docusate	Colace	PO
	Surfak	PO
	Various	PO
PROKINETIC AGENTS		
Cisapride	Propulsid	PO

REVIEW

KEY CONCEPTS

✔ Gastro-intestinal agents address and treat various stomach and intestinal disorders include enzymes, antidiarrheals, antiemetics, antiulcer agents, laxatives and stool softeners.

✔ Other alimentary tract organs (mouth and esophagus), the accessory organs of digestion (salivary, gastric, and intestinal glands, liver, gall bladder, and pancreas), and the organs of elimination (rectum and anus) are often affected by direct GI disorders.

✔ The stomach stores and breaks down food chemically using hydrochloric acid and pepsinogen.

✔ Chyme is the semi-liquid form of food as it enters the duodenum. Peristalsis is the wave-like motion which moves the food products along the intestinal tract.

✔ Most food absorption takes place in the small intestine while the large intestine absorbs water and connects to the rectum and anus for stool evacuation.

✔ Proteolytic enzymes from the pancreas may be used to break down starches and fats. Enzyme therapy includes the use of products that contain pancreatin, an agent prepared from hog pancreas, or pancrelipase.

✔ Antiperistalsis drugs are used to treat diarrhea by slowing the movement of the intestinal contents to allow for greater water and electrolyte absorption.

✔ In cases of infectious diarrhea, antibiotics such as metronidazole and vancomycin may be indicated and ordered in conjunction with other therapies. Note, however, that some antibiotics can kill normal bacterial flora or facilitate regrowth of resistant microorganisms, and so lead to diarrhea.

✔ Antiemetics treat the urge to vomit by reducing the hyperactivity of stimuli receptors and lower the impulse rate.

✔ Antacids are popular antiulcer agents that act to neutralize existing acid, as opposed to inhibiting its production. Antacids are generally composed of inorganic salts such as calcium carbonate, aluminum hydroxide, and magnesium hydroxide.

✔ Histamine receptor antagonists like cimetidine inhibit the secretion of gastric acid by blocking the effects of histamine.

✔ Gastric reflux is a condition in which gastric hyperacidity travels toward the chest and throat area via the esophagus.

✔ Laxatives promote defecation without stress or pain and are often suggested for use prior to certain medical procedures. There are several types: bulk forming, that swell as they mix with intestinal contents; stimulant, that irritate the lining and nerves of the intestine; saline, that rapidly promote watery stool by drawing water into the intestine; and osmotic, that increase the stool's water content using osmosis.

✔ A stool softener, or emollient laxative, promotes the mixing of fatty and watery intestinal substances to soften the stool's contents and ease the evacuation of feces.

SELF TEST

MATCH THE GENERIC AND TRADE NAMES.   *answers are in the back of the book*

1. Bisacodyl	*Dulcolax*	Alka-Seltzer
2. Calcium Carbonate	*AlkaSeltzer*	Citrucel
3. Cimetidine	*Tagamet*	Colace
4. Cisapride	*Propulsid*	Dulcolax
5. Docusate	*Dulcolax Colace*	Maalox
6. Famotidine	*Pepcid*	Metamucil
7. Lansoprazole	*Prevacid*	Pepcid
8. Magnesium Aluminum	*Maalox*	Prevacid
9. Methylcellulose	*Citrucel*	Prilosec
10. Omeprazole	*Prilosec*	Propulsid
11. Psyllium	*Metamucil*	Tagamet
12. Ranitidine	*Zantac*	Zantac

CHOOSE THE BEST ANSWER.   *answers are in the back of the book*

1. Of the following gastrointestinal agents, which one is used specifically for its antiperistalsis action?
   a. cimetidine
   b. docusate
   c. loperamide
   d. trimethobenzamide

2. Which of the following products is not a brand of pancrelipase?
   a. Chronulac
   b. Cotazyme
   c. Creon
   d. Pancrease

3. Which one of the following would most likely be the safest type of laxative?
   a. bulk laxatives
   b. osmotic laxatives
   c. saline laxatives
   d. stimulant laxatives

4. Which of the following gastrointestinal agents is considered an histamine blocker?
   a. cimetidine
   b. docusate
   c. loperamide
   d. trimethobenzamide

HEMATOLOGICAL AGENTS

Blood coagulation or clotting is a complex process in which the protein *fibrinogen* is transformed to an insoluble fiber called *fibrin*. The enzyme thrombin, which comes from prothrombin, acts on fibrinogen in the blood to cause the transformation. Prothrombin and fibrinogen are *clotting factors* or coagulation factors. Other clotting factors, adequate platelets, and healthy blood vessel walls are also essential components to balanced coagulation.

Each stage of clot development can be affected by clotting factors as well as drugs.

For example, patients with hemophilia A have a genetic deficiency in factor VIII (*most clotting factors are denoted by Roman Numerals)* and can be successfully treated with concentrates of Antihemophilic Factor (AHF) that are commercially available. Factor VIII concentrate or cryoprecipitate and desmopressin acetate are other agents that will act to shorten bleeding time. Von Willebrand's disease, a very common congenital coagulation disorder, is also caused by a deficiency in factor VIII. Factor IX concentrates (Christmas factor) are available for patients with hemophilia B, a condition marked by a deficiency in clotting factor IX.

Phytonadione, or Vitamin K$_1$, is a drug that stimulates the liver to produce several clotting factors and mimics the action of Vitamin K (a natural clotting promoter).

Patients who may develop Vitamin K deficiency and require coagulation enhancer therapy include "at risk" infants whose liver and intestines are not fully developed, users of antibiotics that "sterilize" the intestines and prevent vitamin K synthesis, and those with malabsorption disorders such as Whipple's Disease and obstructive jaundice. In addition, patients with liver disease may suffer with bleeding disorders since the liver is responsible for the synthesizing of many clotting factors.

Clotting

The main stages of natural clot formation and dissolution are:

Thromboplastin is formed from blood and tissue (**platelet aggregation** at injury site).

Thrombin is formed from prothrombin and thromboplastin.

The fiber fibrin is formed from thrombin acting on fibrinogen (clot formation).

Fibrinolysin breaks down fibrin (clot breakdown).

Rx Aside from drug therapy, patients with excessive bleeding may receive whole blood and blood products such as packed cells, platelets, and plasma to treat this serious situation.

clotting factors factors in the blood coagulation process.

fibrinogen Factor I.

fibrin the fiber that serves as the structure for clot formation.

Hematopoietics are drugs that treat various forms of anemias by stimulating or helping to stimulate blood cell growth.

Anemias are generally characterized by a decrease in hemoglobin or red blood cells which leads to a series of other disorders manifested by oxygen deficiency. The classifications of anemias include cell shape and structure, cause, and the pathophysiology or disease tract the particular anemia will take.

Most commonly, anemias develop in the elderly from iron deficiency, as a result of genetic predisposition (e.g., Sickle Cell anemia), or due to vitamin B$_{12}$ deficiency (*pernicious anemia*).

An additional type of anemia is associated with chronic disease. Correction of the underlying illness will improve this anemia. Anemias may also occur as a result of cancer or other diseases and treatments that cause bone marrow suppression and decrease of erythropoietin (which stimulates red blood cell production). In addition, a decrease in the granulocyte colony stimulating factor (G-CSF) and granulocyte macrophage colony stimulating factor (GM-CSF), excessive blood loss, infections, and inflammatory processes contribute to anemia. Common drug therapies for anemias include ferrous sulfate for iron-deficiency anemia and cyanocobalmin for vitamin B$_{12}$ deficiency anemia.

Hemostatic drugs are used to treat or prevent excessive bleeding. Used in OR mainly

Patients who have hemophilia or thrombocytic purpura may receive hemostatic medications. They suffer from a lack of platelets and/or blood clotting factors found in the first stage of clotting. Systemic hemostatic agents include aminocaproic acid, tranexamic acid, and aprotinin. Their indications range from preventing hemorrhages during dental procedures to prevention of blood loss in cardiopulmonary bypass surgery. Their primary action is to inhibit the activation of plasminogen. *Topical hemostatics* are used for minor bleeding of small blood vessels when sutures are not appropriate. Examples of topical hemostatics include thrombin powder, microfibrillar collagen hemostat, and oxidized cellulose.

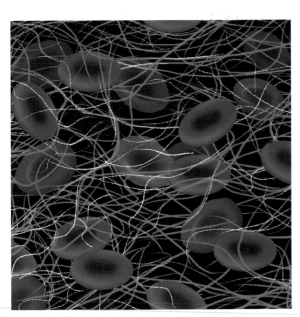

Strands of fibrin interweave and trap red blood cells to form a blood clot.

anemia a decrease in hemoglobin or red blood cells.

hematopoietics drugs used to treat anemia.

hemostatic drugs drugs that prevent excessive bleeding.

topical hemostatics drugs used for minor bleeding when sutures are not appropriate.

COAGULATION ENHANCERS

Desmopressin Acetate (DDAVP)

Action and Indication

Synthetically related to vasopressin (antidiuretic hormone) and indicated to inhibit prolonged bleeding time as well as address platelet dysfunction. It is also used for cases of Hemophilia A and von Willebrand's Disease.

Dosage

A common dosage for bleeding disorders may be 0.3 micrograms per kilogram of body weight, diluted in 50 cc's (ml) of normal saline.

Route

IV infused slowly over a period of 15-30 minutes. The peak levels will be reached in 90-120 minutes and last for about 6 hours. DDAVP can be repeated in 12-24 hours, but the effects are lessened with frequent dosaging. For cases of self-administration, subcutaneous injection is effective and practical. DDAVP is also available as a nasal spray that is used to treat bedwetting and control urination.

Side Effects

GI upset, local irritation at insertion site, possible headaches, and blood pressure changes.

Warnings

The patient's blood pressure and signs of hyponatremia (low sodium) should be monitored during active treatment.

Special Patient Teaching Considerations

Notify the physician of any noted side effects as well as treatment results (absence of bruising or prolonged active bleeding).

Quickens clotting time; Used w/patients w/hemophillia

Phytonadione (Vitamin K$_1$)

Action and Indication

This is the treatment of choice for Vitamin K deficiency or other pathologies relating to coagulation dysfunction.

Dosage

Dependent upon deficiency severity and patient response. For example, 2-25 mg daily for three days for acute "rescue" therapy. Some individuals with abnormal deficiencies may receive 10 mg once monthly or greater, but this is rare.

Route

SQ (subcutaneous), IM, IV or PO. The oral dose will take 6-12 hours to increase blood coagulation factors while even parenteral administration may take up to 48 hours to achieve desired coagulation time results. Note: IV administration has to be cautiously slow, e.g., 1 mg/min. There have been documented deaths when this drug is given IV. Therefore, the preferred routes are SQ or IM.

Side Effects

Hematomas at injection sites, GI distress, rare allergic response.

Warnings

In the event of severe hemorrhage, fresh frozen plasma may be used. If using this treatment for the correction of coumadin overdosage, Vitamin K should be given in low doses only, to make it possible to reinstate effective anticoagulation therapy. Also as an alternative to using Vitamin K, patients should reduce or discontinue their use of drugs that interfere with normal coagulation mechanisms (e.g., salicylates, antibiotics).

Special Patient Teaching Considerations

Notify the physician of any side effects such as prolonged active bleeding.

Injectable form now available

HEMATOPOIETICS

Ferrous Sulfate (Iron, FeSO$_4$)

- toughest on body -

*will cause
constipation
and stools to becoming
very dark.*

*- cause quite a bit
of nausea, recommended
to take it @ night.*

*- take with OJ,
helps with absorption*

Action and Indication

Acts as an iron supplement (element required in red blood cell production) for patients with iron deficiencies, from a variety of causes (anemia and disease-producing anemia related).

Dosage

Dependent upon cause and severity of anemia. For example, for iron deficiency anemia, 325 mg oral iron that is not enteric coated or sustained-release given in 2-3 divided doses a day is suggested. Dietary supplements are also recommended concurrently with this therapy (e.g., meat, fish, and poultry).

Route

PO tablets or elixir. Note: It is possible to receive iron products via Z-tract IM injection or IV for severe cases.

Side Effects

Dark colored stools, cramping, diarrhea, nausea, and constipation.

Warnings

A stool softener such as Colace may be suggested for concurrent use with this drug. Some sources claim that patient tolerance is greater if given twice a day compared to three times a day. Other drugs such as ferrous citrate or ferrous gluconate may be suitable alternative agents.

Special Patient Teaching Considerations

Note that changes in stools are possible and that taking this medication with food would reduce the occurrence of GI upset. In the normal healthy individual, it may take 3-6 months to bring the iron count to a desired level.

tablest or elexirs

Cyanocobalamin (Vitamin B$_{12}$, Cobalamin)

Action and Indication

Used for patients with Vitamin B deficiency such as pernicious anemia.

Dosage

Dependent upon cause of Vitamin B deficiency. For example, for chronic pernicious anemia, the patient may receive a monthly IM injection of 100 micrograms. If the patient has a vitamin malabsorption problem, up to 1000 micrograms IM monthly may be indicated.

Route

IM. Note: PO replacement is rarely indicated unless the individual has a nutritional deficiency.

Side Effects

Local irritation and soreness at injection site, rare allergic response.

Warnings

Be aware of signs and symptoms of Vitamin B deficiency: anemia and neurologic dysfunctioning including ataxia or unsteady gait with reduced mentation.

Special Patient Teaching Considerations

Patient should visit physician for regular check-ups and blood work to monitor this condition and drug therapy.

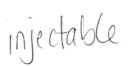

injectable

HEMOSTATIC AGENTS

Aminocaproic Acid (Amicar®)

Action and Indication
Used to treat excessive bleeding through prevention of plasminogen activation.

Dosage
5 gm PO or 1-1.25 gm/hr IV, not to exceed 30 gm in 24 hours.

Route
PO, IV.

Side Effects
GI distress, muscle weakness, dizziness, headache.

Warnings
Oral contraceptives taken concurrently with this drug may cause hypercoagulation.

Special Patient Teaching Considerations
Notify the physician of any signs of adverse effects.

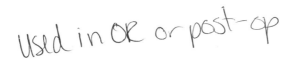
used in OR or post-op

Thrombin Powder

Action and Indication
This agent is used to aid hemostasis of oozing blood and minor bleeding from small vessels.

Dosage
Thin topical application.

Route
Topical

Side Effects
Possible local irritations.

Warnings
Do not inject this product. Do not use in patients with history of allergy to bovine materials. Reconstitute this topical medication with sterile water at 100 U/ml.

Special Patient Teaching Considerations
Notify your physician of bovine allergy history and results of this treatment. Only apply topically.

used in OR or post-op.

DRUG CHART

Generic Name	Trade Name	Route	Generic Name	Trade Name	Route
ANTIANEMIA AGENTS			Protamine	Protamine	Inj.
Cyanocobalamin	Nascobal	PO	Thrombin	Thrombostat	Inj.
(Vitamin B$_{12}$)	Various	PO, Inj.		Thrombinar	Inj.
Folic Acid (Vitamin B$_9$)	Folvite	PO, Inj.			
	Various	PO, Inj.	**PLATELET INHIBITORS**		
			Anagrelide	Agrylin	PO
IRON DEFICIENCY			Cilostazol	Pletal	PO
Iron Dextran	Dexferrum	Inj.	Clopidogrel	Plavix	PO
	INFeD	Inj.	Dipyridamole	Persantine	PO, Inj.
Iron Salts	Fergon	PO		Various	PO, Inj.
	Slow FE	PO	Eptifibatide	Integrilin	Inj.
	Various	PO	Ticlopidine	Ticlid	PO
Sodium Ferric Gluconate	Ferrlecit	Inj.	Tirofiban	Aggrastat	Inj.
Complex					
			PLASMA VOLUME EXPANDERS		
ANTICOAGULANTS			Albumin	Albuminar	Inj.
Antithrombin III	Thrombate III	Inj.	Dextran	Hyskon	Inj.
Ardeparin	Normiflo	Inj.	Hetastarch	Hespan	Inj.
Dalteparin	Fragmin	Inj.			
Danaparoid	Orgaran	Inj.	**THROMBOLYTIC AGENTS**		
Enoxaparin	Lovenox	Inj.	Ateplase, TPA	Activase	Inj.
Heparin	Heparin	Inj.	Anistreplase, APSAC	Eminase	Inj.
	Various	Inj.	Retaplase, r-PA	Retavase	Inj.
Lepirudin	Refludan	Inj.	Streptokinase	Streptase	Inj.
Pentosan	Elmiron	PO		Kabikinase	Inj.
Warfarin	Coumadin	PO, Inj.	Urokinase	Abbokinase	Inj.
COAGULANTS			**COLONY STIMULATING FACTORS**		
HEMOSTATICS			Epoetin Alfa	Epogen	Inj.
Aminocaproic Acid	Amicar	PO, Inj.		Procrit	Inj.
	Various	PO, Inj.	Filgrastim, G-CSF	Neupogen	Inj.
Antihemophilic Factor	Bioclate	Inj.	Glatiramer	Copaxone	Inj.
(AHF)	Hemofil	Inj.	Sargramostim	Leukine	Inj.
	Various	Inj.			
Aprotinin	Trasylol	Inj.	**OTHER**		
Factor IX	Bebulin	Inj.	Desmopressin Acetate	DDAVP	Inj., Nasal Spray
	Various	Inj.			
Phytonadione	Mephyton	PO, Inj.			
	Various	PO, Inj.			

KEY CONCEPTS

✔ Blood coagulation or clotting is a complex process in which the protein fibrinogen is transformed to an insoluble fiber called fibrin. The enzyme thrombin, which comes from prothrombin, acts on fibrinogen in the blood to cause the transformation. Prothrombin and fibrinogen are clotting factors or coagulation factors.

✔ Phytonadione, or Vitamin K_1, is a drug that stimulates the liver to produce several clotting factors and mimics the action of Vitamin K (a natural clotting promoter).

✔ Aside from drug therapy, patients with excessive bleeding may receive whole blood and blood products such as packed cells, platelets, and plasma to treat this serious situation.

✔ Hematopoietics are drugs that treat various forms of anemias by stimulating or helping to stimulate blood cell growth. Anemias are generally characterized by a decrease in hemoglobin or red blood cells which leads to a series of other disorders manifested by oxygen deficiency.

✔ Most commonly, anemias develop in the elderly from iron deficiency, as a result of genetic predisposition (e.g., Sickle Cell anemia), or due to vitamin B12 deficiency (pernicious anemia).

✔ Anemias may also occur as a result of cancer or other diseases and treatments that cause bone marrow suppression and decrease of erythropoietin (which stimulates red blood cell production).

✔ Common drug therapies for anemias include ferrous sulfate for iron-deficiency anemia and cyanocobalmin for vitamin B12 deficiency anemia.

✔ Hemostatic drugs are used to treat or prevent excessive bleeding, e.g., patients who have hemophilia or thrombocytic purpura and suffer from a lack of platelets and/or blood clotting factors found in the first stage of clotting.

CHOOSE THE BEST ANSWER.

answers are in the back of the book

1. Von Willebrand's disease, a very common congenital coagulation disorder, is also caused by a deficiency in
   a. Factor VI
   b. Factor VII
   c. Factor VIII
   d. Factor IX

2) Vitamin B_{12} deficiency would be treated with which vitamin supplementation?
   a. pyridoxine
   b. thiamine
   c. cyanocobalamin
   d. riboflavin

3) Of the following drugs, which one stimulates the liver to produce several clotting factors and mimics the action of Vitamin K?
   a. desmopressin acetate
   b. aminocaproic acid
   c. phytonadione
   d. ferrous sulfate

4) Of the following drugs which one is also available in a nasal formulation used to treat bedwetting?
   a. desmopressin acetate
   b. aminocaproic acid
   c. phytonadione
   d. ferrous sulfate

HORMONES & MODIFIERS

Hormones are secretions of the *endocrine system's* ductless glands.

These substances control or influence a selected organ or set of organs to produce an effect. If a patient does not naturally produce enough or produces too much of a particular hormone, selected drugs can be given to stimulate or inhibit hormone secretion. These hormones and **hormone modifiers** can either be extracted from animals or reproduced synthetically.

The *pituitary gland* is also known as the "master gland" because it regulates the activities of the entire endocrine system.

This pea-sized organ is located deep within the cranium, at the base of the brain. In turn, another major system, the nervous system, greatly controls the pituitary gland and together these two systems are responsible for a large number of our body's regulatory processes.

The *thyroid gland* is located in front of the trachea and secretes hormones that affect metabolism, growth, and central nervous system development.

Thyroxine (T_4) and triiodothyronine (T_3) are thyroid hormones. Their normal secretion is dependent on appropriate amounts of iodine and **TSH (thyroid stimulating hormone)** in the circulating blood. **Hyperthyroidism** is a disorder of overproduction of thyroid hormones that increases the metabolism. Symptoms include increased nervousness and heart rate. Treatment includes surgery and antithyroid medications. **Hypothyroidism** is a disorder of underproduction of thyroid hormone, resulting in a lower metabolism. Symptoms include tiredness, low blood pressure, slow heart rate, and weight gain. Treatment includes thyroid hormone and increased dietary intake of iodine.

---

corticosteroid hormonal steroid substances produced by the cortex of the adrenal gland.

endocrine system the system of hormone secreting glands.

hormone a chemical secretion that influences or controls an organ or organs in the body.

hyperthyroidism overproduction of thyroid hormone.

hypothyroidism underproduction of thyroid hormone.

THE ENDOCRINE SYSTEM

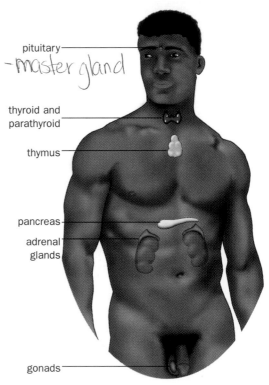

pituitary
– master gland

thyroid and parathyroid

thymus

pancreas

adrenal glands

gonads

Note: the gonads of males are called **testes** and of females, **ovaries**.

Pituitary Gland
➡ Regulation of Endocrine system and growth.

Thyroid and Parathyroid
➡ Metabolic and calcium regulation.

Thymus
➡ Lymphatic regulation.

Pancreas
➡ Blood sugar regulation.

Adrenal Glands
➡ Metabolism and energy regulation.

Gonads
➡ Sexual characteristics.

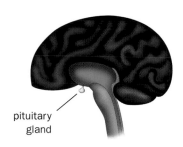

pituitary gland

Pituitary Gland

Divided into posterior and anterior lobes, this organ controls metabolism, growth, water loss and retention, electrolyte balance, and the reproductive cycle. An example of a hormone secreted by the posterior lobe is ADH or antidiuretic hormone. Also known as **vasopressin**, this hormone acts to help the kidneys conserve water and prevent dehydration. Diabetes Insipidus is caused by a deficiency in this hormone and marked by excretion of large amounts of urine (polyuria) and excessive thirst (polydipsia).

Oxytocin is another posterior lobe hormone. It helps stimulate uterine contraction and promote birth or inhibit uterine bleeding post birth.

FSH or follicle stimulating hormone is an anterior lobe hormone called a **gonadatropin** (stimulator of reproductive organ function). It acts to stimulate the egg follicle to produce eggs. Clomiphene is a popular synthetic nonsteroidal agent used to induce ovulation and establish fertility in otherwise unfertile women.

Adrenal Glands

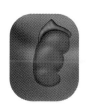

The adrenal glands sit atop the kidneys. They secrete corticosteroids and epinepherine, which influence many aspects of metabolism and energy regulation.

PTH (parathyroid hormone) **and calcitonin are the hormones secreted by the parathryroid glands.**

These hormones regulate the body's serum calcium and phosphorus levels which are integral to normal muscle contraction, bone formation, blood coagulation, milk production in the lactating mother, and nerve impulse conduction. These four small round organs are located behind the thyroid gland and reduction of their function can cause low calcium levels, convulsions, and possible death. Calcitonin-salmon is a common parathyroid gland synthetic hormone.

Located above each kidney, the *adrenal glands* consist of an outer section, the *cortex*, and an inner section, the *medulla*.

The cortex secretes **corticosteroids** which regulate the body's ability to handle stress, resist infection, affect glucose, fat, protein and carbohydrate metabolism and maintain salt and water balance. The adrenal medulla secretes the neurotransmitter **epinephrine** which acts as a stimulator to the sympathetic nervous system. This hormone, referred to as a **catecholamine**, is generally released during stress or activities of "fight or flight." Epinephrine will generally cause a rise in blood pressure, strength and rate of heart beat, blood glucose, metabolic rate, a relaxation of bronchi muscles, coronary and uterine muscles, and dilation of the eye's pupil. Epinephrine is commercially available and used often in serious or medical emergency situations.

Corticosteroids

Hydrocortisone and **cortisone** are two adrenal cortex corticosteroids that act to control anti-inflammatory response and the immune response system. In the 1940's cortisone was recognized as having anti-inflammatory properties. Since then, many synthetic corticosteroids such as prednisone and trimcinolone have been developed and indicated for a number of inflammatory diseases (e.g., arthritis and Crohn's).

The corticosteroid aldosterone helps maintain an adequate supply of serum sodium which accommodates sufficient extracellular fluid or blood volume. A severe deficiency in aldosterone could lead to low blood pressure and circulatory collapse.

HORMONES & MODIFIERS

The pancreas secretes the hormones *insulin* and *glucagon*.

The pancreas is an irregularly shaped organ located between the adrenal glands and behind the stomach. A specialized cluster of pancreatic beta cells called the **Islands (or Islets) of Langerhans** produce insulin, a hormone that controls the body's use of glucose, its normal source of energy. The alpha cells of the pancreas secrete the hormone glucagon which helps convert amino acids (by products of protein digestion) to glucose and raise the level of **serum glucose** (blood sugar). As the serum glucose level increases in a healthy individual, insulin secretion is stimulated. Glucagon and insulin ideally work together to strike a delicate balance and maintain **homeostasis**. Glucagon is available commercially and given to release glucose into the blood stream for severely hypoglycemic patients.

Without adequate insulin levels, serum glucose is not reabsorbed into the intestine, and it spills into the urine for excretion.

Instead of using glucose as it should, the body uses fat and protein as energy sources. This condition, **diabetes mellitus**, is marked by frequent urination, excessive thirst, elevated blood glucose levels, and positive urine glucose and acetone levels. In the early 1920's, Canadian researchers noted a link between the absence of a pancreas and diabetic symptoms. A young boy was subsequently treated with insulin and the diabetic symptoms abated. Insulin, in a variety of types, is given to treat diabetes mellitus, and several oral diabetic agents are also available (e.g., glyburide). Note that insulin does not cure diabetes. It is merely a treatment for it.

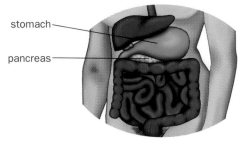

stomach

pancreas

The pancreas is located behind the stomach.

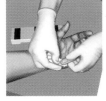 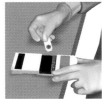

Glucose Monitoring

Patients with diabetes mellitus routinely monitor their blood glucose levels with a **glucometer**. This involves taking a small blood sample, usually from a fingertip, and inserting the sample into the glucometer for analysis. Newer systems that read glucose levels through the skin and do not require blood specimens are being developed.

insulin a hormone that controls the body's use of glucose.

glucagon a hormone that helps convert amino acids to glucose.

diabetes mellitus a condition in which the body does not produce enough insulin or is unable to use it efficiently.

serum glucose blood sugar.

Islands (or Islets) of Langerhans specialized cells of the pancreas that secrete insulin.

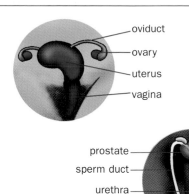

oviduct
ovary
uterus
vagina

prostate
sperm duct
urethra
testes

The *ovaries* are almond shaped organs found on either side of the uterus within the female pelvis.

Under control of the anterior pituitary gland, the ovaries are responsible for the production of ova (eggs) as well as the secretion of the hormones **estrogen** and **progesterone**. These hormones are essential for primary and secondary sex characteristic development, menstruation, healthy pregnancies (gestation), and milk production (lactation).

The *testes* secretes the male hormone testosterone.

Male hormones are called **androgens**. The development and maintenance of the male reproductive tract includes enhancement of secondary sexual characteristics, muscle development, sex organ growth, and body fat distribution. In addition, testosterone also contributes to the building of tissues and prevention of their breakdown. Commercially available testosterone products are often indicated in cases of male hypogonadism or in females for certain breast cancers or engorgement. Fluoxymesterone is a common example of this androgen.

Estrogen

First produced in large quantities at puberty, women secrete estrogens until menopause. Due to their adjunctive role in calcium and phosphorus conservation, many women receive replacement estrogen therapy in their post menopausal years. Women who experience a lack of these hormones during their child bearing years and/or post menopause, may receive them as natural and synthetic products. Synthetic estrogen may also be indicated in cases of breast engorgement, to stunt female growth in height, and for men with prostate cancer. Estrogens are generally contraindicated in cases of breast and/or genital cancer history or if there has been unexplained uterine bleeding.

Progesterone

Progesterone, which is naturally responsible for placenta development and prevention of ovulation, may be indicated in cases of amenorrhea (absence of menstruation), endometreosis (sloughing off of uterine tissue with subsequent attachment to other pelvic organs), dysfunctional uterine bleeding, and for oral contraceptive use.

Oral Contraceptives

There are three types of oral contraceptives:

➡ **monophasic**,

➡ **biphasic**, and *alter amount of estrogen*

➡ **triphasic**. ⟶ *even closer match than biphasic*

Monophasic contraceptives offer a fixed dose of estrogen and progestin (progesterone) while the biphasic and triphasic types deliver the hormones more as they would be naturally secreted by the ovaries. Ortho Novum®, depending on its estrogen/progestin mix, is an example of an oral contraceptive available as any one of the three above mentioned types.

androgens male sex characteristic hormones.

estrogen female sex characteristic hormone that is involved in calcium and phosphorus conservation.

progesterone a female sex characteristic hormone that is involved in ovulation prevention.

testosterone the primary androgen.

ADRENAL

Fludrocortisone (Florinef®)

not used very often
-cause not many
people have
adrenal insufficiencies

Action and Indication

Used to treat hormonal dysfunction of the adrenal cortex and addresses both mineralocorticoid and glucocorticoid insufficiencies.

Dosage

50-200 micrograms per day.

Route

PO tablets.

Side Effects

Edema, hypertension, and possible congestive heart failure.

Warnings

Note that this drug is dosed in micrograms, not milligrams.

Special Patient Teaching Considerations

Notify physician of symptoms such as weight gain, swelling of the ankles, and shortness of breath.

Epinephrine (Adrenalin®)

Action and Indication

For use in serious medical situations such as severe asthma, anaphylactic shock, and cardiac arrest. Stimulates alpha and beta sympathetic nervous system receptors.

Dosage

Dependent upon severity of situation and patient condition For example, for acute asthma: 0.3-0.5 mg of 1:1000 solution SQ or IM.

Route

IV, IM, or SQ.

Side Effects

Tachycardia, hypertension, anxiety, numbness in extremities, flushing, and dypsnea (difficulty in breathing).

Warnings

During a cardiac arrest situation, epinephrine can be administered via an endotracheal tube if IV access cannot be achieved. Other drugs such as monoamine oxidase inhibitors (MAOIs) and tricylic antidepressants may increase the effects. Use with caution if cardiac disease is present or if the asthmatic patient is over 30 years of age.

Special Patient Teaching Considerations

This drug is only to be given in acute medical situations while medical personnel are present. Note: controlled low amounts of epinephrine are available to the public for one time emergency doses in cases of severe allergic reactions, e.g., bee stings.

ANTIDIABETIC

Glyburide (DiaBeta®, Glynase®, Micronase®)

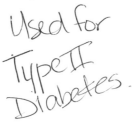

Used for Type II Diabetes.

Diabetes Mellitus

Patients with non-insulin dependent diabetes (NIDDM) may only need a program of diet and weight control as treatment. Patients with insulin dependent diabetes (IDDM) must take insulin injections.

Action and Indication

Glyburide is an oral antidiabetic, hypoglycemic agent used to treat non-insulin dependent (Type II) diabetes. This drug acts to stimulate the pancreas to secrete and strengthen insulin effectiveness.

Dosage

Initial daily dose may be 2.5-5.0 mg every day. The maintenance dose may range from 1.25-20 mg daily, with the higher dose of 20 mg divided as 10 mg and given two times a day.

Route

PO tablets.

Side Effects

Hypoglycemia, heartburn, hives, bloating, dark yellow or brown urine.

Warnings

This drug may worsen the condition of patients with heart disease. The effectiveness of the drug may decrease with time. Hypoglycemia may get worse with prolonged exercise, illness, stress, alcohol use or liver/kidney dysfunction.

Special Patient Teaching Considerations

Take this medication with the morning meal. Notify physician of any signs or symptoms of hypoglycemia (e.g., cold sweats, tachycardia, drowsiness, headache, nervousness, pale skin, and shallow breathing). Avoid direct sun due to increased sensitivity, do not skip meals, and carry a diabetic bracelet or notification.

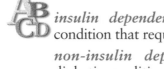 *insulin dependent diabetes (IDDM)* a diabetic condition that requires insulin injections as treatment.

non-insulin dependent diabetes (NIDDM) a diabetic condition that may be treated through diet, exercise, and various oral agents.

Glucagon

Action and Indication

A commercially prepared pancreatic hormone which stimulates the liver to release glucose into the bloodstream. The indication for this drug presumes a healthy and functioning liver.

Dosage

Depending on severity of patient condition. For example, 1 mg or 1 unit per dose and assess results.

Route

IM, SQ, IV.

Side Effects

Rash, nausea/vomiting, possible allergic reaction, and hyperglycemia.

Warnings

Glucagon injection should not be diluted in normal saline.

Special Patient Teaching Considerations

This is a serious medication that is given only under the direct supervision of medical personnel.

Insulin Therapy

Insulin is used to treat Type I Diabetes (also called insulin dependent diabetes mellitus/IDDM). It is calculated in units and usually administered subcutaneously by insulin syringe. There are various types of insulin available, including: regular, semilente, NPH, lente, and ultralente. Each type of insulin works at a specific rate and lasts a specific time. In some cases, two types may be mixed in the same syringe and administered. If a patient receives the wrong insulin or dose, the effects can be serious or even fatal.

Insulin is generally refrigerated. Common sites for insulin injection are the thigh, the deltoid area of the upper arm, the hip, and abdomen.

Insulin is a treatment, not a cure. Dosages may need to be adjusted over time.

ANTIDIABETIC

Troglitazone (Rezulin®)

Action and Indication

Troglitazone is indicated in cases of Type II or non-insulin dependent diabetes. It aids serum glucose transfer from the blood to the muscle cells by potentiating insulin. This drug is not a replacement for insulin, but an assisting agent to it.

Dosage

If taken with insulin or other antihyperglycemic agents, the dose may be 200-400 mg daily, taken with a meal. If taken alone, the dose may be higher at 400-600 mg once daily. In either case, blood glucose will be monitored and the dosage adjusted accordingly.

Route

PO tablets.

Side Effects

Flu-like symptoms, back pain, dark brown or yellow urine, infections, dizziness, diarrhea and possible hypoglycemia (especially when combined with insulin or other oral agents).

Warnings

Female patients should be aware of the nullifying effects on oral contraceptives that troglitazone has. Patients need to follow a recommended diet and exercise program.

Special Patient Teaching Considerations

Follow physician's recommended diet and exercise plan. Continue regular blood and urine testing. Notify physician of any hypoglycemic symptoms such as shakiness, clammy feeling, or blurred vision.

Glipizide (Glucotrol®)

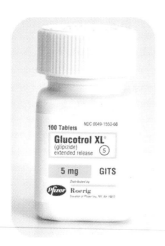

Glucotrol® XL
(glipizide)
Courtesy of Pfizer

Action and Indication
This is an oral **antihyperglycemic agent** that is used to treat non-insulin dependent (Type II) Diabetes. This drug acts to stimulate the pancreas to secrete insulin and reduce hyperglycemic conditions.

Dosage
Initially, 5 mg taken before breakfast. This dosage may be increased to a maximum of 20 mg daily. Some sources claim 40 mg daily maximum), dependent upon patient condition and disease severity. Elderly dosages may be decreased to 2.5 mg daily.

Route
PO tablets.

Side Effects
Hypoglycemia, allergic skin reactions, and GI effects such as diarrhea, abdominal cramping, and possible constipation.

Warnings
The patient's glucose level (blood and urine) should be monitored at regular intervals and inquire as to history of liver, kidney or heart dysfunction requiring beta blockers. Be alert to hypoglycemia conditions in elderly patients.

Special Patient Teaching Considerations
For greatest effectiveness, take this medication 30 minutes before meals. Remember this therapy is not a replacement for the diet suggested by a physician. Follow dietary instructions while taking this drug. Continue with urine and serum blood glucose testing and report any abnormality to the physician.

ANTIDIABETIC

Metformin Hydrochloride (Glucophage®)

Action and Indication

This recently developed oral antidiabetic agent is indicated in cases of non-insulin dependent, Type II Diabetes. It works to decrease glucose production and absorption while promoting optimal use of naturally produced insulin.

Dosage

Initially, 500 mg two times a day, with meals. Daily doses may be increased by 500 mg daily to a maximum of 2500 mg in divided doses, dependent upon patient response and disease severity. Note: This medication has not been recommended for use in children.

Route

PO tablets.

Side Effects

GI effects such as bloating, nausea and loss of appetite.

Warnings

Caution should be used in patients with a history of liver/kidney dysfunction and/or metabolic acidosis. Congestive heart failure may lead to lactic acidosis if taking Glucophage. Caution indicated if patient also is receiving IV contrast for x-rays. Renal function studies should be conducted after prolonged use.

Special Patient Teaching Considerations

Do not take this drug if pregnant. Avoid alcohol. Remember, it is recommended to take this drug with meals, so as to decrease GI side effects. Test your urine and serum regularly for abnormal glucose levels.

Glimepiride (Amaryl®)

Action and Indication

This **oral antihyperglycemic** agent works by stimulating the release of insulin from beta cells in the pancreas. Classified as a **sulfonylurea,** this drug is often indicated in cases of non-insulin dependent or Type II Diabetes.

Dosage

Dependent upon disease severity in adults. For example, 1-2 mg once a day, often with breakfast. This dosage may be increased to a maximum of 8 mg per day, although it is often controlled at 1-4 mg per day.

Route

PO tablets.

Side Effects

Hypoglycemic reactions with symptoms such as cold sweats, blurred vision, dizziness, tachycardia, and GI symptoms such as nausea and stomach pain.

Warnings

Patients should be monitored carefully as to blood glucose levels, hypoglycemic symptoms, diet, and exercise regimes.

Special Patient Teaching Considerations

This medication does not replace diet and exercise routines. It is to be used as an adjunct form of treatment for non-insulin dependent diabetics. Notify the physician of any change in diet or exercise habits and/or any symptoms of hypoglycemia.

THYROID & PARATHYROID

Methimazole (Tapazole®)

Action and Indication

This **antithyroid preparation** is indicated for cases of hyperthyroidism and may be given prior to a thyroidectomy. Methimazole blocks the synthesis of the thyroid hormone by inhibiting iodine entry.

Dosage

Dependent on severity of disease and patient condition. For example, 5-30 mg daily in three divided doses. Some sources suggest one smaller daily dose, if the condition is mild. The maintenance dose may be 5-15 mg once each day.

Route

PO tablets.

Side Effects

Dermatitis, blood dyscrasias (including anemia) and agranulocytosis (drop in the white blood cell count), jaundice, and hypoglycemia.

Warnings

Serum liver enzyme tests should be conducted while taking this drug. Methimazole may prolong the clotting time in patients who are also taking coumadin.

Special Patient Teaching Considerations

Keep appointments for blood work, as ordered and report any sign of infections to the physician.

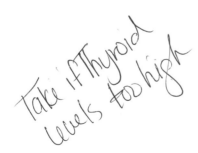

Take if Thyroid levels too high

Levothyroxine Sodium (Synthroid®, Levoxyl®, various)

Action and Indication

This synthetic thyroid hormone is indicated in cases of thyroid disease such as goiter, cancer, or other conditions resulting in low or no thyroid hormone production.

Dosage

Initially 25-50 micrograms daily which may be increased in 25 microgram increments every 2-3 weeks for a maximum of less than 200 micrograms daily.

Route

PO tablets.

Side Effects

Allergic reactions and hyperthyroid symptoms such as tachycardia, sweating, tremors, and weight loss.

Warnings

Monitor thyroxine levels during the course of treatment. Use caution in patients with history of cardiac pathologies, diabetes, adrenocortical insufficiency, and use of drugs such as coumadin.

Special Patient Teaching Considerations

Notify a physician of hyperthyroxine symptoms such as palpitations, chest pain, sweating, and nervousness. Take this medication only as directed and at the same time daily. This drug should not be used as a weight reduction agent.

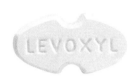

Levoxyl®
(levothyroxine)
Courtesy of JONES PHARMA INC.

Levothyroxine is a synthetic isomer of thyroxine, a hormone of the thyroid gland. It is used in the treatment of hypothyroidism.

Take it if Thyroid levels are too high.

PARATHYROID

Calcitonin-Salmon (Miacalcin®, Calcimar®)

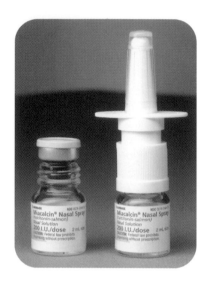

Mlacalcin®
(calcitonin-salmon)
Courtesy of Novartis
Pharmaceutical Corporation

Action and Indication

This synthetic form of calcitonin acts to reduce bone calcium loss and will help keep serum calcium levels lower. A common indication for this agent (Miacalcin) is osteoporosis in post-menopausal women. Calcimar may be prescribed in cases of Paget's disease (abnormal bone growth) and hypercalcemia.

Dosage

Dependent on route of administration. For example, the nasal spray, miacalcin, is frequently ordered as: 1 spray each day, alternating nostrils with each administration, 200 IU per dose. For SQ or IM: 100 IU every day, every other day or 3 times a week in conjunction with oral calcium and Vitamin D.

Route

IM, nasal spray.

Side Effects

Local nostril or injection site irritation, back pain, headache, and possible allergic reaction.

Warnings

The injectable form of this drug (Calcimar) has been known to cause serious allergic reactions. Perhaps an allergy test would be in order prior to ordering the nasal spray as well. Concurrent use of hydrocortisone is recommended. If the patient is hypertensive, the dose must be reduced.

Special Patient Teaching Considerations

Notify the physician of any sign of allergic response or nasal discomfort.

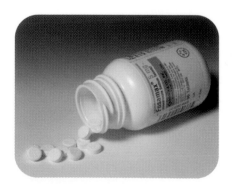

Non-hormonal Therapy for Osteoporosis

Alendronate sodium (Fosamax®) is a relatively new drug used to treat osteoporosis in post-menopausal women, patients using corticosteroids, and Paget's Disease sufferers. Rather than prevent bone loss, it strengthens the bone. The dosage for postmenopausal women is 10 mg daily. For Paget's Disease it is up to 40 mg daily for about 6 months. The dosage for patients taking steroids is 5 mg daily.

Fosamax®
(alendronate sodium)
Courtesy of Merck Archives

Oral Conjugated Estrogen (Premarin®, Premphase®, Prempo®)

Action and Indication

This agent works to replace the natural hormone estrogen in cases of menopause, hysterectomy, or other related conditions.

Dosage

It is suggested that Premarin be administered together with a progesterone drug as it then reduces the risk of endometrial cancer. If Premarin is prescribed alone (perhaps in cases of a hysterectomy where no risk of uterine cancer would exist), this drug may be given for 3 weeks on at 1.25 mg each day and 1 week off the drug entirely. For treatment of osteoporosis, 0.625 mg each day, taken in conjunction with progesterone, would be recommended. For conditions such as hot flashes, the dosage is reduced to 0.3-1.25 mg daily, 3 weeks on and 1 week off and for reduced ovarian function, the dosage may be as high as 7.5 mg daily, in three divided doses for 20 days on and 10 days off. Note: In each case, the physician will decide the necessity of a concurrent progesterone therapy.

Route

PO tablets.

Side Effects

Abnormal vaginal bleeding patterns, abdominal pain, breast tenderness, blood clots (especially if you smoke and/or are over 35), depression, fluid retention, and increased risk of both cardiac related pathologies and gall bladder disease.

Warnings

Without the concurrent administration of a progesterone product, there is an increased risk of uterine cancer. Be aware of patient's history regarding pregnancy and cardiovascular dysfunction.

Special Patient Teaching Considerations

Only take this drug as prescribed. Notify the physician if abnormal uterine bleeding occurs.

Climara®
(estradiol)
0.05mg/day

Climara® (estradiol transdermal system) is a once-weekly translucent estrogen replacement patch.

Courtesy of Berlex Laboratories

CONTRACEPTIVE

Note: In addition to oral, various other forms of contraceptives are available. These include transdermal patches containing estradiol and Norplant® implants containing levonorgestrel that are implanted under the skin.

Norethindrone/Ethinyl Estradiol or Norethindrone/Mestranol (various)

Contraceptives

There are various combinations of estrogens and progestins in contraceptives. Note that the progestins in the compounds shown below are levonorgestrel and norgestimate.

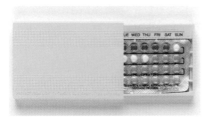

Tri-Levlin® 28
(levonorgestrel and ethinyl estradiol tablets–triphasic system)
Courtesy of Berlex Laboratories

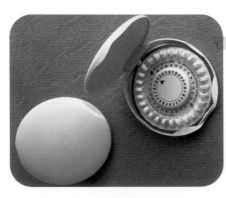

Ortho-Try-Cyclen® 28
(norgestimate and ethinyl estradiol tablets–triphasic system)
Courtesy of Ortho-McNeill Pharmaceutical

Action and Indication

These two oral contraceptives act to prevent pregnancy by inhibiting ovulation, altering the lining of the uterus, thickening the cervical mucus and slowing the movement of an egg down the fallopian tube, should ovulation occur. Norethindrone is a progestin and ethinyl estradiol and mestranol are estrogens.

Most commonly seen components of oral contraceptives

Dosage

Dosing is complex and dependent upon the formulation ordered. There are both 21 and 28 pill preparations, each containing varying amounts of combined hormones. For example, a woman could take one pill every day or take one for three weeks and then none for the last week of the cycle.

Route

PO tablets.

Side Effects

Menstrual changes, vascular pathologies, hypertension, weight and breast changes, depression, and possible liver and/or gallbladder disease.

Warnings

Other agents can decrease this drug's effectiveness: most antibiotics (e.g., ampicillin, sulfonamides, tetracycline, and chloramphenicol), analgesics, barbiturates, and antimigraine medications. These agents are contraindicated in patients with vascular disorders, dysfunctional uterine bleeding, breast or ovarian cancer, liver dysfunction, and suspected pregnancy. Women who smoke, especially over the age of 35, should also not receive these agents.

Special Patient Teaching Considerations

Smoking is highly discouraged while taking these agents due to cardiovascular complications which may occur. Prior to taking this drug, the patient should receive a thorough gynecological examination to include: medical history, BP, breast examination, cervical pap, and pelvic examination. These pills must be taken as directed in order to assure effectiveness.

Fluoxymesterone (Halotestin®)

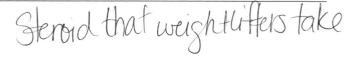

Steroid that weightlifters take

Action and Indication

This androgen is used for males with hypogonadism and delay of puberty. It is also indicated for women who have inoperable breast cancer or are having postmenopausal breast pain.

Dosage

For males, 2.5-20 mg daily. For women, 2.5-10 mg daily. Other medical conditions involving carcinomas are dosed accordingly.

Route

PO tablets.

Side Effects

For males, enlarged breasts and testicular atrophy. For women, loss of menstruation and virilization.

Warnings

This drug can potentiate the anticoagulation effect. Note: At least one state has made this drug a controlled substance level II, due to the abuse potential by athletes. At the national level in the United States, this agent is a level III controlled substance.

Special Patient Teaching Considerations

Notify the physician of any sign of side effects. The dose may be adjusted if necessary.

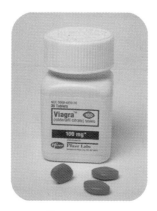

Viagra®
(sildenafil citrate)
Courtesy of Pfizer

Sildenafil Citrate (Viagra)

This very popular drug is not a hormonal agent, but it acts on a process often associated with hormones: male sexual activity. Sildenafil is the first agent developed for cases of male **impotency**, also called **erectile dysfunction**. Its mechanism is a dilation of penile blood vessels that allows the flow of blood necessary to obtain and sustain an erection. Sildenafil is contraindicated for men taking nitrates (e.g., nitroglycerin, isosorbide mononitrate).

PITUITARY

Oxytocin (Pitocin®, Syntocinon®)

Action and Indication

To bring about uterine contractions and hasten birth, help alleviate post birth bleeding, or assist in a spontaneous or therapeutic abortion. These chemically induced contractions help the uterus to return to its normal pre-pregnancy state.

Dosage

IV infusion calculated as per patient's condition (e.g., 10-40 units in 1000 cc's). Nasal spray may be one spray in both nostrils. An IM dose could be 10 units.

Route

IV, IM, or nasal spray.

Side Effects

Nausea, vomiting, cardiac arrhythmias, and possible allergic response.

Warnings

This drug could cause uterine rupture and danger to the fetus. Fetal jaundice, anoxia, and bradycardia could occur.

Special Patient Teaching Considerations

This drug should only be taken under the direct supervision of a physician.

Clomiphene Citrate (Clomid®)

Action and Indication

This drug is often prescribed for infertile women who wish to become pregnant. It acts to promote healthy follicle growth and ovulation. Most women benefit within three cycles and this agent should not be used for long term therapy.

Dosage

50-100 mg once per day, given only for five days in the menstrual cycle.

Route

PO tablets.

Side Effects

Hot flashes, abdominal discomfort, blurred vision, and other visual disturbances, possible abnormal uterine bleeding.

Warnings

Ovarian enlargement and cyst formation may occur. Multiple births and/or birth defects have also been reported from using this infertility drug. The patient's liver function and estrogen levels should be assessed prior to the start of Clomid.

Special Patient Teaching Considerations

Report all side effects to the physician and take precaution in daily activities should vision problems occur. Any signs and symptoms of Ovarian Hyperstimulation Syndrome (e.g., abdominal pain and/or enlargement), labored breathing, and decreased urination, should be reported immediately.

DRUG CHART

Generic Name	Trade Name	Route	Generic Name	Trade Name	Route
ADRENAL AGENTS			**ANTIDIABETIC AGENTS**		
Dexamethasone	Decadron	PO, Inj.	Acarbose	Precose	PO
	Various	PO, Inj.	Insulin	Humulin	Inj.
Methylprednisolone	Medrol	PO, Inj.		Iletin	Inj.
	Various	PO, Inj.		Various	Inj.
Prednisone	Deltasone	PO	Metformin	Glucophage	PO
Metyrosine	Demser	PO	Repaglinide	Actulin	PO
Mitotane	Lysodren	PO		Prandin	PO
Beclomethasone	Beclovent	Inhaler		NovoNorm	PO
	Beconase	Inhaler	Troglitazone	Rezulin	PO
	Various	Inhaler			
Budesonide	Pulmicort	Inhaler	**SULFONYLUREAS**		
	Rhinocort	Inhaler	Acetohexamide	Dymelor	PO
Corticotropin, ACTH	Acthar	Inj.		Varoius	PO
Cortisone	Cortone	PO, Inj.	Chlorpropamide	Diabinese	PO
Fludrocortisone	Florinef	PO		Various	PO
Flunisolide	Aerobid	Inhaler	Glimepiride	Amaryl	PO
	Various	Inhaler	Glipizide	Glucotrol	PO
Prednisolone	Pediapred	PO, Inj., Eye		Glucotrol XL	PO
	Various	PO, Inj., Eye	Glyburide	DiaBeta	PO
Rimexolone	Vexol	Eye		Micronase	PO
				Glynase	PO
ANDROGENS			Tolazamide	Tolinase	PO
Danazol	Danocrine	PO		Various	PO
	Various	PO	Tolbutamide	Orinase	PO
Methyltestosterone	Virilon	PO			
	Various	PO	**ANTI-HYPOGLYCEMIC AGENTS**		
Testosterone	Andro	PO, Inj., Transdermal	Diazoxide	Hyperstat	Inj.
	Androgel	PO, Inj., Transdermal		Proglycem	Inj.
	Testoderm	PO, Inj., Transdermal	**AROMATOSE INHIBITORS**		
			Anastrozole	Arimidex	PO
ANTI ANDROGENS			Letrozole	Femara	PO
Bicalutamide	Casodex	PO			
Finasteride	Propecia	PO			
	Proscar	PO			
Flutamide	Eulexin	PO			
Nilutamide	Nilandron	PO			

GENERIC NAME	TRADE NAME	ROUTE	GENERIC NAME	TRADE NAME	ROUTE
CONTRACEPTIVES			**GONADOTROPIN RELEASING HORMONE ANALOGS**		
Nonoxynol-9	Delfen	Vaginal Gel, Foam, Supp.	Goserelin	Zoladex	Implant
Ethinyl Estradiol / Desogestrel	Desogen	PO	Leuprolide	Lupron	Inj.
	Various	PO	**OXYTOCICS**		
Ethinyl Estradiol / Ethynodiol Diacetate	Demulen 1/35 28 day	PO	Oxytocin	Pitocin	Inj.
	Various	PO			
Ethinyl Estradiol ./ Levonorgestrel	Levlen	PO	**PARATHYROID AGENTS**		
	Various	PO	Calcitonin	Calcimar	Inj., Nas. Spray
Ethinyl Estradiol / Norethindrone	Brevicon	PO		Miacalcin	Inj., Nas. Spray
	Various	PO		Cibacalcin	Inj., Nas. Spray
Ethinyl Estradiol / Norgestimate	Ortho-Cyclen 28	PO	Desmopressin	DDAVP	Inj., Nas. Spray
	Various	PO	Vasopressin, ADH	Pitressin	Inj.
Ethinyl Estradiol / Norgestrel	Lo/Ovral	PO		Various	Inj.
	Various	PO	Somatotropin, rh-GH	Genotropin	Inj.
Levonorgestrel	Norplant	Implants		Various	Inj.
Medroxyprogesterone	Depo-Provera	Inj.			
Norgestrel	Ovrette	PO	**ANTI THYROID AGENTS**		
			Methimazole	Tapazole	PO
ESTROGENS			Potassium Iodide, KI	SSKI	PO
Conjugated Estrogens	Premarin	PO, Inj.		Pima	PO
Conjugated Estrogens / Medroxyprogesterone	Premphase	PO	Propylthiouracil, PTU	PTU	PO
	Prempro	PO			
Diethylstilbestrol, DES	Stilphostrol	PO, Inj.	**THYROID AGENTS**		
	Various	PO, Inj.	Levothyroxine	Synthroid	PO, Inj.
Esterified Estrogens	Estratab	PO		Various	PO, Inj.
	Various	PO	Liothyronine	Cytomel	PO, Inj.
Estradiol	Estrace	PO		Triostat	PO, Inj.
	Various	PO, Inj., Transdermal	Thyroid	Armour	PO
			Thyrotropin, TSH	Thytropar	Inj.
FERTILITY AGENTS					
Clomiphene	Clomid	PO	**TOCOLYTICS**		
	Serophene	PO	Ritodrine	Yutopar	PO, Inj.
Follitropin, r-FSH	Follistim	Inj.			
	Gonal-F	Inj.			
Human Chorionic Gonadotropin (HCG)	Pregnyl	Inj.			
Menotropins	Pergonal	Inj.			
	Humegon	Inj.			
	Repronex	Inj.			

REVIEW

KEY CONCEPTS

- ✔ Hormones are secretions of the endocrine system's ductless glands that control or influence a selected organ or set of organs to produce an effect.
- ✔ The pituitary gland is also known as the "master gland" because it regulates the activities of the entire endocrine system.
- ✔ The thyroid gland secretes the hormones Thyroxine (T_4) and triiodothyronine (T_3) that affect metabolism, growth, and central nervous system development. Their secretion is dependent on iodine and TSH (thyroid stimulating hormone) in the circulating blood.
- ✔ Hyperthyroidism is a disorder of overproduction of thyroid hormones that increases the metabolism. Symptoms include increased nervousness and heart rate. Treatment includes surgery and antithyroid medications.
- ✔ Hypothyroidism is a disorder of underproduction of thyroid hormone, resulting in a lower metabolism. Symptoms include tiredness, low blood pressure, slow heart rate, and weight gain. Treatment includes thyroid hormone and increased dietary intake of iodine.
- ✔ PTH (parathyroid hormone) and calcitonin are the hormones secreted by the parathryroid glands. They regulate the body's serum calcium and phosphorus levels.
- ✔ The adrenal cortex secretes corticosteroids which regulate the body's ability to handle stress, resist infection, effect glucose, fat, protein and carbohydrate metabolism and maintain salt and water balance. Hydrocortisone and cortisone are two adrenal cortex corticosteroids that act to control anti-inflammatory response and the immune response system.
- ✔ The adrenal medulla secretes the neurotransmitter epinephrine (which acts as a stimulator to the sympathetic nervous system.
- ✔ The pancreas secretes the hormone glucagon which helps convert amino acids to glucose and raise the level of serum glucose. As the serum glucose level increases in a healthy individual, insulin secretion is stimulated.
- ✔ Diabetes mellitus is a conditon in which the body does not produce enough insulin or is unable to use it efficiently. Insulin is used to treat Type I Diabetes (also called insulin dependent diabetes mellitus/IDDM). Patients with non-insulin dependent diabetes (NIDDM) may only need a program of diet and weight control as treatment.
- ✔ Estrogen and progesterone are essential for female primary and secondary sex characteristic development, menstruation, healthy pregnancies, and milk production.
- ✔ Women secrete estrogens until menopause. Due to their role in calcium and phosphorus conservation, many women receive estrogen therapy in their post menopausal years.
- ✔ Male hormones are called androgens. The testes secretes the male hormone testosterone.
- ✔ Monophasic contraceptives offer a fixed dose of estrogen and progestin (progesterone) while the biphasic and trpihasic types deliver the hormones more as they would be naturally secreted by the ovaries.
- ✔ Sildenafil Citrate (Viagra®) is not a hormonal agent, but it acts on a process often associated with hormones: male sexual activity. It is the first agent developed for cases of male impotency.

SELF TEST

MATCH THE GENERIC AND TRADE NAMES.   *answers can be checked in the back of the book*

1. Calcitonin-salmon	*Miacalcin*	Clomid
2. Clomiphene	*Clomid*	Desogen
3. Conjugated Estrogens	*Premarin*	Glucophage
4. Ethinyl Estradiol / Desogestrel	*Desogen*	Glucotrol
5. Glipizide	*Glucotrol*	Glynase
6. Glyburide	*Glynase*	Humulin
7. Insulin	*Humulin*	Miacalcin
8. Levothyroxine	*Synthroid*	Pitocin
9. Metformin	*Glucophage*	Premarin
10. Methimazole	*Tapazole*	Rezulin
11. Oxytocin	*Pitocin*	Synthroid
12. Troglitazone	*Rezulin*	Tapazole

CHOOSE THE BEST ANSWER.   *answers are in the back of the book*

1. Of the following medications, which one would be used for NIDDM?
   a. clomiphene
   b. calcitonin
   c. glyburide
   d. norethindone

2. Which disorder below would most likely have the following symptoms: tiredness, low blood sugar, slow heart rate, and weight gain?
   a. diabetes mellitus
   b. Paget's Disease
   c. hypothyroidism
   d. hyperthyroidism

3. Of the following medications, which one can be found in a nasal spray formulation?
   a. clomiphene
   b. calcitonin
   c. glyburide
   d. norethindone

4. Most oral contraceptives are composed of an estrogen and progestin combination. Of the following, which drug would be the progestin component?
   a. clomiphene
   b. calcitonin
   c. glyburide
   d. norethindone

IMMUNOBIOLOGIC AGENTS

Both *passive* and *active immunity* offer the body a defense against pathogens.

Passive immunity is developed by the introduction of preformed antibodies into the body. This provides immediate passive immunity. Active immunity occurs when the body is exposed to a pathogen, develops the disease, and manufactures antibodies against a future invasion. **Acquired active immunity** occurs when the body is purposefully injected with a weakened or even dead pathogen, but still produces antibodies against reoccurring exposures.

One negative aspect of passive immunity is that the life of some of the antibodies is shorter than the life of antibodies found with active immunity.

Another concern is the possibility of allergic reaction that may occur in some individuals. Further, hypersensitization may follow the receipt of passive immunity and render the host more prone to allergic response with each subsequent exposure. Severe anaphylactic reactions are possible.

Immunobiologic agents contain antibodies that have been produced by other humans or animals.

These antibodies are recovered through high tech purification processes and made available commercially through **vaccines, toxoids** (e.g., DPT), and **immune globulins.**

Animal Antibodies

Pathogens for which passive immunity from animals may be used include:

➡ Diphtheria (using Antitoxin, USP
➡ Rabies (using Antirabies serum)
➡ Botulism
➡ Black Widow Spider Venom

Human Antibodies

Human passive immunity is often used in the treatment of:

➡ Measles (using Measles Immune Globulin, USP)
➡ Pertussis (using Pertussis Immune Globulin, USP)
➡ Mumps (using Mumps Immune Globulin, USP)
➡ Tetanus (using Tetanus Immune Globulin, USP)
➡ Hepatitis A and B.

Note: Diphtheria, Tetanus, Hepatitis B, Measles, Mumps and Rabies may also be treated with agents producing active immunity.

VACCINES

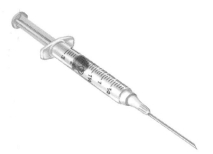

A vaccine is a suspension containing infectious agents used to boost the body's immune system response.

Two forms of vaccines presently exist: one allows **passive immunity** by giving an individual the antibody. This form generally offers a shorter period of protection. The other form stimulates the patient's immune system to produce an antibody, referred to as **active immunity**. This is the longer lasting type of immunity.

The **Smallpox Vaccine** was successfully introduced in Europe in the late 1700's by Dr. Edward Jenner. Since that time, other vaccines such as **DPT** (diptheria, pertussis and tetanus), **MMR** (measles, mumps and rubella), **Polio Typhoid**, **Rabies**, **Hepatitis A and B**, and **BCG** (an antitubercular agent) have been developed and utilized.

Today, most children are required to receive a series of these vaccines prior to attending school and this has resulted in a dramatic reduction in these diseases. Certain childhood diseases such as measles, mumps, and chicken pox, once contracted, should not reoccur due to active immunity created with the antibody formation. **Haemophilus Influenzae Type B** (Hib), a different Hepatitis series and the new **Chicken Pox** vaccine are examples of more recently developed vaccines.

Diphtheria Antitoxin

Action and Indication

Treatment and sometimes prevention of Diphtheria, usually given to adults who had not received the childhood DPT (Diphtheria, Pertussis, Tetanus) immunization.

Dosage

For prevention: 10,000 units. For treatment: 20,000-120,000 units

Route

Dependent on purpose and disease severity. For example, IM for prevention and possibly IV in severe cases.

Side Effects

Local irritation with pain and swelling at injection site. Possible mildly allergic to anaphylactic allergic reactions.

Warnings

Allergic reaction possible. An allergy skin test may be indicated prior to injection.

Special Patient Teaching Considerations

Notify the physician should any allergic responses or disease symptoms occur.

active immunity immunity resulting from the production of antibodies in response to contraction of a disease.

passive immunity immunity resulting from the introduction of preformed antibodies.

antibody (immunoglobulin) a substance in the body that attacks and destroys pathogens.

pathogen viruses or microorganisms that cause disease.

toxoid a toxin that has had its toxicity destroyed but that will stimulate the production of antibodies.

vaccine a suspension containing infectious agents used to boost the immune response.

IMMUNOBIOLOGIC AGENTS

Immune Globulin (Gamastan®, Gammar®)

Action and Indication
To be given as soon as possible following patient exposure to Hepatitis A. This product is also used in prevention of Rubeola/measles and the Varicella/chickenpox viruses.

Dosage
Dependent upon the reason for treatment. For example, 0.02-1.3 ml/kg of body weight, one time injection.

Route
IM.

Side Effects
Fever, local irritation, and itching at injection site.

Warnings
Allergic reactions possible.

Special Patient Teaching Considerations
Report any allergic reaction and/or disease symptom to the physician.

Risks

Despite a stringent purification process, there is a theoretical possibility that an immume globulin may still contain an infectious agent. It is therefore important to monitor patients for any signs of infection.

Hepatitis B Immune Globulin (HBIG)

Action and Indication

This immunization is given after a person has been exposed to Hepatitis in an effort to prevent them from developing the disease.

Dosage

0.06 ml/kg of body weight, as soon as possible after the exposure. A follow-up of this dose may be repeated in 28-30 days.

Route

IM.

Side Effects

Fever, local skin irritation, and itching at injection site.

Warnings

Allergic reaction and interactions with certain vaccines possible.

Special Patient Teaching Considerations

Allergic reactions and/or disease symptoms should be reported to the physician.

IMMUNOBIOLOGIC AGENTS

Rabies Immune Globulin (Human RIG, Imogam®)

Action and Indication

To be given to those patients who were or suspect they were exposed to Rabies. This immunization would help prevent the development of this disease in the exposed individual.

Dosage

20 IU/kg. Half of this dose may be used to infiltrate the wound.

Route

IM.

Side Effects

Local injection site irritation, and soreness. Possible fever and allergic response.

Warnings

Rabies immune globulin should be given in conjunction with Rabies Vaccine or up to 8 days after the first vaccine dose.

Special Patient Teaching Considerations

Notify the physician should any allergic response or disease symptoms develop.

Tetanus Immune Globulin (Hyper-Tet®)

Action and Indication

To provide passive immunity for Tetanus should a possible Tetanus producing event occur (injury or cut from an unclean source).

Dosage

Adults: 250U – 500U (higher doses used for severe wounds when a delay in administering the prophylaxis has occurred). Children's dose is calculated according to body weight in kg (4U per kg). The Tetanus Antitoxin can be given prophylactically at 1500 – 5000U or 50,000 – 100,000 U for active treatment.

Route

IM for the Immune Globulin and IV for the Antitoxin. (These routes are split 50/50.) SQ and IM are preferred for prophylaxis.

Side Effects

Muscle stiffness, pain, and irritation at the injection site.

Warnings

Allergic reaction possible.

Special Patient Teaching Considerations

The importance of the patient's vaccination history and also of receiving this immunization in the event of a potential Tetanus producing occurrence should be emphasized. Patients should notify their physician immediately should any allergic response or disease symptom appear. Note: Do not take other vaccinations 2 weeks prior or up to 3 months after any other vaccinations.

DPT (Diptheria-Pertussis-Tetanus)

Tetanus immunization is included in the childhood immunization DPT and may be given as a booster every 5-10 years.

DRUG CHART

GENERIC NAME	TRADE NAME	ROUTE
ANTITOXINS		
Diptheria Antitoxin		Inj.
IMMUNOGLOBULINS		
Cytomegalovirus Immune Globulin, CMV-IGI	Cytogam	Inj.
Hepatitis B Immune Globulin, HBIG	BayHep Nabi-HB	Inj. Inj.
Immune Globulin IM, IGIM	Gammar-P IM	Inj.
Immune Globulin IV, IGIV	Gamimune Various	Inj. Inj.
Rho [D] ImmuneGlobulin	RhoGAM	Inj.
Rabies Immune Globulin, human RIG	Hyperab Imogam	Inj. Inj.
	Human RIG	Inj.
Tetanus Immune Globulin	Hyper-Tet	Inj.
MONOCLONAL ANTIBODIES		
Abciximab	ReoPro	Inj.
Basiliximab	Simulect	Inj.
Daclizumab	Zenapax	Inj.
Digoxin Immune Fab	Digibind	Inj.
Infliximab	Remicade	Inj.
Muromonab-CD3	Orthoclone OKT3	Inj.
IMMUNOSUPPRESIVES		
Antithymocyte Globulin	Atgam	Inj.
	Thymoglobulin	Inj.
Azathioprine	Imuran	PO, Inj.
Cyclosporine	Neoral	PO, Inj.
	Various	PO, Inj.
Mycophenolate	CellCept	PO, Inj.
Tacrolimus	Prograf	PO, Inj.
Dexamethasone	Decadron	PO, Inj.
Methylprednisolone	Solu-Medrol	PO, Inj.
Prednisone	Orasone	PO
	Deltasone	PO
	Various	PO

GENERIC NAME	TRADE NAME	ROUTE
INTERFERONS		
Interferon Beta	Avonex	Inj.
	Betaseron	Inj.
Interferon Gamma-1b	Actimmune	Inj.
INTERLEUKENS		
Oprelvekin, rh-IL-11	Neumega	Inj.
TOXOIDS		
Diptheria/Tetanus Toxoids & Pertussis Vaccine	Acel-Imune	Inj.
Tetanus Toxoid	Various	Inj.
VACCINES		
Haemophilus b Conjugate Vaccine	HibTITER	Inj.
Hepatitis A Vaccine, Inactivated	Havrix VAQTA	Inj. Inj.
Hepatitis B Vaccine, Recombinant	Engerix-B Recombivax HB	Inj. Inj.
Influenza Virus Vaccine	Fluogen	Inj.
	FluShield	Inj.
	Fluviron	Inj.
	Fluzone	Inj.
Lyme Disease Vaccine	Immulyme	Inj.
	LYMErix	Inj.
Measles/Mumps/Rubella, MMR	M-M-R	Inj.
Pneumococcal Vaccine, Polyvalent	Pneumovax 23 Pnu-Imune 23	Inj. Inj.
Poliovirus Vaccine Live Oral, OPV	Orimune	PO
Rotavirus Vaccine	RotaShield	Inj.
Varicella Virus Vaccine Live	Varivax	Inj.

KEY CONCEPTS

✔ Immunobiologic agents are used to provide passive or active immunity. Passive immunity is provided by the introduction of preformed antibodies into the body. Active immunity occurs when the body is exposed to a pathogen, develops the disease, and manufactures antibodies against a future invasion. Acquired active immunity occurs when the body is injected with a weakened or even dead pathogen, but still produces antibodies against reoccurring exposures.

✔ An antibody (immunoglobulin) is a substance in the body that attacks and destroys pathogens.

✔ Immunobiologic agents contain antibodies that have been produced by other humans or animals. These antibodies are recovered through high tech purification processes and made available commercially through vaccines, toxoids (e.g., DPT), and immune globulins.

✔ Despite a stringent purification process, there is a theoretical possibility that an immmue globulin may still contain an infectious agent, so it is important to monitor patients for signs of infection.

✔ Pathogens for which passive immunity from animals may be used include: diphtheria (using Antitoxin, USP), rabies (using Antirabies serum), botulism, and Black Widow Spider venom.

✔ Human passive immunity is often used in the treatment of: measles (using Measles Immune Globulin, USP), pertussis (using Pertussis Immune Globulin, USP), mumps (using Mumps Immune Globulin, USP), tetanus (using Tetanus Immune Globulin, USP), and hepatitis A and B.

✔ One negative aspect of passive immunity is that the life of some of the antibodies is shorter than the life of antibodies found with active immunity.

✔ A toxoid is a toxin that has had its toxicity destroyed but that will still stimulate the production of antibodies.

CHOOSE THE BEST ANSWER.   *answers are in the back of the book*

1. Of the following antibodies which one is derived from an animal source?
   a. diphtheria
   b. measles
   c. mumps
   d. tetanus

2. Of the following, which one is not available as a vaccine?
   a. diphtheria
   b. measles
   c. mumps
   d. tetanus

3. Of the following products, which one is for Rabies Immune Globulin (RIG)?
   a. Hyper-Tet®
   b. Gammar®
   c. Gamastan®
   d. Imogam®

4. Hepatitis B Immune Globulin (HBIG) immunization is most often given
   a. to children prior to attending school.
   b. prior to exposure
   c. immediately after exposure
   d. only if there is a family history or genetic predisposition of this disease.

MUSCULOSKELETAL AGENTS

Rheumatoid arthritis is a chronic and often progressive inflammatory condition linked to the dysfunction of the immune system. Antibodies called **rheumatoid factors** contribute to the course of the disease. Inflammation caused by the release of histamine and prostaglandins leads to swelling, feelings of warmth, and pain in joints (especially in the hands, wrists, feet, hips, knees, and ankles). As the disease progresses, a decrease in range of motion and an increase in bony fusion and muscle deformity may occur. Patients often show fatigue, low-grade fever, stiffness, and joint pain, especially in the morning.

There is no known cure or method of prevention for rheumatoid arthritis.

Treatment may include drug therapy, physical therapy, occupational therapy, weight reduction, rest, and the use of adaptive or assistive devices. Drug therapy primarily consists of NSAIDs that inhibit prostaglandins synthesis and reduce inflammation. They are also the first line drug of choice due to their analgesic properties. However, as the condition progresses, **disease modifying antirheumatic drugs (DMARD's)** such as methotrexate (see chapter 13, Antineoplastics) as well as gold preparations such as gold sodium thiomate (aqueous) and aurothioglucose (suspended in oil) are indicated.

Gout **is an inflammatory condition in which an excess uric acid and urate crystals accumulate in** *synovial fluids* **of the joints.**

This leads to joint swelling, redness, warmth, and pain. The cause of the gout may be dietary or due to a metabolism dysfunction. A patient may experience an acute attack of gouty arthritis with severe pain, fever, swelling of joints, and inflammation. Stress, diet (e.g., foods high in iodine such as shellfish), alcohol, and infection can precipitate an attack. A first line drug used to treat gouty arthritis would be colchicine. **Uricosuric** drugs (e.g., probenecid) increase elimination of uric acid and **xanthine oxidase inhibitors** (e.g., allopurinol) interfere with uric acid synthesis.

gout a painful inflammatory condition in which excess uric acid accumulates in the joints.

rheumatoid arthritis a chronic and often progressive inflammatory condition with symptoms that include swelling, feelings of warmth, and joint pain.

MUSCULAR SYSTEM

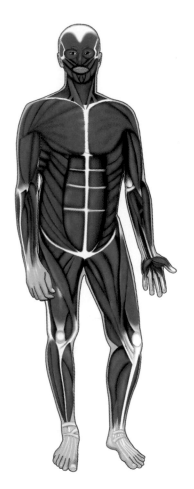

The muscular system is a complex system of connecting and overlapping muscles that completely cover the body. There are **cardiac muscles** in the heart and **smooth muscles** in the arteries and digestive tract, but most muscles are **skeletal muscles** attached to the skeleton by **tendons**. These muscles are made up of long muscle fibers that expand and contract to push and pull bones and cause body movement.

SKELETAL SYSTEM

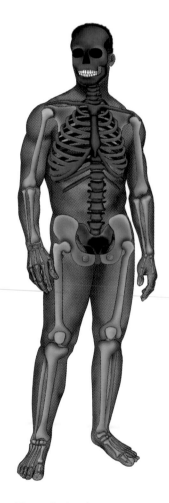

The skeletal system works with the muscular system to provide precise and powerful movement. The system's 206 bones are called **axial** (brain and spinal column) or **appendicular** (arms, legs, and connecting bones). They are held together at **joints** by connective tissue called **ligaments** and **cartilage**. Joints range from rigid to those allowing full motion. The **hinge joints** of the knee, elbow and ankle allow motion along a single axis. The **ball-and-socket joints** of the hips and shoulders allow a much broader range of movement.

Osteoarthritis is marked by weight-bearing bone deterioration, decreasing range of motion, and increasing pain, deformity, and disability.

Water content changes in the bone cartilage weakens the bones, causes cartilage damage and prevents repair. Inflammation may occur. Deep aching and local pain is experienced but can initially be relieved by rest. However, as the disease progresses, pain becomes chronic. Deformity also occurs in the later stages and bony enlargements (**osteophytes**) develop on the fingers and toes.

Drug therapy, physical therapy, adaptive or assistive devices, patient education, and possibly surgery are part of a comprehensive treatment approach.

Drug therapy primarily consists of analgesics, NSAID's, and corticosteroids. Since the majority of patients are elderly, drug treatment is directed at pain relief and is traditionally more conservative than aggressive.

Muscle spasms **are painful occurrences that can be infrequent, chronic, or acute, depending on their origin and the patient's underlying medical condition.**

Trauma, overwork, or a disorder such as connective tissue irritation can cause painful muscle contractions and involuntary spasms. Severe **spasticity** is usually linked to central nervous system disorders. Traditionally, treatment of muscle spasms is directed at muscle relaxation, pain relief, ability to exercise the muscle, and prevention of motion loss. Centrally acting **antispasmodics** (e.g., diazepam) eliminate contracture and cramps without affecting normal muscle activity. The sedative action of agents such as carisoprodol, chlorzoxazone, and chlorphenesin helps relieve acute musculoskeletal pain while cyclobenzapine decreases muscle tone and reduces spasm.

---

osteoarthritis a disorder characterized by weight-bearing bone deterioration, decreasing range of motion, pain, and deformity.

uricosuric drugs drugs used to treat gout that increase the elmination of uric acid.

MUSCULOSKELETAL AGENTS

Gold Sodium Thiomalate

Action and Indication

These gold preparations are used to treat rheumatoid arthritis, but may take 3-6 months to become effective. They act to prevent joint damage and preserve function.

Dosage

A test dose is often tried before the actual doses are given. For example, 10 mg one time as a test. If therapy is to be continued, 25-50 mg may be given weekly. Dosage may be cumulative up to 1 gm or when the patient's toxicity has been reached.

Route

IM.

Side Effects

GI upset, rash, anemia, hematuria, possible hypotension, palpitations, and headache

Warnings

Monitoring the patient's blood counts and urine while taking this drug is recommended.

Special Patient Teaching Considerations

Patients should be advised that the positive effects of this treatment may not be realized for several months. They should keep appointments for blood and urine monitoring and notify the physician of side effect occurrence.

Colchicine

Action and Indication

This is an anti-inflammatory agent used to treat gout by protecting the synovial (joint) cell from urate crystal damage. It is the preferred agent for gouty arthritis.

Dosage

For gout prevention: 1 tablet (0.5-1.8 mg) per day. For acute attacks: 1-2 tablets initially followed by 1-2 tablets every 2 hours until pain resolves, with a maximum of 8 tablets per attack. For very severe attacks: IV colchicine may be given at 2 mg infusing slowly over 2-5 min. with a repeat of 0.5 mg every 6 hours if necessary, up to a maximum of 4 mg IV.

Route

PO, IV.

Side Effects

GI distress such as nausea/vomiting, diarrhea, and stomach pain.

Warnings

The IV site should be monitored for signs of infiltration that can cause tissue damage. This drug is most effective if used within 24 hours of an attack of gout.

Special Patient Teaching Considerations

Report continuing diarrhea to a physician. Notify physician of attacks of gout as soon as possible to achieve optimal effect of this treatment. Avoid the use of alcohol while taking this medication as alcohol will increase uric acid levels.

MUSCULOSKELETAL AGENTS

Allopurinol (Zyloprim®)

Action and Indication

This agent acts to decrease uric acid production and reduce the precipitating factor in gout development. Colchicine may be given along with allopurinol to reduce the chances of precipitating a gout attack.

Dosage

The initial dosage may be 100 mg, given daily and may increase to 200-300 mg daily to reach the desired serum uric acid levels.

Route

PO tablets.

Side Effects

Nausea/vomiting, elevated liver function tests, diarrhea, drowsiness, and possible severe allergic reaction.

Warnings

Gastrointestinal distress and severe allergic reaction possible. Patients with a history of renal disease may need to receive a reduced dose of this drug.

Special Patient Teaching Considerations

It is imperative that patients experiencing any signs of allergic response (fever, chills, nausea/vomiting rash, hematuria or swelling of mouth and/or lips), should report this event immediately to their physician. A condition known as **Stevens-Johnson Syndrome**, a very severe systemic allergic reaction, can occur. Patients taking this drug should also drink 10-12 glasses of water daily, avoid alcohol, and avoid vitamin C as vitamin C increases the chances of kidney stones.

Carisoprodol (Soma®)

Action and Indication

This drug is indicated in cases of muscular discomfort including strain, spasm and aching pain.

Dosage

Dependent upon severity of pain, patient age, weight, and general medical condition. For example, 350 mg 3-4 times a day.

Route

PO.

Side Effects

Dizziness and drowsiness, vertigo, nausea/vomiting.

Warnings

This agent has the potential for abuse.

Special Patient Teaching Considerations

This product may produce drowsiness and an inability to conduct normal daily activities.

MUSCULOSKELETAL AGENTS

Cyclobenzaprine Hydrochloride (Flexeril®)

Action and Indication

This product reduces muscle tone, eases muscle spasm and the pain which results from general musculoskeletal discomfort. It is closely related to the tricyclic antidepressants in chemical structure.

Dosage

Dependent upon severity of injury and general medical condition. For example, 20-60 mg per day in divided doses.

Route

PO.

Side Effects

Drowsiness, dry mouth, headache, ringing in the ears, increased heart rate, and dizziness.

Warnings

Should not be used concurrently with monoamine oxidase inhibitors or within fourteen days of their use. Contraindicated for patients with hyperthyrodism, arrhythmias, heart block, or congestive heart failure. This drug has the potential for abuse.

Special Patient Teaching Considerations

This product may produce drowsiness and an inability to conduct normal daily activities. Avoid the use of alcohol while taking this drug.

Diazepam (Valium®)

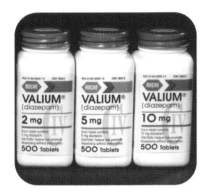

Valium®
(diazepam)
Courtesy of Hoffman LaRoche Inc.

Action and Indication

This antianxiety drug also has antispasmodic properties. It is used to relieve skeletal muscle spasm due to inflammation or trauma, spasticity resulting from various disorders (e.g., cerebral palsy or paraplegia), and tetanus. It is also indicated in cases of status epilepticus and is administered IV for this event.

Dosage

2-10 mg PO three to four times a day. 5-10 mg IM or IV initially and 5-10 mg in three to four hours. Higher doses may be necessary for tetanus

Route

PO, IM, or IV.

Side Effects

CNS depression leading to drowsiness, fatigue, disorientation, confusion, and constipation. Phlebitis or thrombosis may also occur.

Warnings

Some patients may be hypersensitive to diazepam. This drug is contraindicated for patients with glaucoma, who are pregnant, and in pediatric patients under six months of age.

Special Patient Teaching Considerations

Patients could abuse this drug, as well as other benzodiazepines. *Abrupt discontinuation could cause withdrawal symptoms which may be new or worse than those occurring prior.* Avoid use during preganancy, OTC cough or cold preparations, alcohol, and other CNS depressants when taking this drug. Avoid abrupt discontinuation after prolonged use.

DRUG CHART

Generic Name	Trade Name	Route	Generic Name	Trade Name	Route
Anti-Gout Agents			**Skeletal Muscle Relaxants**		
Colchicine	Various	PO, Inj.	Baclofen	Lioresal	PO
Allopurinol	Zyloprim	PO		Various	PO
Probenecid	Benemid	PO	Carisoprodol	Soma	PO
				Rela	PO
Corticosteroids				Various	PO
Dexamethasone	Decadron	PO, Inj.	Chlorzoxazone	Parafon Forte	PO
	Various	PO, Inj.		Paraflex	PO
Methylprednisolone	Medrol	PO		Various	PO
	Depo-Medrol	Inj.	Cyclobenzaprine	Flexeril	PO
	Various	PO, Inj.		Various	PO
Prednisone	Deltasone	PO	Dantrolene	Dantrium	PO, Inj.
	Orasone	PO	Metaxalone	Skelaxin	PO
	Various	PO	Methocarbamol	Robaxin	PO, Inj.
				Marbaxin	PO, Inj.
Salicylates			Orphenadrine	Norflex	PO, Inj.
Aspirin / Oxycodone	Percodan	PO		Myophen	PO, Inj.
	Percodan Demi	PO		Flexoject	Inj.
	Roxiprin	PO			
			Neuromuscular Blockers		
Bone Resorption Inhibitors			Atracurium	Tracrium	Inj.
Biphosphonates			Cisatracurium	Nimbex	Inj.
Alendronate	Fosamax	PO	Doxacurium	Nuromax	Inj.
Etidronate	Didronel	PO, Inj.	Mivacurium	Mivacron	Inj.
Pamidronate	Aredia	Inj.	Pancuronium	Pavulon	Inj.
Risedronate	Actonel	PO	Rocuronium	Zemuron	Inj.
Tiludronate	Skelid	PO	Succinylcholine	Anectine	Inj.
				Sucostrin	Inj.
Vitamin D Analogs				Quelicin	Inj.
Calcitriol	Rocaltrol	PO	Tubocurarine	Tubocurarine	Inj.
	Calcijex	Inj.	Vecuronium	Norcuron	Inj.
Ergocalciferol, Vitamin D2	Calciferol	PO			
	Drisdol	PO	**Reverse Neuromuscular Blockers**		
	Various	PO	Edrophonium	Enlon	Inj.
				Reversol	Inj.
Disease Modifying Antirheumatic Drugs				Tensilon	Inj.
Immunosuppresives			Neostigmine	Prostigmin	Inj.
Hydroxychloroquine	Plaquenil	PO			
Gold Compounds					
Auranofin	Ridaura	PO			
Aurothioglucose	Solganal	Inj.			

Note: for NSAIDs, see the Analgesics Drug Chart on page 166.

KEY CONCEPTS

✔ Rheumatoid arthritis is a chronic and often progressive inflammatory condition linked to the dysfunction of the immune system. Antibodies called rheumatoid factors contribute to the course of the disease. Inflammation caused by the release of histamine and prostaglandins leads to swelling, feelings of warmth, and pain in joints. As the disease progresses, a decrease in range of motion and an increase in bony fusion and muscle deformity may occur.

✔ There is no known cure or method of prevention for rheumatoid arthritis.

✔ Drug therapy primarily consists of NSAIDs that inhibit prostaglandins synthesis and reduce inflammation. As the condition progresses, disease modifying antirheumatic drugs (DMARD's) such as methotrexate are used.

✔ Gout is an inflammatory condition in which an excess uric acid and urate crystals accumulate in synovial fluids of the joints.

✔ Uricosuric drugs (e.g., probenecid) increase elimination of uric acid and xanthine oxidase inhibitors (e.g., allopurinol) interfere with uric acid synthesis.

✔ Osteoarthritis is marked by weight-bearing bone deterioration, decreasing range of motion, and increasing pain, deformity, and disability.

✔ Trauma, overwork, or a disorder such as connective tissue irritation can cause painful muscle contractions and involuntary spasms. Traditionally, treatment of muscle spasms is directed at muscle relaxation, pain relief, ability to exercise the muscle, and prevention of motion loss. Centrally acting antispasmodics (e.g., diazepam) eliminate contracture and cramps without affecting normal muscle activity.

CHOOSE THE BEST ANSWER. *answers are in the back of the book*

1. Of the following drugs, which one is closely related to tricyclic antidepressants?
   a. carisoprodol
   b. cyclobenzapine
   c. diazepam
   d. probenecid

2. Of the following drugs, which one is not only used as an antispasmodic agent but as an antianxiety agent as well?
   a. carisoprodol
   b. cyclobenzapine
   c. diazepam
   d. probenecid

3. Which following trade names does not match with the generic name?
   a. carisoprodol / Soma®
   b. cyclobenzapine / Flexeril®
   c. diazepam / Valium®
   d. probenecid / Zyloprim®

4. Of the following drugs below, which one is used to increase elimination of uric acid?
   a. carisoprodol
   b. cyclobenzapine
   c. diazepam
   d. probenecid

NEUROLOGICAL AGENTS

Since nerve cells do not contact other neurons and the muscles they affect directly, nerve impulses are communicated by chemical transmission.

These chemical mediators are **neurotransmitters** or **neurohormones.** They cross the **synapses** (the junctions between nerve cells) and allow transmission of impulses from one neuron to another. Two common peripheral nerve neurotransmitters are **acetylcholine** and **norepinephrine.**

Several common neurological disorders are affected by abnormalities in neurotransmitter release and/or response.

This includes the following disorders: Parkinson's Disease, Alzheimers Disease, epilepsy, and migraine headaches.

NERVOUS SYSTEM

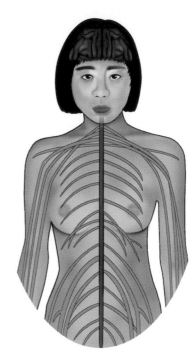

The Nervous System

The nervous system is divided into two main subsystems: the **central nervous system (CNS)** and the **peripheral nervous system.** The central nervous system consists of the brain and spinal cord. The peripheral nervous system carries information throughout the body and links the body's systems together. It is made up of the **somatic nervous system** and the **autonomic nervous system.**

The somatic nervous system is associated with voluntary movements of the musculoskeletal system and sensations (heat, cold, pressure and pain). The autonomic nervous system is responsible for automatic movements (breathing, digestion, etc.).

The autonomic nervous system is divided into the **sympathetic** and **parasympathetic** systems. The sympathetic branch works with the adrenal

gland's medulla and regulates energy in times of stress such as danger, emotional tensions and severe illness. The parasympathetic branch influences bodily functions to slow down and conserve energy. The sympathetic and parasympathetic nervous systems effect a delicate balance and maintain homeostasis on a daily basis within the human body. Drugs referred to as mimics act upon these systems to affect this balance and force a reaction.

fight or flight

parasympathetic

sympathetic

slows metabolism

A Delicate Balance

The balance between the sympathetic and parasympathetic systems is illustrated in the "fight or flight" response. In the event of being threatened and frightened, the sympathetic system reacts to increase heart rate, deep breathing, and blood pressure (increases circulation of oxygen), dilate pupils (provides extra light for vision), increase liver glycogen breakdown (supplies glucose and oxygen to muscles for energy), and halt peristalsis. The parasympathetic system will restart digestive and peristaltic actions, constrict the pupils, slow the heart and respiratory rates, and lower blood pressure when the threat is removed.

DISORDERS

THERAPIES

Parkinson's Disease

Parkinson's Disease is a progressive neuromuscular condition that usually affects patients above 50 years of age and is characterized by flat emotionless expression, bent posture, shuffling and unsteady gait, fine tremors, and difficulty chewing and swallowing. Early symptoms may include muscle aches, numbness, coldness, and loss of sensation or tingling. It is associated with low levels of the neurotransmitter **dopamine** in the brain and increased levels of acetylcholine. Brain tumors, arteriosclerosis, severe infectious processes, and excessive use of some antipsychotic drugs may also cause this disease.

Drug therapy will not stop the progress of this disease. Instead, an increased quality of life, decreased side effects, and minimization of disabilities are the goals of chemical treatment. Levodopa, carbidopa and levodopa together, amantadine, and selegiline hydrochloride are commonly prescribed antiparkinsonian drugs. In addition, dopamine agonists (e.g., pergolide and bromocriptine) are indicated when patients are experiencing a decrease in L-dopa's responsiveness. Anticholinergics are used for the treatment of tremors and decreased muscle tone.

Alzheimer's Disease

Alzheimer's, a progressive **dementia** often classified as a psychiatric disorder, has been linked to neurotransmitter abnormalities. It primarily affects the elderly. Loss of memory is often one of the first signs of this condition, with speech impairment, frustration, depression and decreased socialization soon occurring. These symptoms are generally followed by an inability to conduct the activities of daily living as well as a loss of spatial relationships. Ultimately, an inability to recognize familiar people and surroundings, wandering, combative aggression and incontinence occur.

Drug therapy can be divided into treatment for cognitive symptoms most closely associated with dementias and noncognitive symptoms such as depression. Tacrine and donepezil are examples of cognitive symptom agents while secondary amine tricyclic antidepressants (e.g., nortriptyline and desipramine) and SSRI's (e.g., paroxetine and sertraline) are indicated for symptoms such as depression in the Alzheimer patient.

Epilepsy

Epilepsy is a neurologic disorder associated with neuron transmission instability and characterized by recurrent seizure activity. Though there are other causes for seizures (trauma, fever, stress, etc.), the excess excitability seen in seizures may be linked to an imbalance of dopamine and acetylcholine release coupled with factors such as improper pH balance or an inadequate supply of glucose, oxygen, potassium, calcium or amino acids.

Common antiepileptic drugs include phenytoin and phenobarbital. Other drugs include valproic acid and carbamazepine. With anticonvulsant agents, the diagnosis needs to be conclusive and the most appropriate drug for the specific seizure type is chosen.

Migraine Headaches

There are two common theories on the causes of migraine headaches: the *vascular* and *nerve theories*. The vascular theory is that arterial vasoconstriction causes loss of oxygen and inflammation that stimulates sensory nerves in the head and results in possible auras and pain. An aura is an unusual sensation that can include hallucination. Stress, intense lights, colors, and sounds, and sleep deprivation are all considered stimulants of vasoconstriction. The nerve theory is that inflammation of nerve endings in the brain by inflammatory neurotransmitters (i.e., prostaglandins) causes pain.

Aspirin is considered the drug of choice (with caution used when treating children), and NSAID's are especially useful if the patient is female and menstruating. Other drug therapies include: ergotamine, sumatriptan, and midrin. Prophylactic treatment may include: betablockers, antidepressants, calcium channel blockers and anticonvulsants.

ANTIPARKINSONIAN

Carbidopa + Levodopa (Sinemet®)

Action and Indication

Levodopa causes antiparkinsonian effects by converting to dopamine. Carbidopa prevents the reversal of levodopa's effects caused by Vitamin B_6 (pyroxidine). Sinemet helps to relieve muscular tremor, weakness, and stiffness found in Parkinson's patients.

Dosage

Dosing of this medication can be complex. Initially, 1 tablet of 25 mg of carbidopa and 100 of levodopa may be given 2-3 times a day, with hourly spacing of 4-8 hours. The usual long term dose is 2-8 tablets a day, dependent upon patient response. Note: This is also available in other dosage combinations, i.e., 25/250 and 10/100. Sinemet is available in a standard and a **controlled release** form. The standard form is often used for initial dosing and then converted to CR once ideal levels are reached.

Route

PO, tablets.

Side Effects

Uncontrolled motor movements such as twitching (dyskinesia), confusion, depression, and nausea.

Warnings

Caution should be used in patients with a history of cardiac arrhythmias, peptic ulcer, asthma, COPD (chronic obstructive pulmonary disease), narrow-angle glaucoma, melanoma, and liver or kidney dysfunction. Levodopa should be stopped at least 8 hours before Sinemet CR is given.

Special Patient Teaching Considerations

Do not abruptly stop taking this drug as it may cause tachycardia, fever, and blood pressure changes. The patient's saliva, urine or sweat may become discolored (red, brown or black). Discoloration is not an event of concern.

Permax®

Permax is usually given as adjunctive treatment with Sinemet. It is a **dopamine receptor agonist** and will support the antiparkinsonian effects of the dopamine converted from levodopa.

Benztropine Mesylate (Cogentin®)

Actions and Indications

An **anticholinergic agent** that acts to reduce muscular spasm associated with Parkinson's.

Dosage

Dependent on severity of disease and patient condition. For example, 0.5-1 mg, at bedtime initially and followed by 1-2 mg, one to three times a day.

Route

PO tablets, IM, IV (dosages will be different for IV route).

Side Effects

Possible CNS effects such as depression, confusion, dilated pupils, and nervousness and atropine-like effects such as dry mouth, rapid heart rate, urine retention, and constipation.

Warnings

Caution should be used in patients with history of cardiac disease, especially tachycardia, and enlarged prostate, and wide-angle glaucoma. Serious drug interactions can occur in patients taking antipsychotics, antihistamines, doxepin hydrochloride, and amantadine hydrochloride. Antacids may decrease this drug's effectiveness. The dosage should be lowered in times of severe heat.

Special Patient Teaching Considerations

Do not take this medication within one hour of taking antacids such as Maalox or Tums. Avoid overheating. Drink plenty of fluids.

ANTIALZHEIMER'S

Tacrine Hydrochloride (Cognex®)

Action and Indication

This medication is used for mild to moderate cognitive related Alzheimer's symptoms. Tacrine acts to increase available acetylcholine for binding to certain receptors. Tacrine also increases the release of norepinepherine and dopamine. These neurotransmitters will help improve the patient's memory, thinking, and behavior processes.

Dosage

To start, 10 mg four times a day and increased over a 6 week period to 40 mg daily, as tolerated, with an increase to the maximum of 20-40 mg, four times a day.

Route

PO.

Side Effects

Nausea/vomiting, diarrhea, abdominal pain, anxiety, confusion, and agitation. Tacrine has also been known to cause seizures and difficulty in urination.

Warnings

Tacrine may cause liver enzyme elevation. Caution should be used in patients with history of liver dysfunction, stomach ulcers, or asthma.

Special Patient Teaching Considerations

Tacrine is most effective when taken between meals, though if GI upset occurs, notify the physician and he/she may suggest you take it with meals. Do not abruptly stop taking this drug as symptoms of forgetfulness and agitation could get worse. Keep appointments for liver function studies.

Gabapentin (Neurontin®)

Action and Indication

An antiseizure medication that is indicated in the treatment of epilepsy and epilepsy-like conditions. The mechanism of action is not clearly defined although this agent has been successful in cases of partial seizures which do not involve loss of consciousness.

Dosage

The doses are stepped from 300 mg the first day to 600 mg the second day and 900 mg the third day. Each 300 mg is given separately, so 900 mg would be divided into three doses. The suggested daily maintenance dose ranges from 900-1800 mg, divided into 3 doses. This drug is not recommended for use in children and should be discontinued gradually over a week period.

Route

PO capsules.

Side Effects

Sleepiness, dizziness, blurred vision, poor muscular coordination, and fatigue.

Warnings

Caution should be used in patients with a history of renal dysfunction. Antacids such as maalox could cause an unwanted drug interaction. This drug could cause a false positive urine protein reading. *Patients should not abruptly discontinue gabapentin as status epilepticus could occur.*

Special Patient Teaching Considerations

Do not abruptly stop taking this drug. Gabapentin may cause drowsiness and use of alcohol, dangerous machinery or activities requiring optimal mental alertness should be avoided. Do not take antacids without conferring with a physician.

ANTIEPILEPTIC

Phenytoin Sodium (Dilantin®)

Seizures

Seizures may be categorized as **petit mal**, a less severe form (i.e., staring and a trance-like state), and **grand mal,** a more severe form in which the patient may experience an auditory or visual aura, a loss of consciousness, convulsions, loss of bladder and/or bowel control, and foaming of the mouth. Following a grand mal episode, the patient will experience a **post-ictal** period of exhaustion and a need to sleep. They may also be confused and frightened at this time. Other seizure activity includes pyschomotor seizures which are hallmarked with bizarre and often repetitive behavior and **focal** or **Jacksonian seizures**, in which a specific part of the body will react with tremorous activity (i.e., hand or foot).

Action and Indication

An anticonvulsant used primarily to treat seizure activity such as in epileptic grand mal, temporal lobe, and post-surgery seizures.

Dosage

Dosage depends on the severity of the condition and the patient's age and weight. For example, an adult may initially take 100 mg three times daily. This may be followed by 1-2 capsules three times daily or one dose of 300 mg daily. Children may take 5 mg/kg per day, divided into 2-3 equal doses. The maximum should not exceed 300 mg per day.

Route

PO tablets, chewables, liquid suspension or IV for serious cases.

Side Effects

Allergic reactions, nystagmus (involuntary eye movements), decreased coordination, confusion, slurred speech, and possible elevated glucose and liver enzymes.

Warnings

Patient should be sensitive to signs of Stevens-Johnson syndrome, particularly red or purple scaly rash development. Caution should be used in patients with a history of liver dysfunction.

Special Patient Teaching Considerations

Do not take alcohol while taking this drug. Practice good oral hygiene and do not change from one form of Dilantin to another without speaking to your doctor. Do not stop taking this agent abruptly as prolonged seizure activity (status epilepticus) could occur.

 Status Epilepticus is a serious condition in which the patient is in a constant state of grand mal seizure activity. It is imperative in this case for the patient to receive immediate drug therapy treatment (i.e., diazepam IV) to end the seizure and restore the respiratory function of the patient.

Phenobarbital

Action and Indication

This **barbiturate** is often indicated for epileptic patients due to its anticonvulsant and sedative properties.

Dosage

Dependent upon route, severity of seizure activity and patient's condition. For example, 100-300 mg PO, every day for chronic therapy and ranges from 200-320 mg to 10 mg/kg. IV for status epilepticus.

Route

PO tablets, liquid elixir and IV.

Side Effects

Sleepiness, exaggerated thought patterns and emotional responses, possible respiratory depression, and severe allergic reaction.

Warnings

Not indicated in patients with respiratory insufficiency or sensitivity to barbituates. Frequent complete blood count assessments should be performed and patient should be monitored for withdrawal symptoms. Phenobarbital decreases clotting time in patients taking warfarin.

Special Patient Teaching Considerations

Since this agent may cause a sleepy or drowsy state, do not operate machinery or conduct business which requires complete alertness. Do not drink alcohol while taking this drug and be aware that phenobarbital may be habit forming and cause withdrawal symptoms if discontinued.

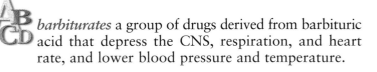

barbiturates a group of drugs derived from barbituric acid that depress the CNS, respiration, and heart rate, and lower blood pressure and temperature.

ANTIMIGRAINE

Ergotamine Tartrate, with Caffeine (Cafergot®)

More Than A Simple Headache

Migraines most often manifest in the morning and will peak in about 1 hour from onset. The pain can be severe causing such events as vomiting, diarrhea, irritability, anxiety and personality change. These headaches can last from 4 hours to a number of days and are often addressed with analgesics and NSAID's. Migraines may occur with or without auras, although the majority occur without them.

Action and Indication

This medication is indicated in cases of vascular headaches such as migraines. The action of ergotamine is thought to be that of a vasoconstrictor of cranial blood vessel smooth muscle. Ergotamine works most effectively if taken when the migraine symptoms first appear.

Dosage

This agent comes in 1 and 2 mg tablets, with or without 100 mg of caffeine. The 2 mg tablets may be regular or sublingual. It is also available in 2 mg suppositories with caffeine and as an inhaler and IM or IV solution. A common dosage may be 1-2 tablets at onset with 1 tablet every 30 minutes until a maximum of 6 tablets a day or 10 tablets a week is reached.

Route

PO tablets, suppositories, inhaler, IM, and IV.

Side Effects

Hypertension, peripheral ischemia, including numbness and coldness, fluid retention, and vertigo.

Warnings

This agent is a vasconstrictor and abuse could cause serious effects such as chest pain and severe hypertension. This medication should be taken at the onset of symptoms. Patients should also lie down in a dark and quiet environment and avoid exposure to the cold. Discontinuance may cause withdrawal symptoms such as severe and sudden rebound headaches. Certain other drugs, such as beta blockers, nicotine, and selected antibiotics may cause an effect on this agent.

Special Patient Teaching Considerations

Notify the physician of any known allergy to this drug or caffeine, history of hypertension, cardiac pathologies, and liver or kidney dysfunction. Psychological dependence could occur with prolonged use or abuse of this drug. Do not exceed the recommended dosage.

Sumatriptan Succinate (Imitrex®)

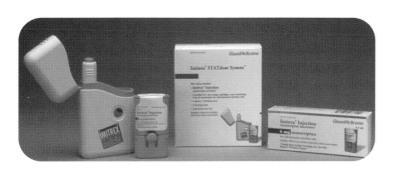

Imitrex®
(sumatriptan succinate)
Courtesy of Glaxo Wellcome Inc.

Action and Indication

This drug is used in the treatment of migraine headches by acting as an agonist, vasoconstrictor and blocker of inflammation. It is thought by many sources to be more effective than ergotamine with caffeine.

Dosage

Upon onset, 6 mg SQ or 1 tablet (25 mg) PO with a maximum of 2, 6 mg injections, or 300 mg PO daily. The injections should be separated by at least one hour and the oral tablets by 2 hours.

Route

PO, SQ.

Side Effects

From tablets: nausea/vomiting, dizziness, and vertigo. From SQ injection: chest tightness, pressure, and injection site irritation.

Warnings

This drug is contraindicated in patients with heart attack and ischemic heart disease history. Also, caution should be used if patient has a history of liver or kidney dysfunction.

Special Patient Teaching Considerations

Notify the physician if any side effects occur or if headache persists in a different form. The physician should be notified if the patient smokes, is pregnant, has hypertension, cardiac disease, diabetes and/or high cholesterol. Note: Imitrex is to be used in cases of an attack and not for regular or chronic headaches. Its action is to shorten an attack, not prevent one.

DRUG CHART

GENERIC NAME	TRADE NAME	ROUTE
ANTIPARKINSONS AGENTS		
Bromocriptine	Parlodel	PO
	Ergoset	PO
Levodopa / Carbidopa	Sinemet	PO
	Atamet	PO
	Various	PO
Pergolide	Permax	PO
Pramipexole	Mirapex	PO
Ropinirole	Requip	PO
Tolcapone	Tasmar	PO
ANTIMIGRAINE		
SEROTONIN-RECEPTOR AGONISTS		
Naratriptan	Amerge	PO
Rizatriptan	Maxalt	PO
Sumatriptan	Imitrex	PO, Inj., Nasal Spray
Zolmitriptan	Zomig	PO
ERGOT ALKALOIDS		
Dihydroergotamine	D.H.E. 45	Injection
	Migranal	Nasal Spray
Methysergide	Sansert	PO
ANTIVERTIGO AGENTS		
Scopolamine	Scopace	PO
	Various	PO, Inj., Transdermal
Meclizine	Dramamine Non Drowsy	PO
	Bonine	PO
	Antivert	PO
	Various	PO
Dimenhydrinate	Dramamine	PO
	Various	PO

KEY CONCEPTS

✔ Nerve impulses are communicated by chemical transmission since nerve cells do not contact other neurons or the muscles they affect. These chemicals are neurotransmitters or neurohormones. They cross the synapses and allow transmission of impulses from one neuron to another.

✔ Two common peripheral nerve neurotransmitters are acetylcholine and norepinephrine.

✔ Common neurological disorders affected by abnormalities in neurotransmitter release and/or response include Parkinson's Disease, Alzheimers Disease, epilepsy, and migraine headaches.

✔ The sympathetic and parasympathetic nervous systems maintain homeostasis on a daily basis within the body. When frightened, the sympathetic system causes a "fight or flight" response (increased heart rate, deep breathing, blood pressure, etc.). Once the threat is gone, the parasympathetic system will slow the heart and respiratory rates, lower blood pressure, etc.

✔ Parkinson's Disease is a progressive neuromuscular condition that usually affects patients above 50 years of age. Its symptoms include flat emotionless expression, bent posture, and fine tremors. It is associated with low levels of dopamine in the brain and increased levels of acetylcholine.

✔ Alzheimer's, a progressive dementia often classified as a psychiatric disorder, has been linked to neurotransmitter abnormalities.

✔ Epilepsy is a neurologic disorder associated with neuron transmission instability and characterized by recurrent seizure activity.

✔ The vascular theory of migraines is that arterial vasoconstriction causes loss of oxygen and inflammation that stimulates sensory nerves in the head and results in possible auras and pain. The nerve theory is that inflammation of nerve endings in the brain by inflammatory neurotransmitters (i.e., prostaglandins) causes pain.

CHOOSE THE BEST ANSWER.

answers are in the back of the book

1. Of the following neurotransmitters, which one is needed in the treatment of Parkinson's?
   a. acetylcholine
   b. dopamine
   c. norepinephrine
   d. serotonin

2) Of the following drugs, which one comes in a nasal spray formulation?
   a. carbidopa / levodopa
   b. gabapentin
   c. sumatriptan
   d. tacrine

3. Of the following brand name drugs, which one would not be indicated in the treatment of migraines?
   a. Cafergot®
   b. Cognex®
   b. Imitrex®
   c. Midrin®

4. Which of the following is an antiseizure medication which is indicated in the treatment of epilepsy and epilepsy-like conditions?
   a. carbidopa / levodopa
   b. gabapentin
   c. sumatriptan
   d. tacrine

OPHTHALMIC AGENTS

Ophthalmic agents are used to treat various conditions or disorders of the eye.

Disorders include **glaucoma**, infection, pain, and inflammation, but agents may also be used for eye examinations and in preparation for surgery. Ophthalmic agents are generally applied topically as drops or ointments.

Due to the special requirements for ophthalmic formulations, there are often many ingredients in a product besides the active ingredient.

Preservatives, antioxidants, buffers, and wetting agents that control such factors as pH, sterility, and proper isotonic percentages are often included.

Glaucoma represents several disorders characterized by abnormally high pressure within the eye that leads to optic nerve damage and progressive loss of vision.

The onset of glaucoma can be a slow process that may not be apparent to the patient and may only be detected during an eye examination. Early detection is essential for successful treatment and prevention of vision loss.

Although infection and inflammation can increase *intraocular pressure* **temporarily, the common cause of glaucoma is a structural defect in the eye.**

This form is called **primary glaucoma** and is divided into two types: **narrow or closed angle** and **wide or open angle**. Narrow angle glaucoma is corrected with surgery. Open angle glaucoma can be successfully treated with antiglaucoma drugs such as cholinergic receptor agonists, acetylcholinesterase inhibitors, carbonic anhydrase inhibitors, beta-adrenergic receptor antagonists, and adrenergic receptor agonists.

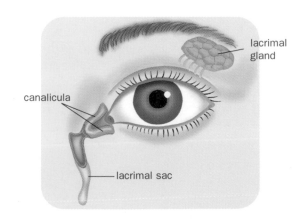

THE EYE

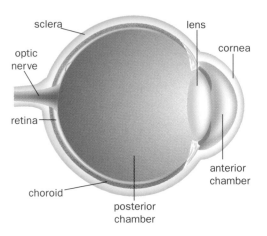

The eyeball has three layers:

➡ the outer layer contains the **sclera** (white part) and the **cornea** (clear);

➡ the middle vascular layer called the **choroid** contains the **iris** and **pupil**;

➡ the inner layer contains the **retina,** responsible for visual reception.

Both the anterior and posterior optic chambers are filled with a liquid called **aqueous humor**. The **lens** is located behind the **iris**. Ocular muscles control the movement of the eyeball and accommodate focusing. The thickness of the lens helps determine the distance at which one can see an object. Behind the lens, a jelly-like substance called the **vitreous body** helps maintain the shape of the eyeball.

Similar to a camera, the pupil allows light to enter. The lens focuses the light, and the retina receives the image. A complex chemical reaction within the retina processes the picture. The optic nerve then carries the image to the visual area of the brain.

Accessory structures to the eyeball include eyelids, ocular muscles, conjunctiva, eyelashes, and lacrimal glands.

Ophthalmic Administration

- ➡ Hands should always be washed prior to drug administration.

- ➡ If more than one agent is to be instilled, wait the suggested time (5 minutes between solutions, 10-15 minutes before ointments) between administrations.

- ➡ Do not rub eyes. Carefully instill, as per order, onto conjunctiva, one eye at a time.

- ➡ Do not touch the applicator to the eye at any time.

- ➡ Replace the applicator cap carefully and do not touch the top of the applicator.

- ➡ Be aware that temporary vision distortion may occur and encourage the patient accordingly.

- ➡ The physician should be notified if condition symptoms do not alleviate.

Note: The incidence of adverse reactions to ophthalmic agents is small. Systemic absorption may cause allergic response and steroidal side effects in some cases.

Antiglaucoma Agents

Cholinergic receptor agonists such as **pilocarpine** and **acetylcholine** were the first antiglaucoma drugs developed. More recently, acetylcholinesterase agents such as **physostigmine** and **demecarium** are preferred, since they are more potent, longer acting, and include both reversible and irreversible properties.

Beta-adrenergic receptor antagonists are also now used more commonly than the cholinergic receptor agonists as they are considered more effective and have fewer side effects. Examples of this type include: **betaxolol, carteolol, metipranolol,** and **timolol.**

Adrenergic receptor agonists such as **epinepherine, atropine,** and **dipivefrin** are used to lower intraocular pressure by increasing outflow of aqueous humor from the eye.

Conjunctivitis ("pink eye") is a common eye infection resulting from conjuctival irritation due to infectious organism or allergy. Conjunctivitis infections are highly contagious. Symptoms are redness of the conjunctiva and pus-like crusty exudate that often leads to the eyelid closing. Antibiotics such as gentamicin, bacitracin, neomycin, sodium sulfacetamide, norfloxacin, and ciprofloxacin are indicated if the infection is bacterial. For viral infections such as herpes simplex and cytomegalovirus retinitis, idoxuridine, vidarabine, and trifluridine are used. If the conjunctivitis is caused by an allergy, histamine blocking agents such as levocabastine, olopatadine, and emedastine may be ordered.

Inflammation of the eye may be treated with both NSAID's and corticosteriods.

Agents such as medrysone, prednisolone, and loteprednol are common ophthalmic corticoseriods while flurbiprofen, suprofen, and ketorolac are NSAID's available for ophthalmic application. Note: flurbiprofen and ketorolac are often used following cataract extraction surgery.

Other drugs include *mydriatics*, anesthetics, and lubricating agents.

Mydriatics are drugs that dilate the pupil and are commonly indicated prior to eye exams. When the pupil is dilated, more light is allowed in and visualization into the eye is enhanced. Phenylephrine and hydroxyamphetamine are popular examples. For optic related pain, a topical anesthetic such as proparacaine (also known as ophthaine) or tetracaine may be prescribed. To provide lubrication to the eyes if abnormal drying is occurring, the isotonic solution Artificial Tears® is available as an over-the counter agent. Lacrisert® is a prescription lubricating drug.

conjunctivitis inflammation of the conjunctiva (eyelid lining).

glaucoma disorders characterized by abnormally high pressure within the eye that leads to optic nerve damage and loss of vision.

intraocular inside the eye.

mydriatics drugs that dilate the pupil.

OPHTHALMIC AGENTS

Physostigmine Sulfate (Isopto® Eserine)

Action and Indication

This **parasympathomimetic** (a drug whose actions mimic those of the parasympathetic nervous system) **cholinesterase inhibitor** is indicated in the treatment of glaucoma as it increases outflow of aqueous humor and therefore reduces intraocular pressure.

Dosage

1-2 gtts (0.25-0.5% solution), every 8-12 hours.

Route

Eye drop instillation.

Side Effects

Rare.

Warnings

Related to administration of product more so than the product itself. See "Ophthalmic Administration" on preceding page.

Special Patient Teaching Considerations

See "Ophthalmic Administration" on preceding page.

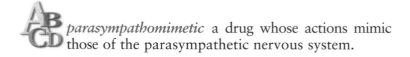 *parasympathomimetic* a drug whose actions mimic those of the parasympathetic nervous system.

Betaxolol Hydrochloride (Betoptic®)

Action and Indication

This **beta adrenergic blocker** acts to reduce intraocular pressure and is indicated in cases of open angle glaucoma.

Dosage

1-2 gtts (0.5% solution), two times a day in divided doses (every 12 hours)

Route

Eye drop instillation.

Side Effects

Temporary eye discomfort, possible allergic reactions and changes in taste or smell.

Warnings

Since this product is a beta blocker and has a possibility of being systemically absorbed, caution should be used if the patient has any medical history that could cause side effects such as cardiac pathology, asthma, thyroid dysfunction, or diabetes. *Other beta blockers such as propanolol and atenolol may be contraindicated for concurrent use with this product.*

Special Patient Teaching Considerations

See "Ophthalmic Administration" at beginning of chapter. Note: Do not rinse the dropper after an application. The eye drop solution is sterile and tap water is not. Also, water residue may dilute the medication.

OPHTHALMIC AGENTS

Timolol Maleate (Timoptic®)

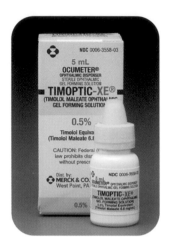

Timoptic®
(timolol)
Courtesy of Merck Archives

Action and Indication

This **beta adrenergic blocker** is used in the treatment of glaucoma to lower intraocular pressure.

Dosage

1 gtt (0.25-0.5% solution), once every 12-24 hours.

Route

Eye drop instillation.

Side Effects

Temporary eye discomfort including burning upon instillation, blurred vision, overflow of tears, possible allergic response.

Warnings

This product is a beta blocker and caution needs to be exercised if the patient's medical history includes cardiac pathologies, asthma, thyroid dysfunction, or diabetes. *Other beta blockers such as propanolol and atenolol may be contraindicated with concurrent use of this product.*

Special Patient Teaching Considerations

Advise your physician regarding your medical history and current medications.

Dipivefrin Hydrochloride (Propine®)

Action and Indication

This **adrenergic agonist** increases the outflow of aqueous fluid and thus reduces intraocular pressure. Dipivefrin is known as a **prodrug,** which means it does not become active until within the body. Prodrugs generally offer increased absorption and reduced side effects. Propine is indicated for treatment in cases of chronic open angle glaucoma.

Dosage

1 gtt (0.1% solution), once every 12 hours.

Route

Eye drop instillation.

Side Effects

Temporary eye discomfort including stinging and redness, possible allergic response and adrenergic events such as increase in heart rate and/or blood pressure and extreme pupil dilation.

Warnings

See proper administration techniques at beginning of chapter. Note: This product may come with a dose numbered cap for easy recall of application number.

Special Patient Teaching Considerations

Be aware that Dipivefrin may cause a temporary blurred vision following the instillation. Do not attempt to drive or conduct activity requiring clear vision until the condition abates.

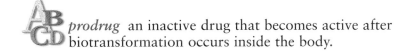 *prodrug* an inactive drug that becomes active after biotransformation occurs inside the body.

OPHTHALMIC AGENTS

Gentamicin Sulfate (Garamycin Ophthalmic®, Genoptic®)

Action and Indication

This antibiotic is available in an ophthalmic solution or ointment and is indicated for cases of eye infections, such as conjunctivitis.

Dosage

1-2 gtts of 0.3% solution every 4 hours. More severe infections may require up to 2 gtts per hour. Ointment dosage is 0.5 inches of 0.3% ointment to be applied 2-3 times a day.

Route

Eye drop instillation, eye ointment.

Side Effects

Eye irritation, stinging, possible allergic responses related to systemic absorption.

Warnings

There is the possibility of the development of a secondary infection following prolonged use of this drug.

Special Patient Teaching Considerations

Complete the entire course of treatment, even if symptoms subside and you are feeling better. A mutant strain or secondary infection could develop otherwise. Store this product away from heat and light.

Dexamethasone 0.1%, Tobramycin 0.3% (Tobradex®)

Action and Indication

Indicated in cases of bacterial conjunctivitis. Dexamethasone is a **glucocorticoid** used to reduce inflammation and the antibiotic, tobramycin, fights the infectious process.

Dosage

One centimeter of ointment or 1-2 drops every 3-4 hours.

Route

Solution or ointment.

Side Effects

Local irritation at application site (redness, itching of periorbital area).

Warnings

Allergic reaction possible.

Special Patient Teaching Considerations

Use only as directed and notify your physician if the condition does not get better in a few days after starting this medication.

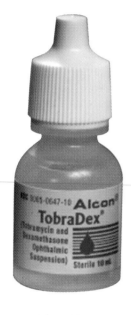

Tobradex®
(tobramycin/dexamethasone)
Courtesy of Alcon Laboratories

OPHTHALMIC AGENTS

Prednisolone Acetate (Pred Forte®, various)

Action and Indication

This ophthalmic **corticosteroid** preparation is indicated in cases of eye irritation, swelling, and inflammation.

Dosage

For the first 1-2 days, the dosage may be increased, due to condition severity. Regularly, the dosage may be 1-2 gtts, 2-4 times a day.

Route

Eye drop instillation.

Side Effects

Eye irritation and stinging, blurred vision, possible allergic response, dilated pupils, increased intraocular pressure.

Warnings

Prolonged use of this drug could lead to eye damage and/or increase in side effects, including side effects which occur with prolonged steroidal use (e.g., swelling). Patient should be assessed for signs of glaucoma following a course of 10 days or greater.

Special Patient Teaching Considerations

Use this drug only as prescribed. Notify the physician of any side effects, especially allergic reactions and/or worsening of symptoms.

Ketoralac Tromethamine (Acular®)

Action and Indication

This ophthalmic **NSAID** preparation is indicated in cases of eye irritation, swelling, and inflammation caused by seasonal allergy.

Dosage

One drop 0.25 mg four times a day for up to one week.

Route

Eye drop instillation.

Side Effects

Eye irritation and stinging, blurred vision, possible allergic response.

Warnings

This agent is for short term use only. Should not be used in patients with known allergies to aspirin or NSAIDs. Should not be used in pregnant or breast feeding women. Do not wear contact lenses while taking.

Special Patient Teaching Considerations

Do not take for more than seven days. Use this drug only as prescribed. Notify the physician of any side effects, especially allergic reactions, nausea, or if symptoms do not improve after two to three days.

DRUG CHART

GENERIC NAME	TRADE NAME	ROUTE
ANTIGLAUCOMA AGENTS		
ADRENERGIC RECEPTOR AGONISTS		
Atropine	Isopto Atropine	Eye drops
Dipivefrin	Propine	Eye drops
Epinephrine	Epifin	Eye drops
MIOTICS		
Demecarium	Humorsal	Eye drops
Physostigmine	Isopto Eserine	Eye drops
Pilocarpine	Isopto Carpine	Eye drops
	Pilocar	Eye drops
	Salagen	Eye drops
BETA BLOCKERS		
Betaxolol	Betoptic	Eye drops
Carteolol	Ocupress	Eye drops
Dorzolamide / Timolol	Cosopt	Eye drops
Levobunolol	Betagan	Eye drops
Metipranolol	OptiPranolol	Eye drops
Timolol	Timoptic	Eye drops
OTHERS		
Brimonidine	Alphagan	Eye drops
Brinzolamide	Azopt	Eye drops
Dorzolamide	Trusopt	Eye drops
STEROIDAL (ANTI-INFLAMMATORY)		
Prednisolone	Pred Forte	Eye drops
	Various	Eye drops
Dexamethasone	Decadron	Eye drops, ointment
	Maxidex	Eye drops, ointment
Fluorometholone	Flarex	Eye drops
	FML Forte	Eye drops
	Various	Eye drops
ANTI-INFECTIVE		
Tobramycin	Tobrex	Eye drops, ointment
	AKTob	Eye drops, ointment
Dexamethasone/Tobramycin	Tobradex	Eye drops, ointment
Gentamicin	Garamycin	Eye drops, ointment
	Genoptic	Eye drops, ointment
	Various	Eye drops, ointment
ANESTHETICS		
Tetracaine	Opticaine	Eye drops, ointment
	Pontocaine	Eye drops, ointment

See the Anti-infectives Drug chart on pages 198-199 for additional ophthalmic agents.

KEY CONCEPTS

✔ Ophthalmic disorders include glaucoma, infection, pain, and inflammation, but ophthalmic agents may also be used for eye examinations and in preparation for surgery. Ophthalmic agents are generally applied topically as drops or ointments.

✔ Due to the special requirements for ophthalmic formulations, there are often many ingredients in a product besides the active ingredient. Preservatives, antioxidants, buffers, and wetting agents are often included.

✔ Glaucoma represents several disorders characterized by abnormally high pressure within the eye that leads to optic nerve damage and progressive loss of vision. Although infection and inflammation can increase intraocular pressure temporarily, the common cause of glaucoma is a structural defect in the eye.

✔ Narrow angle glaucoma is corrected with surgery. Open angle glaucoma can be successfully treated with antiglaucoma drugs.

✔ Conjunctivitis ("pink eye") is a common eye infection resulting from conjuctival irritation due to infectious organism or allergy. Conjunctivitis infections are highly contagious and are treated with anti-infectives.

✔ Inflammation of the eye may be treated with both NSAID's and corticosteriods.

✔ Mydriatics are drugs that dilate the pupil and are commonly indicated prior to eye exams.

✔ For optic related pain, a topical anesthetic such as proparacaine (also known as ophthaine) or tetracaine may be prescribed.

✔ To provide lubrication to the eyes if abnormal drying is occurring, the isotonic solution Artificial Tears® is available as an over-the counter agent. Lacrisert® is a prescription lubricating drug.

CHOOSE THE BEST ANSWER.

answers are in the back of the book

1. Of the following ophthalmic agents, which one below not only comes in an eye drop formulation but also an eye ointment formulation?
   a. Betoptic®
   b. Propine®
   c. Garamycin®
   d. Isopto Tears®

2. Of the following types of primary glaucoma, which type can be treated with medication?
   a. narrow angle glaucoma
   b. closed angle glaucoma
   c. open angle glaucoma
   d. all of the above

3. A mydriatic agent is used to:
   a. decrease intraocular inflammation
   b. decrease intraocular pressure
   c. dilate the pupil
   d. dilate the lens

4. Of the following ophthalmic agents, which one would be most likely used in the treatment of conjunctivitis or pink eye?
   a. Betoptic®
   b. Propine®
   c. Garamycin®
   d. Isopto Tears®

PSYCHOTROPIC AGENTS

Psychotropic agents are drugs that affect behavior, psychiatric state, and sleep.

They act on specialized areas of the brain to suppress or control the symptoms of common psychological disorders such as bipolar disorder, anxiety, depression, schizophrenia, and drug abuse. The primary drug types in this class are **antidepressants**, **antipsychotics**, and **antianxiety agents**. Other related psychotropic agents include **sedatives** and **hypnotics**.

THE BRAIN

The brain is an incredibly versatile and complex organ responsible for a vast number of the body's functions. To a great extent, the structures or areas of the brain are specialized by function. These specialized structures are shown below.

Cerebrum

➡ concerned mostly with learned behavior, thought, memory, sensation and voluntary motion. It is divided into lobes: Frontal, Occipital (back) Parietal (top) and Temporal (side).

Cerebellum

➡ controls balance and muscle coordination.

Medulla Oblongata (brain stem)

➡ controls processes that affect the heart, breathing, temperature control and circulation.

Pons

➡ bridges from the medulla oblongata to the cerebellum and also works on muscle coordination.

Thalamus

➡ above the Pons, receives sensations such as heat, cold, pressure and pain.

Hypothalamus

➡ below the Thalamus, controls blood sugar levels, body temperature, emotions, appetite and sleep.

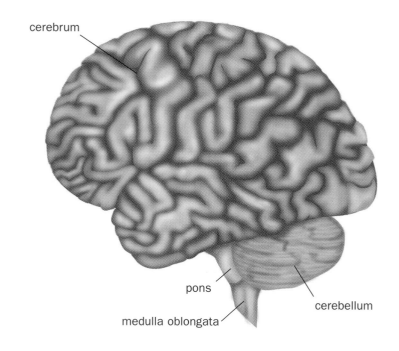

cerebrum

pons

medulla oblongata

cerebellum

Midbrain

➡ works to control blood pressure and the Pineal Gland secretes the hormone melatonin which effects the body's biological rhythms.

Limbic System

➡ an interconnecting network of brain cells inside the brain that affects behavior, emotions, sociosexual drives, motivation, learning, and memory storage and retrieval.

Sedatives and Hypnotics

Sedatives are drugs that are intended to relax and calm. They reduce restlessness and may produce mild drowsiness. Antianxiety medications that include benzodiazepines (e.g., diazepam and chlordiazepoxide) are included in this group.

Hypnotics are often referred to as "sleeping pills" and are designed to induce and, in some cases, prolong sleep. This group includes barbiturates such as secobarbital and pentobarbital. Nonbarbituate sedative-hypnotics include chloral hydrate and meprobamate.

DISORDERS

THERAPIES

Bipolar Disorder

Also known as **Manic-Depression**, this disorder is characterized by mood, energy, and behavior swings from periods of elation to episodes of depression. These swings are found to occur in a cyclical and recurring pattern. Theories of cause include chemical imbalance and neurotransmitter alterations in the brain. There is a high degree of family history associated with this disorder.

Although pychotherapy is included in the suggested treatment, antipsychotic drugs such as lithium combined with benzodiazepines such as lorazepam are commonly prescribed. Carbamazepine and valproic acid are often added to this therapy to treat seizure activity secondary to psychotropic agents.

Lithium carbonate - most popular choice

Anxiety

People experiencing anxiety may appear abnormally tired or energetic, withdrawn, tremorous, tense and restless and may suffer from insomnia, phobias and panic attacks. Theories of cause include a hypersensitive sympathetic nervous system, excessive serotonin release, and an inability to chemically receive the body's natural calming agents.

In conjunction with psychotherapy and various relaxation techniques, the commonly prescribed drugs include antianxiety agents such as the benzodiazapines (diazepam, lorazepam, and alprazolam).

Depression

Depression is characterized by mood disturbances that may be mild (e.g., lack of interest or inability to experience joy) or severe (e.g., physical aggression or suicide attempts). Sleep disturbances, crying episodes, gastro-intestinal upset and heart palpitations may occur. Theories of cause include: experience of trauma (real or perceived), loss, as well as poor neurotransmitter response of norepinephrine.

serotonin↑

While psychotherapy and even shock therapy are often prescribed treatment, antidepressants such as amitriptyline, paroxetine, and sertraline are common drug suggestions

3 classes of antidepressants
1. Tricyclic
2. Monoamine oxidase Inhibitors (MAOI)
→ levels are lowered
3. Selective Serotonin Reuptake Inhibitors (SSRI)

Schizophrenia

This is characterized by extreme and inappropriate behavior and dysfunctional daily routine. Hearing "voices," experiencing delusions, becoming agitated or hostile and perhaps a lack of response at all (flat affect) are examples of schizophrenic behavior. Theories of cause include: family history and chemical imbalances, especially norephinephrine and serotonin, noted in the limbic system.

Patients experiencing schizophrenia must undergo a complete medical and psychological examination. The drug therapy selected will result from the findings. Antipsychotic agents commonly used may include: chlorpromazine, trifluoperazine, and haloperidol.

Drug Dependency

Addiction to drugs and alcohol may occur for various reasons, including chronic usage without adequate physician supervision, chemical intolerance, error in personal judgement or purposeful abuse. Family history and social situation may be contributing factors.

Treatment for dependency often encompasses an on-site treatment program designed to identify and address the patient holistically. Adjunct drug therapy may or may not be included in this. For example, disulfiram and naltrexone may be used to dissuade the alcoholic from drinking, desipramine curbs cocaine desire, and methadone is prescribed for narcotic detoxification.

PSYCHOTROPIC AGENTS

Carbamazepine and valproic acid are often used for treatment of seizure activity secondary to psychotropic agents.

Carbamazepine, CBZ (Tegretol®)

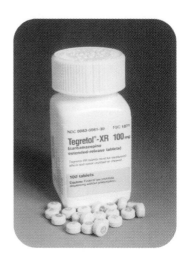

Tegretol®
(carbamazepine)
Courtesy of Novartis
Pharmaceutical Corporation

Action and Indication

Mood stabilizer. Preferred with patients who also have dementias. Acts as an antimanic and antidepressant by decreasing the release of norepinephrine. Note: also used as an anticonvulsant and for neurological disorders.

Dosage

If symptoms are acute, may be started at 200 -400 mg per day with increase to 600-1200 mg per day. The dose changes should be gradual and given in divided doses 2-4 times per day. If given in combination with other antipsychotics, the recommended dose would be less.

Route

PO as chewable tabs or liquid suspension.

Side Effects

Central Nervous System effects may be noted, such as dizziness, ataxia, confusion, tiredness, mood swings and blurred vision. Mild GI upset, rash, and anemia may also occur.

Warnings

Yearly liver enzyme testing and initial white blood count (WBC) monitoring is recommended. This drug should be given with food to minimize GI upset and abrupt discontinuence could precipitate seizures.

Special Patient Teaching Considerations

If a patient is pregnant, she should notify her physician immediately, as fetal developmental delays could occur. Patients should not abruptly stop taking this drug and should tell their physician if any side effects occur. Avoid alcohol while taking this drug. Carbamazepine may cause impotence and birth control should be non-hormonal. Avoid exposure to UV light.

Very effective for bipolar disorder

Divalproex Sodium, (Depakote®)

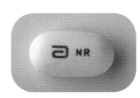

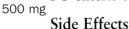 250 mg

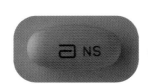 500 mg

Depakote®
(divalproex sodium)
Courtesy of Abbott Laboratories

Valproic Acid

Divalproex sodium (Depakote®), valproate sodium (Depacon®) and valproic acid (Depakene®) are closely related compounds that circulate in the body as the same ion. As a result, they have similar effects, uses, and characteristics.

Action and Indication

Recommended for rapid cycling manias or manias also exhibiting depressions and panic attacks. Also used for certain types of epilepsy.

Dosage

An initial dose of 750 mg per day , with the amount increased gradually, as needed, but not to exceed 60 mg/kg/ per day.

Route

PO enteric coated tablets.

Side Effects

Mild GI effects, drowsiness, confusion, mood swings, lethargy, hair loss, itching, and prolonged bleeding with liver toxicity leading to possible hepatic failure.

Warnings

Should not be used in pregnant patients, children, or those with hepatic disorders. Drug is taken with food to minimize GI upset. Lower doses may be used if symptoms become great. Avoid brand/generic interchange or dosage form changes.

Special Patient Teaching Considerations

Patients should be monitored regularly by their physician and be aware of the effects of this therapy. Liver function tests and platelet evaluations are especially important with this drug choice. Avoid alcohol when taking this drug. Patients should not engage in activities that require alertness.

ANTIANXIETY AGENTS

Diazepam (Valium®)

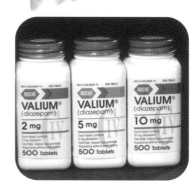

Valium®
(diazepam)
Courtesy of Hoffman La Roche

Action and Indication

An **antianxiety drug** that has calming effects as well as anticonvulsive and antispasmodic properties. Used for management of anxiety disorders, the short term relief of anxiety symptoms, alcohol withdrawal, convulsive disorders, and pre-surgery medication. This agent is indicated in cases of status epilepticus and is administered IV for this event.

Dosage

Acute anxiety may necessitate 2-10 mg IV or IM. For chronic anxiety, 2-10 mg PO bid-qid.

Route

PO for less severe symptoms and IM or IV for acute symptoms.

Side Effects

CNS depression leading to drowsiness, fatigue, disorientation, confusion, and constipation. Phlebitis or thrombosis may also occur.

Warnings

Some patients may be hypersensitive to diazepam. This drug is contraindicated for patients with glaucoma, who are pregnant, and in pediatric patients under six months of age.

Special Patient Teaching Considerations

Patients could abuse this drug, as well as other benzodiazepines. *Abrupt discontinuation could cause withdrawal symptoms which may be new or worse than those occurring prior.* Avoid use during preganancy, OTC cough or cold preparations, alcohol, and other CNS depressants when taking this drug. Avoid abrupt discontinuation after prolonged use.

Lorazepam (Ativan®)

Action and Indication

Used to treat more severe anxiety and act as a sedative. Potentiates GABA (gamma-aminobutyric acid)

Dosage

1 mg bid-tid to 2mg bid-tid, not to exceed 6 mg per day.

Route

PO, IM or IV.

Side Effects

CNS depression with symptoms such as drowsiness, confusion, disorientation, and over sedation or sleepiness.

Warnings

Elderly and otherwise debilitated patients need to be dosed with caution. In addition, attention needs to be paid to related physical symptoms (e.g., cardiovascular and musculo-skeletal) that could contribute to the anxiety. This drug may be contraindicated for patients with narrow angle glaucoma, liver or kidney failure.

Special Patient Teaching Considerations

Patients should use caution in operating machinery, driving a car, taking care of others, and making legal decisions when undergoing antianxiety drug therapy. Avoid OTC cough/cold preparations and alcohol when taking this medication.

ANTIANXIETY AGENTS

Alprazolam (Xanax®)

Action and Indication

A **benzodiazapine** commonly used to treat anxiety.

Dosage

0.75-4 mg per day, for anxiety with a higher dose of 1.5-10 mg per day for panic attacks. Initial doses could be as low as 0.25-0.50 mg, tid. The elderly may be treated with one-half of the above suggested dose. The dosage may be given tid and should not exceed 6 mg per day.

Route

PO tablets.

Side Effects

CNS depression manifested by drowsiness, impaired memory, decrease of coordination, and confusion.

Warnings

As with other benzodiazapines, this drug should not be used by pregnant or breast feeding women. Drug interactions are possible with various agents and all drug therapies must be reported to the physician. Caution should be observed when treating the elderly or debilitated patient. When discontinuing use, the dosage should be gradually decreased to avoid serious withdrawal reactions.

Special Patient Teaching Considerations

This class of drug should not be taken if mentally alert work is required (e.g., driving, operating machinery, legal decisions, dedicated personal care). *Do not take this drug or other benzodiazapines with alcohol. Avoid OTC cough/cold preparations when taking this drug.*

benzodiazepines a group of CNS depressing agents with the potential for abuse and/or dependence. These agents should not be taken by pregnant or breast feeding women or taken along with alcohol consumption.

Buspirone Hydrochloride (Buspar®)

Action and Indication

An anti-anxiety medication that is indicated in cases of short term use and mild symptoms. This drug does not exhibit anticonvulsant or muscular relaxant effects of typical benzodiazepine anxiolytics.

Dosage

7.5 mg two times a day., initially, and may be increased by 5 mg per day to a maximum daily dosage of 60 mg per day.

Route

PO tablets.

Side Effects

CNS effects such as dizziness and nervousness. Also, dry mouth and headache may occur.

Warnings

Taking this drug with selected MAO inhibitors is not recommended. Caution should be used if patient has a history of kidney or liver dysfunction.

Special Patient Teaching Considerations

It may take 1-2 weeks to realize the optimal potential of this agent. Do not operate potentially dangerous machinery while taking Buspar. Notify physician of any allergic response or history of anti-depressant drug therapy. Avoid drinking alcohol while taking this drug.

Monoamine Oxidase Inhibitors

MAOIs are a group of drugs used to treat depression that can have toxic interactions with other drugs and with certain foods containing tyramine. These interactions can be fatal. Tyramine is found in cheeses, sausages, and red wine, among other foods. Example of MAOIs are:

➡ phenelzine (Nardil®)

➡ tranylcypromine (Parnate®)

➡ isocarboxazid (Marplan®)

Does not have additive qualites

ANTIDEPRESSANTS

Paroxetine Hydrochloride (Paxil®)

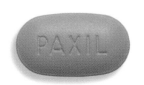

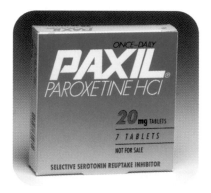

Paxil®
(paroxetine hydrochloride)
Courtesy of Smith, Kline, Beecham

Action and Indication

An antidepressant **selective serotonin reuptake inhibitor** (*SSRI*) drug which is used for debilitating depression that interferes with the functioning of a patient's daily life.

Dosage

20 mg per day, single dose in the morning. This may increase to a maximum of 50 mg per day. For elderly or those with impaired liver/kidney function, the dosage is about half.

Route

PO, tablets.

Side Effects

Could cause mania in those with a manic disorder. Common side effects include: dry mouth, mild GI upset, dizziness, drowsiness, impotence, restlessness, agitation, and weakness.

Warnings

Contraindicated for patients taking or who have recently taken MAO inhibitors. Severe reactions could occur. Elderly, children, pregnant or nursing mothers, or those with impaired liver or kidney failure should receive special consideration if receiving this medication.

Special Patient Teaching Considerations

Take this drug early in the morning to avoid insomnia. This drug may work quickly to lift depression (1-2 weeks). Do not discontinue taking this medication without first consulting with a physician. Notify the physician of any mania, seizure, or other antidepressant usage history.

MAOI's and SSRI drugs should never be used together, as severe interactions could occur. The taking of OTC's (except for acetaminophen and aspirin) and SSRI drugs should also be avoided.

Sertraline Hydrochloride (Zoloft®)

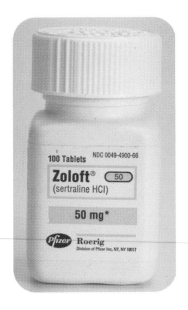

Zoloft®
(sertraline)
Courtesy of Pfizer

Action and Indication

Like Paxil, Zoloft is a **selective serotonin reuptake inhibitor** prescribed for depression. It is often chosen for the elderly due to its decreased sedative and cardiovascular side effects.

Dosage

Initial dose may be 25-50 mg per day. This may be increased to a maximum of 200 mg per day.

Route

PO tablets.

Side Effects

Dry mouth, mild GI upset, insomnia or sleepiness, restlessness, agitation, and impotence.

Warnings

Check history of patient to *assure MAO inhibitors were not recently taken.* Severe reactions could occur. Also cimetidine will increase the blood levels of this drug.

Special Patient Teaching Considerations

Take this drug early in the morning to avoid insomnia. Notify physician of any side effects.

 selective serotonin reuptake inhibitor antidepressant agents that inhibit the reuptake of serotonin and are generally better tolerated than tricyclic agents.

ANTIDEPRESSANTS

Fluoxetine Hydrochloride (Prozac®)

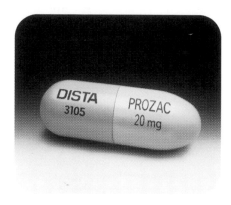

Prozac®
(fluoxetine)
Courtesy of Eli Lilly & Company

Action and Indication

An antidepressant classified as a **serotonin reuptake inhibitor** and indicated for cases of serious depression, obsessive-compulsive disorder, and sometimes seen in the treatment of eating disorders.

Dosage

To start, 20 mg taken daily in the am, is recommended. This dosage may be increased dependent upon condition being treated. The dosage may also be lowered if the patient is elderly or has a history of liver and/or kidney dysfunction.

Route

PO pulvules or liquid solution.

Side Effects

GI effects such as weight and appetite loss, insomnia, anxiety, tremor, and possible rash.

Warnings

Taking this drug with MAOI drugs is strongly contraindicated. The gap between taking the two agents should be at least 2 weeks after taking MAOI drugs or 5 weeks after taking fluoxetine. Caution should be used in patients with history of cardiac disease (including recent heart attacks), liver dysfunction, seizures, and/or diabetes.

Special Patient Teaching Considerations

Notify the physician of dizziness, a skin rash, or pregnancy. Do not drink alcohol and avoid work with dangerous machinery while taking this medication. Take fluoxetine at the same time each day and remember that it may take up to 4 weeks to experience depression relief. Continue to take fluoxetine as directed. The effects will be long lasting.

— doesn't affect pregnancy

Amitriptyline Hydrochloride (Elavil®)

Action and Indication
This is a **tricyclic antidepressant** that also has sedative effects. Though its mechanism of action is not known, its interference with the reuptake of norepinephrine is thought by some to be the cause of its antidepressant activity. Note: Although not an approved indication, it may also be used in cases of chronic pain (such as herpes zoster).

Dosage
Dosages vary based on patient and condition. An initial dose may be as little as 5 mg a day. This dose may increase every several days to a maximum of 100-300 mg daily. Doses greater than 150 mg are recommended only for hospitalized patients.

Route
PO tablets or IM.

Side Effects
Dry mouth, cardiovascular conduction changes, multiple CNS effects (blurred vision, lack of coordination), orthostatic hypotension, and mild GI upset. Male and female breast enlargement may also occur.

Warnings
Contraindicated for patients using monoamine oxidase inhibitors. If MAOI therapy is discontinued, allow at least 14 days before administration of amitriptyline. Caution should be used in patients with a history of seizures, urinary retention, angle-closure glaucoma, and cardiac disease. The elderly, children, and pregnant women need special dosaging considerations if taking this drug.

Special Patient Teaching Considerations
Notify a physician if abnormal heart rhythms or dizziness upon standing up occur. Note: It may take two to four weeks for the positive effects of this drug to be experienced. In diabetic patients, blood glucose levels should be monitored at the onset of therapy. Avoid other agents that cause sedation such as alcohol or OTC cough/cold preparations.

 tricyclic antidepressants common antidepressant agents with side effects that include dry mouth, blurred vision, constipation, sedation, and sexual dysfunction.

ANTIDEPRESSANTS

Trazodone Hydrochloride (Desyrel®)

Action and Indication

The chemical action of this antidepressant in humans is not fully understood. This drug is indicated in cases of major depressive episodes present for at least two weeks on a daily or almost daily basis that are characterized by events such as insomnia, loss of appetite, fatigue, lost interest, feelings of worthlessness, and thoughts of suicide.

Dosage

150 mg daily, to start, with a possible increase to a maximum of 400-600 mg taken daily in divided doses. The dose may be increased every 3-4 days, in increments of 50 mg and then reduced as the depression lightens.

Route

PO tablets.

Side Effects

Anger, confusion, lightheadedness, hypotension, dizziness, muscle pain, and GI effects such as abdominal pain, constipation, and/or diarrhea. Anticholinergic effects may also occur such as dry mouth and blurred vision.

Warnings

Caution should be exercised for patients with heart disease. This drug has been known to aggravate ventricular arrhythmias. Unwanted drug interactions may result when used with other drug therapy such as Prozac, seconal, thorazine, digoxin, and warfarin. Male patients may experience priapism or painful prolonged erection.

Special Patient Teaching Considerations

This medication may cause drowsiness and caution should be used if operating dangerous machinery. Patients should accurately relate cardiac history to their physician and notify him/her of any irregular cardiac rhythm which may occur. Take with food. Do not drink alcohol while taking this medication.

Bupropion Hydrochloride (Wellbutrin®)

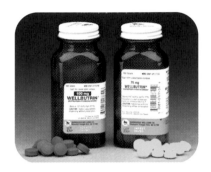

Wellbutrin®
(bupropion hydrochloride)
Courtesy of Glaxo Wellcome

Action and Indication

An antidepressant agent that works by inhibiting dopamine uptake and is used to treat cases of depression. Note: 150 mg sustained release tablets of bupropion hydrochloride (Wellbutrin SR® and Zyban®) are also used as a non-nicotinic aid to treating smoking cessation.

Dosage

100 mg two times a day to start with a possible increase to 100mg three times a day. Certain cases may require a higher and maximum dosage of 150 mg three times a day. Note: Allow at least 6 hours between each dose. Gradual dosing is important to lower the risk of seizures.

Route

PO tablets.

Side Effects

Weight loss, confusion, blurred vision, agitation, headache, palpitations, and possible auditory or taste disturbance.

Warnings

Caution should be used with patients having a history of seizure disorder, liver/kidney dysfunction, eating disorder, and cardiac pathology. *Concurrent usage of monoamine oxidase inhibitors (MAOIs) could result in serious hypertension.* High doses of Wellbutrin may cause seizure activity especially if the patient has a seizure disorder or history of drug addiction.

Special Patient Teaching Considerations

Notify physician of any sign or symptom of seizure activity. Do not drink alcohol while taking this product. If this drug does impair your judgement, do not operate dangerous machinery during the therapy.

ANTIPSYCHOTICS

Olanzapine (Zyprexa®)

Action and Indication

This antipsychotic medication inhibits dopamine and serotonin receptors and is indicated in cases of psychological disorders such as schizophrenia.

Dosage

Available in various dosages. Initial dosage could be 5-10 mg once daily, increased every 7 days to a maximum of 20 mg daily. Patients who have slower metabolisms may receive lower doses.

Route

PO, tablets.

Side Effects

Agitation, anxiety, back pain, blurred vision, dry mouth, hypotension, chest pain and GI effects such as abdominal pain and constipation.

Warnings

Caution should be used in patients with Alzheimer's disease, narrow angle glaucoma, enlarged prostate, heart disease and/or seizures. Can lead to development of tardive dyskinesia or symptoms such as high fever, muscle rigidity, and tachycardia. This agent should be used for short periods only.

Special Patient Teaching Considerations

Avoid exposure to overheating and drink plenty of fluids while taking olanzapine. Do not drink alcohol as this combination could cause serious hypotension. Olanzapine could also cause drowsiness, therefore avoid use of dangerous machinery. *Report any signs of neuroleptic malignant syndrome to the physician (muscle rigidity, high fever, tachycardia).*

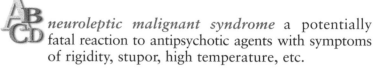

— cannot drink alcohol while on this medication

ABCD *neuroleptic malignant syndrome* a potentially fatal reaction to antipsychotic agents with symptoms of rigidity, stupor, high temperature, etc.

Chlorpromazine Hydrochloride (Thorazine®)

Action and Indication

Used to treat psychotic disorders, namely schizophrenia. Therapeutic effects are thought to occur in the limbic system where it acts on dopamine.

Dosage

25 mg IM for acute psychotic episode. This may be repeated in 1 hour. Initial doses may range from 30-75 mg per day taken in 3-4 divided doses. When prescribing for the elderly, the dosage will be significantly decreased.

Route

IM or PO tablets, sustained release capsules or syrup.

Side Effects

Tardive dyskinesia (involuntary muscle twitches and spasms of the face and body), dry mouth, drowsiness, protruding tongue, and drooling.

Warnings

Caution should be used with patients having respiratory disorders such as asthma or emphysema and brain tumor or intestinal blockage. *Be aware of neuroleptic malignant syndrome symptoms (high body temperature, irregular pulse and muscle rigidity). This could be fatal.*

Special Patient Teaching Considerations

This medication could cause urine discoloration. Avoid hot tubs and saunas as the body's sensitivity to heat or cold could be effected. Also avoid UV light exposure. Do not dilute medication with alcohol. Report side effects to the physician. Notify the physician of pregnancy.

ANTIPSYCHOTICS

Trifluoperazine Hydrochloride (Stelazine®)

Action and Indication

This drug is used to treat severe psychotic disturbances, such as schizophrenia. It is from the Phenothiazine class of drugs, which are thought to effect dopamine in the limbic system and help to alter behavior.

Dosage

2-5 mg bid for maintenance dosing, with higher doses required for acute episodes. Maximum amount for a healthy adult, not in an acute or elderly state, would be 40 mg daily. Psychotic children 6-12 years may start 1 mg per day, with a gradual increase of perhaps 15 mg per day.

Route

PO tablets or IM for more severe cases.

Side Effects

CNS depression manifested by drowsiness, dizziness, and blurred vision. Dry mouth and tardive dyskinesia may also occur.

Warnings

Caution should be used in patients with history of blood dyscrasias, liver disease, and concurrent use of methyldopa (could raise blood pressure) or other CNS depressants.

Special Patient Teaching Considerations

Notify the physician of pregnancy or breast feeding, have a history of heart problems, respiratory distress, glaucoma, or breast cancer. Do not drink alcohol while taking this drug. Urine discoloration may occur. Avoid use of hot tubs, saunas or UV light exposure.

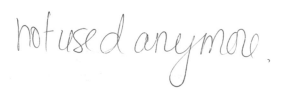

not used anymore.

Haloperidol (Haldol®)

Action and Indication

This drug is used to treat a variety of mental disorders, such as schizophrenia. A member of the antipsychotic class **butyrophenones**, Haldol also works on the limbic system to alter behavior.

Dosage

1-6 mg daily, with an increase to 15 mg daily for more severe symptoms. This dosage may be divided into 2-3 doses per day.

Route

PO tablets or liquid, IM.

Side Effects

Depression, confusion, headache, high or low blood pressure, high or low blood sugar and breast pain. Parkinsonian symptoms may occur as well as CNS depression, cardiac (ECG) changes, Neuroleptic Malignant Syndrome, and Tardive Dyskinesia.

Warnings

Caution should be used in patients with history of heart condition, allergies, or who are taking anticoagulants or anticonvulsants. Check for other drug therapy to assure against drug incompatabilities. Haloperidol should not be given to children.

Special Patient Teaching Considerations

Skin may be more sensitive to sunlight. Keep this in mind while outside. Since haloperidol may interfere with your body's temperature regulation, avoid exposure to extreme heat or cold.

ANTIPSYCHOTICS

Risperidone (Risperdal®)

Action and Indication

An antipsychotic drug that is indicated in cases of schizophrenia and other selected mental illnesses. The mechanism of action is related to antagonism of dopamine and serotonin receptor sites.

Dosage

Doses will be increased daily to start. For example, 1 mg two times a day, for the first day and increasing to 2 mg the second day and 3 mg the third day. Once a therapeutic level is reached, 4-6 mg daily divided into 2 doses is suggested. Patients who are elderly or have liver/kidney dysfunction may receive a lesser dose.

Route

PO tablet or liquid.

Side Effects

Insomnia, restlessness, chest pain, and possible GI effects such as abdominal pain and nausea.

Warnings

Patient must be monitored for signs and symptoms of neuroleptic malignant syndrome such as tachycardia, irregular heart rhythm, muscle stiffness and change in blood pressure. Caution should be used in patients with liver, kidney, cardiac, thyroid disease, or seizure history.

Special Patient Teaching Considerations

Caution should be exercised while operating dangerous machinery while taking this medication as drowsiness could occur. Avoid alcohol and drugs such as demerol and valium while taking Risperdal.

Zolpidem Tartrate (Ambien®)

Action and Indication

This recently developed hynotic agent is indicated for short term use in cases of insomnia. Reacting with the GABA receptor complex found in CNS neurons, zolpidem will decrease excitability and functional activity of the brain.

Dosage

Usual dose is 10 mg at bedtime. This dosage may be decreased for elderly or otherwise medically weakened patients.

Route

PO tablets.

Side Effects

Drowsiness, headache, GI effects such as nausea, and possible allergic response.

Warnings

Caution should be used in patients with history of respiratory distress and/or liver dysfunction.

Patient Teaching Considerations

Do not stop taking this medication abruptly. Do not drink alcohol while taking this medication. Note that taking a sleeping aid could become habit forming, decrease mental alertness, and that it is possible to experience personality and behavioral changes. Notify the physician if any of the above should occur.

DRUG DEPENDENCY

Disulfiram (Antabuse®)

Action and Indication

Used to dissuade the alcoholic from drinking by causing symptoms such as nausea, vomiting, palpitations, and fever. Acetaldehyde is formed due to blocked oxidation of the alcohol by this drug and the patient becomes sick.

Dosage

250-500 mg per day. The patient may start at a higher dose for a couple of weeks and then be decreased to a lower dose.

Route

PO scored tablets.

Side Effects

Flushing, nausea, vomiting, throbbing headache, hypotension, respiratory difficulty, and CNS effects. Although these are desired responses, they are very unpleasant for the patient to experience.

Warnings

With the use of this **aversion therapy**, a patient could become very ill or even die. Alcohol use is strictly prohibited and alcohol should be avoided for up to two weeks after discontinuing therapy with this drug. Care should be taken to assure cardiovascular status and sensitivity to thiuram derivatives prior to starting this medication. *Health care workers and pharmacy techs handling this drug or inhaling its dust could be prone to the same reaction.*

Special Patient Teaching Considerations

A patient needs to be aware of this treatment plan and the ramifications of it. The physical effects caused by drinking alcohol and taking this drug can be very severe. Avoidance of alcohol would also include refraining from mouthwashes, cough and cold preps, toiletries, liniments, and food or sauces containing alcohol. Note: this is only a deterrent to alcohol abuse and not a cure.

- helps an alcoholic stay sober.

Naltrexone Hydrochloride (ReVia®)

Action and Indication

This drug is used to treat alcohol and narcotic addictions. It blocks the euphoric effects of opiates and will reduce alcoholic cravings.

Dosage

25-50 mg per day. The lower dose is used while the physician is watching for symptoms of withdrawal.

Route

PO.

Side Effects

Dizziness, nausea, fatigue, headache, abdominal pain, and cramps.

Warnings

Patients must be drug free for at least 7-10 days prior to use and monitored for signs of withdrawal and liver toxicity. This drug is not recommended for children under 18 years of age.

Special Patient Teaching Considerations

Patient needs to be aware of the drug therapy they are on and the effects they may incur. Any signs of liver toxicity (clay colored stools, brown urine, jaundice or severe abdominal pain) should be reported immediately to the physician.

℞ Related drug therapies include: Despiramine (Norpramin®), a tricyclic antidepressant found in some cases to curb cocaine cravings, and Methadone, a synthetic narcotic analgesic used to treat narcotic addiction.

DRUG CHART

Generic Name	Trade Name	Route	Generic Name	Trade Name	Route
ANTIDEPRESSANTS			SELECTIVE SEROTONIN REUPTAKE INHIBITORS		
HETEROCYCLIC			Citalopram	Celexa	PO
Amoxapine	Asendin	PO	Fluoxetine	Prozac	PO
	Various	PO	Fluvoxamine	Luvox	PO
Bupropion	Wellbutrin	PO	Paroxetine	Paxil	PO
	Zyban	PO	Sertraline	Zoloft	PO
Maprotiline	Ludiomil	PO	MONOAMINE OXIDASE INHIBITORS		
Mirtazapine	Remeron	PO	Phenelzine	Nardil	PO
Trazodone	Desyrel	PO	Isocarboxazid	Marplan	PO
	Various	PO	Selegiline	Carbex	PO
Venlafaxine	Effexor	PO		Eldepryl	PO
TRICYCLIC			Tranylcypromine	Parnate	PO
Amitriptyline	Elavil	PO	OTHER		
	Endep	PO	Nefazodone	Serzone	PO
	Various	PO			
Clomipramine	Anafranil	PO	ANTIMANICS		
	Various	PO	Carbamazepine	Tegretol	PO
Desipramine	Norpramin	PO		Carbatrol	PO
	Various			Various	PO
Doxepin	Sinequan	PO,	Valproic Acid	Depakene	PO
Topical				Depakote	PO
	Various	PO		Depacon	Inj.
Imipramine	Tofranil	PO, Inj.	Lithium	Eskalith	PO
	Various	PO, Inj.		Lithobid	PO
Nortriptyline	Pamelor	PO		Various	PO
	Aventyl	PO			
	Various	PO			
Protriptyline	Vivactil	PO			
	Various	PO			

GENERIC NAME	TRADE NAME	ROUTE	GENERIC NAME	TRADE NAME	ROUTE
ANTIPSYCHOTICS			**ANTIANXIETY AGENTS**		
PHENOTHIAZINES			**BENZODIAZEPINES**		
Chlorpromazine Supp.	Thorazine	PO, Inj.,	Alprazolam	Xanax	PO
			Clorazepate	Tranxene	PO
	Various	PO, Inj.		Various	PO
Fluphenazine	Prolixin	PO, Inj.	Chlordiazepoxide	Librium	PO
Perphenazine	Trilafon	PO, Inj.		Various	PO
Thioridazine	Mellaril	PO	Clonazepam	Klonopin	PO
	Various	PO	Diazepam	Valium	PO, Inj.
Trifluoperazine	Stelazine	PO, Inj.		Various	PO, Inj.
	Various	PO, Inj.	Lorazepam	Ativan	PO, Inj.
OTHER				Various	PO, Inj.
Clozapine	Clozaril	PO	Oxazepam	Serax	PO
Haloperidol	Haldol	PO, Inj.		Various	PO
	Various	PO, Inj.	**OTHER**		
Loxapine	Loxitane	PO, Inj.	Buspirone	Buspar	PO
	Various	PO, Inj.			
Mesoridazine	Serentil	PO	**DRUG DEPENDENCY**		
Molindone	Moban	PO	Disulfiram	Antabuse	PO
Olanzapine	Zyprexa	PO		Others	PO
Quetiapine	Seroquel	PO	Naltrexone	Depade	PO
Risperidone	Risperdal	PO		ReVia	PO
Thiothixene	Navane	PO, Inj.		Trexan	PO
	Various	PO, Inj.	Naloxone	Narcan	Inj.
			Nalmefene	Revex	Inj.

REVIEW

KEY CONCEPTS

✔ Psychotropic agents are drugs that affect behavior, psychiatric state, and sleep. They act on specialized areas of the brain to suppress or control the symptoms of common psychological disorders such as bipolar disorder, anxiety, depression, schizophrenia, and drug abuse.

✔ The primary psychotropic agents are antidepressants, antipsychotics, and antianxiety agents. Other related psychotropic agents include sedatives and hypnotics.

✔ Also known as Manic-Depression, Bipolar Disorder is characterized by mood, energy, and behavior swings from periods of elation to episodes of depression. Antipsychotic drugs combined with benzodiazepines are commonly prescribed. Carbamazepine and valproic acid are often added to this therapy to treat seizure activity secondary to psychotropic agents.

✔ People suffering from anxiety may appear abnormally tired or energetic, withdrawn, tremorous, tense, and restless and may suffer from insomnia, phobias and panic attacks. In conjunction with psychotherapy and various relaxation techniques, the commonly prescribed drugs include antianxiety agents such as the benzodiazapines.

✔ Depression is characterized by mood disturbances that may be mild (e.g., lack of interest or inability to experience joy) or severe (e.g., physical aggression or suicide attempts). While psychotherapy and even shock therapy are often prescribed treatment, tricylcic antidepressants and SSRIs are commonly used.

✔ Schizophrenia is characterized by extreme and inappropriate behavior and dysfunctional daily routine. Hearing "voices," experiencing delusions, becoming agitated or hostile and perhaps a lack of response at all are examples of schizophrenic behavior. Antipsychotic agents commonly used may include: chlorpromazine, trifluoperazine, and haloperidol.

✔ Sedatives are drugs that are intended to relax and calm. They reduce restlessness and may produce mild drowsiness. Antianxiety medications that include benzodiazepines (e.g., diazepam and chlordiazepoxide) are included in this group.

✔ Hypnotics are often referred to as "sleeping pills" and are designed to induce and, in some cases, prolong sleep. This group includes barbiturates such as secobarbital and pentobarbital. Nonbarbituate sedative-hypnotics include chloral hydrate and meprobamate.

✔ Carbamazepine and valproic acid are often used for treatment of seizure activity secondary to psychotropic agents.

✔ Benzodiazepines are a group of CNS depressing agents with the potential for abuse and/or dependence. These agents should not be taken by pregnant or breast feeding women or taken along with alcohol consumption.

✔ Monoamine oxidase inhibitors (MAOIs) are agents used to treat depression that can have toxic or fatal interactions with other drugs and with foods containing tyramine. Tyramine is found in cheeses, sausages, and red wine, among other foods. Example of MAOIs are: phenelzine (Nardil®), tranylcypromine (Parnate®), isocarboxazid (Marplan®).

✔ MAOI's and SSRI drugs should never be used together, as severe interactions could occur. Taking OTC's (except for acetaminophen and aspirin) and SSRIs should also be avoided.

SELF TEST

MATCH THE GENERIC AND TRADE NAMES.   *answers can be checked in the back of the book*

1. Alprazolam	*Xanax*	~~Ativan~~
2. Amitriptyline	*Elavil*	Depakene
3. Carbamazepine	*Tegretol*	~~Elavil~~
4. Chlorpromazine	*Thorazine*	Nardil
5. Diazepam	*Valium*	~~Paxil~~
6. Doxepin	*Sinequan*	Prozac
7. Fluoxetine	*Prozac*	~~Sinequan~~
8. Lorazepam	*Ativan*	~~Tegretol~~
9. Olanzapine	*Zyprexa*	~~Thorazine~~
10. Paroxetine	*Paxil*	~~Valium~~
11. Phenelzine	*Nardil*	~~Xanax~~
12. Valproic Acid	*Depakene*	~~Zyprexa~~

CHOOSE THE BEST ANSWER.   *answers are in the back of the book*

1. Which classification of drugs is most commonly used in the treatment of anxiety disorders?
   a. benzodiazepines *(circled)*
   b. phenothiazines
   c. tri-cyclics
   d. none of the above

2. Which of the following drugs is the first drug marketed as an SSRI and is still one of the top drugs dispensed in the retail setting today?
   a. amitriptyline
   b. chlorpromazine
   c. fluoxetine *(circled)*
   d. naltrexone

3) Of the following drugs, which one would be most likely used in the treatment of opiate dependency?
   a. amitriptyline
   b. chlorpromazine
   c. fluoxetine
   d. naltrexone *(circled)*

4) Of the following drugs, which one is most likely to have anticholinergic effects such as dry mouth?
   a. amitriptyline *(circled)*
   b. chlorpromazine
   c. fluoxetine
   d. naltrexone

RESPIRATORY AGENTS

Balancing oxygen and carbon dioxide levels correctly is essential to health.

The cells of the body use oxygen for energy and produce carbon dioxide as waste. The respiratory system is responsible for exchanging oxygen from the air with carbon dioxide from the body. High carbon dioxide levels alert the medulla of the brain to signal **inspiration** (breathing in) to the **diaphragm** and **intercostal muscles** of the rib cage. It is their action that drives normal respiration. There are two phases of respiration: the **mechanical phase** which involves the diaphragm and the rib cage and allows air to enter the lungs, and the **physiologic phase** in which oxygen and carbon dioxide are exchanged between the lungs and the blood cells. Dysfunction can occur at any time during either phase.

Emotional stimuli as well as medical disorders may alter gas exchange and breathing patterns.

Abnormal breathing patterns can occur for a variety of reasons and include **dyspnea** (labored breathing), wheezing, hyperventilation, and **apnea** (absence of breathing). Common respiratory disorders include: asthma, emphysema, bronchitis, COPD, croup, pneumonia, and allergy (see below).

Drugs commonly indicated in the treatment of respiratory diseases and disorders include *antihistamines, decongestants, antitussives,* **and** *bronchodilators.*

These agents act in a variety of ways to clear the airways and restore normal respiration.

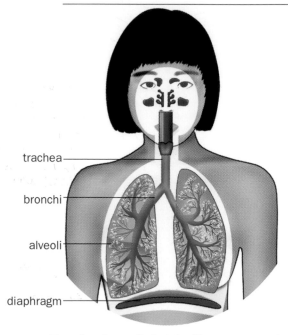

trachea

bronchi

alveoli

diaphragm

The **trachea** ("windpipe") connects the larynx or "voicebox" and the **bronchi**, the two airway branches that carry air to the lungs. The smaller bronchial tubes are called **bronchioles**, They carry the air to the **alveoli** (air sacs) of the lungs where gas exchange takes place.

[handwritten] Steroid Inhaler pulmicort + fluticazone

Common Respiratory Disorders

[handwritten] Huge w/ children

➡ **Asthma**: chronic airway inflammation related to stimuli hyperresponsiveness, resulting in airflow obstruction with symptoms such as wheezing and potentially acute spasms and breathlessness.

➡ **Allergy**: allergic response to food, drugs, animals, insect bites, pollens, or dust.

➡ **Emphysema:** chronic airway obstruction due to lung hyperinflation and diminished oxygen intake, characterized by breathlessness and flushed color.

➡ **Croup** (bronchiolitis): an infection of the bronchioles occurring in young children and resulting in airway obstruction and labored breathing.

➡ **Bronchitis**: infection producing excess mucus in the bronchial tree that makes breathing difficult.

➡ **COPD** (chronic obstructive pulmonary disease): also termed COLD (lung) or COAD (airway) by some sources. Abnormal lung function that generally encompasses both emphysema and chronic bronchitis that is present at least for 3 months a year for 2 consecutive years.

➡ **Pneumonia**: infectious process of either bacterial or viral origin whereby fluid accumulates in the lungs causing inadequate or in severe cases, impossible, air exchange at the alveolar level.

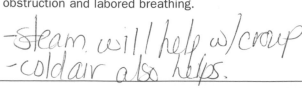

[handwritten] -Steam will help w/croup
[handwritten] -cold air also helps.

AGENTS

Antihistamines

Antihistamines act to respond to the release of **histamine** or inflammation producing substance from white blood cells that occurs with an injury or allergic reaction. Antihistamine agents replace histamine at the inflammation receptor sites to reduce inflammation, swelling, and irritation. Additional properties of antihistamines include: antipruritic (anti-itching), antiemetic, and sedative. Common antihistamines listed by chemical structure are **alkylamines** (e.g., triprolidine), **piperizines** (e.g., hydroxyzine), **phenothiazines** (e.g., promethazine), **piperidines** (e.g., loratidine), **ethanolamines** (e.g.,), and **ethylenedramines** (e.g., pyrilamine).

Decongestants

Decongestants cause mucous membrane vasoconstriction, reduction of nasal passage drainage and relief of stuffiness. These products are available as both oral agents (e.g., pseudoephedrine) and nasal sprays (e.g., phenylephrine).

Antitussives

Antitussives are products which treat both productive (with phlegm) and non-productive (without phlegm) coughs. These agents are available in both narcotic and non-narcotic preparations. Dextromethorphan is the most widely used antitussive agent. Codeine sulfate is a widely used narcotic antitussive agent. **Mucolytic** drugs that act to liquefy thickened bronchial mucous and assist in clearing airways are included in this category by some sources. Acetylcysteine is a commonly indicated mucolytic agent. The **expectorant** guaifenesin is often used with antitussives. It increases the production of respiratory secretions and decreases irritation caused by dryness in the airways.

Bronchodilators

Bronchodilators are drugs which act to relieve **bronchospasm** (a narrowing of the bronchi, accompanied by wheezing and coughing, i.e, an "asthma attack," as seen in disorders such as asthma, emphysema and bronchitis). **Sympathomimetics** (e.g., proventil and metaproterenol) dilate the bronchi. **Xanthine derivatives** (e.g., amoline and theopylline) directly relax the smooth muscle of the bronchi. Both categories of bronchodilators increase the opening of the bronchi and allow more airflow to occur. Note: corticosteroids such as prednisone and anticholinergics such as Atrovent may be used to decrease respiratory airway inflammation and produce some bronchodilation in cases where bronchodilators have failed.

[handwritten margin note: Sympo xxx ventolin]

[handwritten note: Steroid Inhalers. Antibiotics are used for a respiratory agent as well]

ANTIHISTAMINES

Diphenhydramine Hydrochloride (Benadryl®)

most popular antihistamine on the market - makes you very drowsy.

Action and Indication

This **antihistamine** is indicated in cases of allergic response from a number of sources (food, insect bites, drugs, pollens) and acts to reduce mucous membrane inflammation and fluid accumulation. Benadryl also relieves itching, redness, coughing, and runny nose and/or eyes.

Dosage

25-50 mg, 3-4 times a day.

Route

PO capsules, liquid.

Side Effects

Dizziness, sleepiness, excitability (especially in children), nausea, and possible chest congestion.

causes excitability.   *Children paradorial effect,*

Warnings

Use caution in patients with history of asthma, glaucoma, hypertension, hyperthyroidism, cardiovascular disease, and prostate hypertrophy. *This product is contraindicated if the patient is taking monoamine oxidase inhibitors.*

Special Patient Teaching Considerations

Since this product may cause drowsiness, do not operate machinery or conduct daily activities that require complete alertness. Avoid alcohol consumption while taking this drug.

Fexofenadine Hydrochloride (Allegra®)

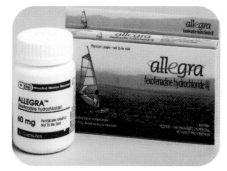

Allegra®
(fexofenadine hydrochloride)
Courtesy of Hoechst Marion
Roussell

Action and Indication

This recently developed **antihistamine** is often prescribed for relief of allergy symptoms such as runny nose, itchy watery eyes, and sneezing.

Dosage

This medication is not recommended for children under the age of 12. The usual adult dosage is 60 mg twice a day.

Route

PO capsules.

Side Effects

Drowsiness, nausea, fatigue, and possible mild GI symptoms such as indigestion.

Warnings

This drug may cause an allergic reaction. Although some sources say there are no drug interaction risks associated with this new agent, others believe it may interact with certain antibiotics such as erythromycin and/or antifungals such as ketoconazole. Patients with kidney dysfunction may need to receive a decreased dosage of this drug.

Special Patient Teaching Considerations

You may not experience a desired effect from Allegra for 1 hour after taking it, with a peek effect felt after 2-3 hours. The overall therapeutic effect should last about 12 hours. Notify your physician of other drugs you are taking to avoid a drug interaction.

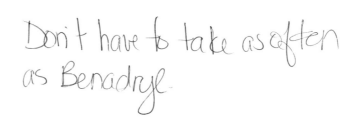

Don't have to take as often as Benadryl.

ANTIHISTAMINES

Loratadine (Claritin®)

Action and Indication

An **antihistamine** which is long acting and indicated in the treatment of respiratory allergy symptoms (e.g., runny nose, itchy eyes and sneezing).

Dosage

This recommended dosage is for children over the age of 12 and adults: 10 mg once a day. Dosage should be reduced if patients have liver or kidney dysfunction.

Route

PO tablets.

Side Effects

Dry mouth, insomnia, and possible tachycardia (especially in cases of overusage).

Warnings

Drug interactions may occur if the patient is concurrently taking selected antibitotics such as erythromycin or related drugs such as fluconazole or metronidazole.

Special Patient Teaching Considerations

For optimal effect, take this drug on an empty stomach. This drug may cause sleepiness in the elderly.

take on empty stomach.

Cetirizine Hydrochloride (Zyrtec®)

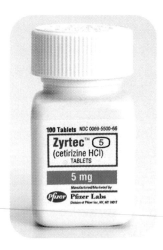

Zyrtec®
(cetirizine hydrochloride)
Courtesy of Pfizer

Action and Indication

This **antihistamine** is indicated in cases of allergy symptom relief such as from hay fever, hives, dust, mold and animal dander. Itchy runny noses and eye irritation are examples of symptoms that can be relieved with cetirizine. This drug acts as a selective histamine receptor antagonist.

Dosage

5-10 mg daily for both adults and children over the age of 12.

Route

PO tablets and syrup.

Side Effects

Drowsiness, headache, cough, dry mouth, and fatigue.

Warnings

May cause allergic reaction. Caution must be used in patients with liver or kidney dysfunction.

Special Patient Teaching Considerations

Avoid drinking alcohol, muscle relaxants and/or sedatives while taking this agent. Severe drowsiness could occur. Zyrtec can be taken without regard to meals and sucking hard candy or ice chips could help avoid dry mouth.

DECONGESTANTS

Pseudoephedrine Hydrochloride (Sudafed®)

Action and Indication
This drug is indicated for cases of nasal and sinus congestion. Pseudoephedrine stimulates the release of catecholamines and acts on adrenergic receptors to cause vasoconstriction and reduce swollen mucosa.

Dosage
60 mg every 4-6 hours and 120 mg every 12 hours for sustained release application.

Route
PO tablets.

Side Effects
Nervousness, nausea, vomiting, blurred vision, and possible arrhythmias.

another side effect: anxious people get reved up fight or flight

Warnings
This medication should not be taken by patients using MAOIs and/or tricyclic drugs, or by patients with a history of hypertension or cardiovascular disease. Avoid excessive caffeine while taking this drug as caffeine is an added stimulant.

Special Patient Teaching Considerations
Report any side effects, particularly irregularity of heart rate.

closely related chemically to epinephren.

Phenylephrine Hydrochloride (Neo-Synephrine®, Alconefrin®)

Action and Indication

A topical decongestant nasal spray, this drug is used to treat nasal decongestion by acting as an alpha agonist and causing vasoconstriction of nasal blood vessels.

Dosage

1-2 sprays into each nostril, every 4 hours.

Route

Nasal spray.

Side Effects

Rebound congestion, local irritation including burning, redness, and stinging.

Warnings

If this product would be systemically absorbed (most sources agree that there is often little or no systemic absorption), concurrent use with MAOI's and/or tricyclics would be contraindicated. Contraindicated for use by patients with history of hypertension, hyperthyroidism, prostatic hypertrophy, and diabetes.

Special Patient Teaching Considerations

Report side effects.

ANTITUSSIVES

↗ narcotic ↗ expectorant

Codeine Phosphate + Guaifenesin (Robitussin A-C®)

Action and Indication

Robitussin AC is guaifenesin 100 mg plus codeine 10 mg per 5 ml. Due to its sedative property, this narcotic antitussive is used in cases of severe and/or persistent coughing and acts as a cough suppressant.

Dosage

10-20 mg, every 4-6 hours for tablet form and a corresponding dose of 5-10 ml every 4-6 hours, as needed, for liquid form.

Route

PO liquid.

Side Effects

Sedation, lightheadedness, nausea/vomiting, constipation, and possible respiratory depression.

Warnings

This product should be used with caution in patients with liver or kidney dysfunction.

Special Patient Teaching Considerations

This agent is a narcotic and capable of producing sedation. Do not operate machinery or conduct activities of daily living which demand complete alertness. Avoid alcohol consumption while taking this drug.

used when wanting to deal w/flem in chest + calm cough

Benzonatate (Tessalon® Perles)

Action and Indication
This non-narcotic antitussive is a peripherally acting agent which decreases coughing by dulling stretch receptors in the respiratory passages.

Dosage
100 mg, three times a day with a recommended maximum dosage of 600 mg or 6 perles a day.

Route
PO perles (soft capsules to be swallowed whole and not chewed).

Side Effects
Allergic response, dizziness, headache, constipation, sedation, and possible numbness in chest.

Warnings
Possible confusion or bizarre behavior could occur as a reaction to this drug being taken concurrently with certain other medications.

Special Patient Teaching Considerations
Always swallow these perles whole. If chewed, it may cause throat numbness that could lead to choking.

Dextromethorphan (Robitussin DM®, Benalyn®, various)

Dextromethorphan is a widely used non-narcotic antitussive that suppresses the cough reflex. It is available in various forms (e.g., capsules, lozenges, syrup, etc.). It should not be used for chronic coughs caused by smoking or emphysema. It should not be used with monoamine oxidase inhibitors or CNS depressants.

MUCOLYTIC

Acetylcysteine (Mucomyst®)

Action and Indication

This mucolytic agent decreases respiratory distress by decreasing the viscosity of respiratory secretions. Acetylcysteine is often indicated in cases of emphysema.

Dosage

3-10 ml of a 20% solution, 3-4 times a day or 6-20 ml of a 10% solution, 3-4 times a day.

Route

Nebulizer (inhaled mist). Note: This product may also be instilled into a tracheostomy tube.

Side Effects

Nausea/vomiting and possible bronchospasm.

Warnings

If this drug is used for a tracheostomy patient, use of suction equipment may be necessary. With all other patients, it is important to stay with patients during their first treatment course to reduce anxiety. Observe for side effects.

Special Patient Teaching Considerations

Use this product only as directed and notify the physician of any side effect occurrences. Ask for instruction regarding proper use of the nebulizer equipment and instillation of the medication if this agent is indicated for home use. Drink plenty of water to help thin secretions.

Chronic Bronchitis
Emphyseema
Cystic Fibrosis

Guaifenesin (Robitussin®, Organidin® NR)

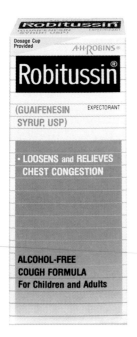

Robitussin®
(guaifenesin syrup)
Courtesy of Whitehall-Robins

Action and Indication

This agent is used to treat persistent coughs by liquefying and loosening viscous respiratory mucous and promoting its expulsion.

Dosage

PO 200-400 mg tablets every 4 hours, with a suggested maximum of 2400 mg in a 24 hour period. Robitussin syrup is recommended at 2 tsp. every 4 hours as needed.

Route

PO tablets and syrup.

Side Effects

Possible GI distress, including diarrhea.

Warnings

Guaifenesin is well tolerated in most individuals.

Special Patient Teaching Considerations

Do not exceed the suggested daily maximum dosage. Drink plenty of water to help thin secretions. If symptoms persist for more than one week, notify the physician.

Guaifenesin + Phenylpropanolamine (Entex LA) — *taken off market 10 yr safe. caused hemmorrhagic strokes in young females*

This product is a popular combination of the decongestant phenylpropanolamine with guaifenesin. It contains 75 mg of phenylpropanolamine and 400 mg of guaifenesin and is indicated for the treatment of sinusitis, bronchitis, and pharyngitis resulting from nasal and lower respiratory congestion. It should not be taken with monoamine oxidase inhibitors.

effective w/ wet productive coughs.

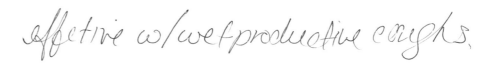

BRONCHODILATORS

Metaproterenol Sulfate (Alupent®, Metaprel®)

Action and Indication

Metaproterenol is a bronchodilator used to treat respiratory disorders such as reactive airway disease, asthma, emphysema, and bronchitis.

Dosage

20 mg PO three to four times a day or 2-3 puffs of inhaled metaproterenol every 3-4 hours, with a maximum of 12 puffs per day. Nebulizer dose may be 0.3 mL of 5% solution in 2.5 ml of normal saline. Note: Children's doses may be less and are calculated according to body weight and medical condition.

Route

PO tablets or liquid, inhaler, nebulizer.

Side Effects

Palpitations, tachycardia, fear, hypertension, nervousness, and possible nausea/vomiting.

Warnings

Caution should be used in patients with history of coronary artery disease and other cardiovascular disorders (e.g., tachycardia), as well as hypertension and anxiety.

Special Patient Teaching Considerations

While taking this drug, avoid the use of alcohol and smoking. Notify the physician if the condition does not improve or worsens or if side effects occur.

- used primarily w/ chronic bronchitis,

Ipratropium Bromide (Atrovent®)

Atrovent is a bronchodilator used as maintenance therapy for bronchospasm associated with chronic bronchitis, emphysema, and obstructive pulmonary disease. It is not used for a rapid response to bronchspasm. It is not used in patients with soy or peanut allergy or hypersensitivity to atropine.

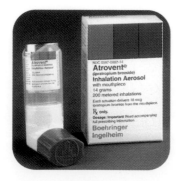

Atrovent®
(ipratropium bromide)
Courtesy of Boehringer Ingelheim, Inc.

Albuterol Sulfate, Salbutamol (Proventil® HFA, Ventolin®, Volmax®)

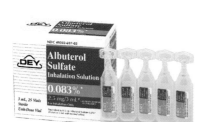

Albuterol Sulfate
Courtesy of Dey, L.P.

Action and Indication

This is a **beta stimulant** used in the prevention and treatment of bronchial spasms often associated with reactive airway disease and asthma.

Dosage

Dependent on the route. For example, regular acting 2-4 mg three to four times a day PO, or 2 puffs every 4-6 hours by inhaler.

Route

PO liquid, tablets, and extended release tablets. Inhalation by aerosol and nebulizer.

Side Effects

Cardiac effects such as tachycardia and/or palpitations, tremors, restlessness, labored breathing, light-headedness and anxiety.

Warnings

Drug interactions could occur with agents such as certain beta blockers, antidepressants, and diuretics that are used by patients with a history of cardiac conditions, high blood pressure, seizure disorder or Diabetes.

Special Patient Teaching Considerations

Do not take more of this medication than prescribed. Respiratory distress symptoms could become worse with increased doses. Notify your physician of your medical history and present drug therapy.

most popular bronchodialator on market.

) Can worsen the situation

BRONCHODILATORS

Salmeterol Xinofoate (Serevent®)

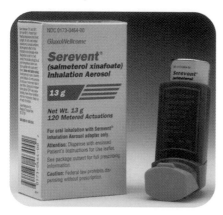

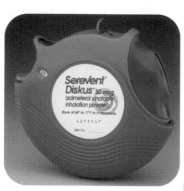

Serevent®
(salmeterol xinafoate)
Courtesy of Glaxo Wellcome

Action and Indication

Serevent is a long acting beta receptor agonist **bronchodilator** indicated in cases of asthma where maintenance therapy and prevention of exercise-induced episodes are required.

Dosage

For maintenance, 2 puffs divided equally two times a day. For prevention of exercise induced asthma, 2 puffs 30-60 minutes before exercise.

Route

Inhalation aerosol and powder.

Side Effects

Palpitations, tachycardia, and possible allergic response such as rash, itching, and bronchospasm

Warnings

Do not take for acute episodes of asthma. Shorter acting agents are prescribed. Patients receiving tricyclic antidepressants or monoamine oxidase inhibitors should not take salmeterol.

Special Patient Teaching Considerations

Do not take for acute episodes of asthma. Use shorter acting bronchodilators instead. Notify the physician of any signs of adverse effects.

→ takes too long to become effective

Theophylline (Slo-Phyllin®, Elixophyllin®, Theo-24®, various)

Action and Indication

This bronchodilator is chemically classified as a **xanthine derivative**. It acts by directly relaxing the bronchial smooth muscle. This relieves bronchospasm and allow for easier air exchange in the bronchioles and related air passages. Reactive airway disease and asthma are examples of respiratory disorders that may be treated with this class of drug. Aminophylline is another example of a popular xanthine derivative bronchodilator.

Dosage

Dependent upon patient condition and body weight. For example, a dose might be 2-6 mg/kg of body weight PO daily. This could be increased every 3 days up to 25% to a maximum of 900 mg daily.

Route

PO tablets, capsules, and liquid.

Side Effects

Palpitations, tachycardia, nausea/vomiting, restlessness, and anxiety.

Warnings

Caution should be used in patients with history of peptic ulcers, seizures, and cardiac arrhythmias (excluding bradyarrhymias) as it may aggravate the condition.

Special Patient teaching Considerations

Notify the physician should the condition not improve, worsen, or if side effects occur. Take only the ordered dose and avoid alcohol and smoking while taking this medication. Avoid caffeine and chocolate as they may cause an increase in side effect activity.

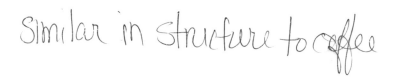

Similar in structure to coffee

ANTI-INFLAMMATORY

Triamcinolone Acetonide (Azmacort®, Nasacort®, various)

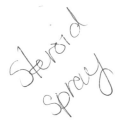
Steroid spray

Action and Indication

This **anti-inflammatory steroidal** is prescribed for long term therapy in cases of bronchial asthma or as short term use to treat nasal polyps or allergies. Note: This product is not a bronchodilator and is not indicated for asthma symptoms needing immediate relief.

Dosage

Dependent upon disease severity. For example, two inhalations 3-4 times a day, equal to about 200 micrograms.

Route

Oral inhalant. Note: it is available in other delivery forms for allergic rhinitis and other conditions.

Side Effects

Headache, flu-like symptoms, and possible back pain.

Warnings

This drug is not indicated for quick relief of asthma-associated respiratory distress. Optimal effect may not be noted for about one week after beginning use of this drug.

Special Patient Teaching Considerations

If possible steroidal side effects occur, notify your physician. Also be alert for oral fungal infection development, depression, or joint/muscle pain. If asthma symptoms do not improve in about one week, notify the physician.

Have a habit of draining down back of throat.

-this can set up throat for thrush candida infection

patients should rinse mouth & throat out

Beclomethasone Dipropionate (Beclovent®, various)

Action and Indication

A **steroid inhaler or nasal spray** used in cases of mild to moderate recurring asthma symptoms, hay fever, and post surgical removal of nasal polyps. Note: This product is not a bronchodilator and is not indicated for asthma symptoms needing immediate relief.

Dosage

For the oral inhalant: adults and children 12 years old and older may take 2 inhalations two to four times a day. This dosage may be increased depending on the severity of asthma and the patient's condition. For children 6-12 years old, 1-2 inhalations three to four times a day is recommended. The suggested maximum for children is 10 inhalations daily. Beclomethasone is not recommended for use in children under the age of 6.

Route

Oral inhalation or nasal spray.

Side Effects

Local irritation to nostrils, allergic symptoms such as rash and hives, dry mouth, hoarseness, possible fluid retention, and increased intraocular pressure.

Warnings

Possible immune system suppression and steroidal side effects such as weight gain, fluid retention, and possible cataract development. In children, this includes the possibility of abnormally slow growth.

Special Patient Teaching Considerations

Spray the inhaler into the air first before using it for the first time or if you have not used it regularly. The inhaler will lose it's effectiveness if not used within 6 months. Take this drug only as directed. Remember this is not a bronchodilator and will not quickly relieve serious asthma symptoms. Rinse mouth after each administration to help alleviate hoarseness. Notify physician if you don't experience improvement of asthma symptoms within 3 weeks after initial dose.

steroid spray.

ANTI-INFLAMMATORY

Fluticasone Propionate (Flovent®)

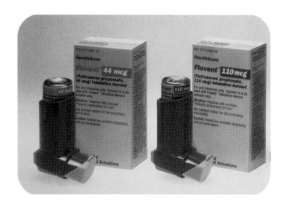
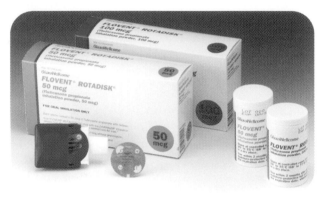

Flovent®
(fluticasone propionate)
Courtesy of Glaxo Wellcome

Action and Indication

A synthetic **anti-inflammatory glucocorticoid** used to treat asthma. The effects of this drug are not immediate and it may take 24 hours to realize improvement in the condition. Optimal therapeutic benefit may not occur for 1-2 weeks. However, the effects are long lasting.

Dosage

Recommended for patients 12 years and older. The doses are based on previous use, suggested starting dose and highest recommended dose. For example, if bronchodilators were used before, 88 mcg two times a day, not to exceed 440 mcg two times a day, is recommended. If the patient received oral corticosteroids before, 880 mcg two times a day, not to exceed 880 mcg two times a day, is recommended.

Route

Inhalation aerosol and powder.

Side Effects

Irritation of the eyes or sinus, GI effects such as nausea and diarrhea, headache and fatigue.

Warnings

This drug should not be stopped abruptly. There are possible steroidal side effects. Adolescents taking this medication should be closely monitored regarding their growth.

Special Patient Teaching Considerations

Rinse your mouth following inhalation administration. Store inhaler at room temperature and shake before using.

Fluticasone Propionate (Flonase®)

Action and Indication

A synthetic anti-inflammatory glucocorticoid used to treat allergic rhinitis It reduces inflammation in nasal passages therefore relieving allergy symptoms such as stuffed or runny nose and itchy eyes.

Dosage

This medication is not recommended for children below 4 years of age. The suggested adult dosage is 1 spray in each nostril every 12 hours, for a maximum of 2 sprays in each nostril per day.

Route

Intranasal.

Side Effects

Local irritation to nostrils, bad taste in mouth, and possible respiratory congestion.

Warnings

Possible steroidal side effect. Should not be used for non-allergic rhinitis.

Special Patient Teaching Considerations

It is possible to develop chicken pox or measles more easily when taking steriodal drugs. If a patient is exposed to either and has not been vaccinated or had the disease, they should immediately notify their physician. Patients should not take more than the recommended dose and if there is no improvement in a few days, should notify their physician.

Same as flovent, made into a nasal spray.

DRUG CHART

Generic Name	Trade Name	Route
Antihistamines		
Histamine 1 Blockers		
Azelastine	Astelin NS	Nas. Spray
Cetirizine	Zyrtec	PO
Chlorpheniramine	Chlor-Trimeton	PO, Inj.
	Teldrin	PO
	Various	PO
Clemastine	Tavist-1	PO
Cyproheptadine	Periactin	PO
	Various	PO
Diphenhydramine	Benadryl	PO
	Banophen	PO
	Diphedryl	PO
	Various	PO
Emedastine	Emadine	Eye
Fexofenadine	Allegra	PO
Hydroxyzine	Atarax	PO, Inj.
	Vistaril	PO
	Vistazine	PO
	Various	PO, Inj.
Loratadine	Claritin	PO
Loratadine / Psuedoephedrine	Claritin-D	PO
Phenylephrine	Neo-Synephrine	Inh., Inj., Eye
Promethazine	Phenergan	PO, Inj.
	Various	PO, Inj.

Generic Name	Trade Name	Route
Antitussives		
Chlorpheniramine/ Hydrocodone	Tussionex	PO
Dextromethorphan	Benylin Adult Formula	PO
	Benylin Pediatric	PO
	Robitussin Ped. Cough	PO
	Sucrets Cough Conrol	PO (Loz.)
	Various	PO
Guaifenesin / Codeine	Robitussin AC	PO
	Various	PO
Benzonatate	Tessalon Perles	PO
Bronchodilators		
Beta 2 Agonists		
Albuterol	Proventil	PO, Inhaler
	Ventolin	PO, Inhaler
	Volmax	PO
	Xopenex	Inhaler
	Various	PO, Inhaler
Metaproterenol	Alupent	PO
	Metaprel	Inhaler
	Various	Inhaler
Salmeterol	Serevent	Inhaler
Xanthine Deriviatives		
Theophylline	Slo-Bid	PO
	Theo-Dur	PO
	Theobid	PO
	Various	PO, Inj.
Aminophylline	Aminophylline	PO.
Antimuscarinics		
Ipratropium	Atrovent	Inhaler
Other		
Epinephrine	Adrenalin (1:1000)	Inj.
	EpiPen	Inj.

GENERIC NAME	TRADE NAME	ROUTE	GENERIC NAME	TRADE NAME	ROUTE
ANTI-INFLAMMATORY AGENTS			**EXPECTORANTS**		
Cromolyn Sodium	Gastrocom	PO	Acetylcysteine	Mucomyst	PO
	Intal	Inhaler	Guaifenesin	Breonesin	PO
	Nasalcrom	Inhaler		Fenesin	PO
	Various	PO, Eye		Humibid	PO
Nedocromil	Tilade	Inhaler		Organidin	PO
				Robitussin	PO
LEUKOTRIENE RECEPTOR ANTAGONIST				Various	PO
Montelukast	Singulair	PO	Potassium Iodide	Pima	PO
Zafirlukast	Accolate	PO		SSKI	PO
				Various	PO
CORTICOSTEROIDS					
Beclomethasone	Beclovent	Inhaler	**RESPIRATORY ENZYMES**		
	Beconase AQ	Inhaler	Dornase Alfa	Pulmozyme	Inhaler
	Vanceril	Inhaler			
	Vancenase	Inhaler	**SURFACTANTS**		
Budesonide	Pulmicort	Inhaler	Beractant	Survanta	Intratracheal
	Rhinocort	Inhaler	Calfactant	Infasurf	Intratracheal
Dexamethasone	Decadron	Inh., Inj., Eye	Colfosceril/Cetyl Alcohol/ Tyloxapol	Exosurf Neonatal	Intratracheal
	Various	Inh., Inj., Eye			
Fluticasone	Flonase	Inhaler			
	Flovent	Inhaler			
LIPOOXYGENASE INHIBITOR					
Zileuton	Zyflo	PO			

REVIEW

KEY CONCEPTS

✔ Balancing oxygen and carbon dioxide levels correctly is essential to health.

✔ The respiratory system is responsible for exchanging oxygen from the air with carbon dioxide from the body. High carbon dioxide levels alert the medulla of the brain to signal inspiration (breathing in) to the diaphragm and intercostal muscles of the rib cage.

✔ Abnormal breathing patterns can occur for a variety of reasons and include dyspnea (labored breathing), wheezing, hyperventilation, and apnea (absence of breathing). Common respiratory disorders include: asthma, emphysema, bronchitis, COPD, croup, pneumonia, and allergy.

✔ Drugs commonly indicated in the treatment of respiratory diseases and disorders include antihistamines, decongestants, antitussives, and bronchodilators.

✔ Asthma is a disorder of chronic airway inflammation related to stimuli hyperresponsiveness, resulting in airflow obstruction with symptoms such as wheezing and potentially acute spasms and breathlessness.

✔ Emphysema is a disorder of chronic airway obstruction due to lung hyperinflation and diminished oxygen intake, characterized by breathlessness and flushed color.

✔ COPD (chronic obstructive pulmonary disease) is a disorder of abnormal lung function that generally encompasses both emphysema and chronic bronchitis that is present at least for 3 months a year for 2 consecutive years.

✔ Pneumonia is an infectious process of either bacterial or viral origin in which fluid accumulates in the lungs, inhibiting air exchange at the alveolar level.

✔ Antihistamines act to respond to the release of histamine or inflammation producing substance from white blood cells that occurs with an injury or allergic reaction. Antihistamine agents replace histamine at the inflammation receptor sites to reduce inflammation, swelling, and irritation.

✔ Decongestants cause mucous membrane vasoconstriction, reduction of nasal passage drainage and relief of stuffiness

✔ Antitussives are products which treat both productive (with phlegm) and non-productive (without phlegm) coughs. These agents are available in both narcotic and non-narcotic preparations. Dextromethorphan is the most widely used antitussive agent. Codeine sulfate is a widely used narcotic antitussive agent.

✔ Mucolytic drugs that act to liquefy thickened bronchial mucous and assist in clearing airways are included in this category by some sources. Acetylcysteine is a commonly indicated mucolytic agent.

✔ The expectorant guaifenesin is often used with antitussives. It increases the production of respiratory secretions and decreases irritation caused by dryness in the airways.

✔ Bronchodilators are drugs that act to relieve bronchospasm, i.e, an "asthma attack."

✔ Corticosteroids and anticholinergics may be used to decrease respiratory airway inflammation and produce some bronchodilation in cases where bronchodilators have failed.

SELF TEST

MATCH THE GENERIC AND TRADE NAMES.   *answers can be checked in the back of the book*

1. Acetylcysteine   *Mucomyst*   Adrenalin

2. Albuterol   *Proventil*   Allegra

3. Cetirizine   *Zyrtec*   Alupent

4. Diphenhydramine   *Benadryl*   Atrovent

5. Epinephrine   *Adrenalin*   Benadryl

6. Fexofenadine   *Allegra*   Claritin

7. Fluticasone   *Flonase*   Flonase

8. Guaifenesin   *Robitussin*   Mucomyst

9. Ipratropium   *Atrovent*   Neo-Synephrine

10. Loratadine   *Claritin*   Proventil

11. Metaproterenol   *Alupent*   Robitussin

12. Phenylephrine   *Neo-Synephrine*   Zyrtec

CHOOSE THE BEST ANSWER.   *answers are in the back of the book*

1. Which of the following respiratory agents comes in a perle formulation and should not be chewed?
   a) benzonatate
   b. cetirizine
   c. diphenhydramine
   d. guaifenesin

2. Which one of the following generic and trade name combinations is not correct?
   a. acetylcysteine / Mucomyst®
   b. albuterol / Alupent®
   c. fexofenadine / Allegra®
   d. guaifenesin / Organidin®

3) Which of the following disorders generally occur in children resulting in airway obstruction and dyspnea?
   a. bronchitis
   b. bronchiolitis
   c. emphysema
   d. pneumonia

4) Of the following agents, which one is an expectorant?
   a. benzonatate
   b. cetirizine
   c. diphenhydramine
   d. guaifenesin

VITAMINS

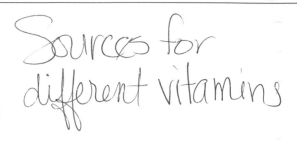

It has long been known that eating certain foods could help prevent some diseases from occurring.

For example, eating oranges can prevent scurvy and drinking milk can prevent rickets. However, substantial research of vitamins as nutrients did not begin until the late 19th century. During the 1930's and 1940's, great strides were made in discovering and isolating the value of vitamins, and today we are aware of the vitamin contents of a great number of specific foods as well as their contribution to health.

The body generally only needs those vitamins found in a balanced daily diet.

However, there are situations (especially with certain GI disorders) in which supplements may be required. In addition, not everyone maintains a balanced daily diet. Populations at risk include young children, teenagers, adults on the run, and the elderly.

The function of these organic substances is mainly that of a *coenzyme* that can effect many biochemical reactions in the body.

In this function, vitamins are considered essential to many body processes. For this reason, daily intake of minimum amounts of vitamins is recommended. RDA's (recommended daily allowances) are calculated to address both males and females and include a breakdown according to age.

There are two categories of vitamins: *water-soluble* and *fat-soluble*.

Examples of the water-soluble vitamins include vitamin C (ascorbic acid) and the B-complex vitamins such as Vitamin B_1 (thiamin), Vitamin B_2 (riboflavin), Vitamin B_3 (niacin), and Vitamin B_{12} (cyanocobalamin). Fat-soluble vitamins include Vitamins A, D, E, and K. These vitamins, as a class, are stored by the body in fat and used as needed.

---

coenzyme a substance that activates enzymes.

fat-soluble vitamins vitamins stored in body fat for later use (e.g., A, D, E, K).

RDA's recommended daily allowances for intake of vitamins and other nutrients.

water-soluble vitamins vitamins stored in water for quick usage by the body (e.g., C and B-Complex).

RDA's

Four organizations that are recognized as official references for recommended daily allowances are:

➡ The Food and Nutrition Board of the National Academy of Sciences,

➡ The United States Food and Drug Administration,

➡ The United Nations Food and Agriculture Organization,

➡ The World Health Organization.

Note: The recommended daily allowances of vitamins may vary according to the specific reference.

Examples of Suggested RDA's

Vitamin C

➡ 35 mg for infants.

➡ 45 mg for children.

➡ 50-60 mg for adults.

➡ 60 mg for pregnant females.

Thiamin

➡ 0.3-0.5 mg for infants.

➡ 0.7-1.2 mg for children.

➡ 1.1 mg for adult females.

➡ 1.2-1.5 mg for adult males.

➡ 1.0-1.1 for pregnant females.

Vitamin A

➡ 400-420 mcg for infants.

➡ 400-700 mcg for children.

➡ 800 mcg for adult females.

➡ 1000 mcg for adult males.

➡ 800 mcg for pregnant females.

VITAMIN

SOURCE / DOSAGE

Vitamin C

Vitamin C, also known as **ascorbic acid** and trade name **Cevalin**, is used to prevent and treat Vitamin C deficiencies. For example, the condition scurvy occurs when the diet is deficient in fruits and vegetables for an extended period of time. Traditionally those who lived in colder climates, the poor, and sailors out to sea for prolonged periods would fall victim to this disorder. Today, with fresh produce available to most everyone, scurvy is less of a concern. Other vitamin C indications may include: post-surgical healing, cold sore and bed sore prevention and treatment, and the controversial common cold cure. The chemical element hydroxyproline, a building block of collagen (the main element of connective tissue) is synthesized with the help of Vitamin C. Therefore, lack of Vitamin C may result in abnormal tooth and bone development, increased capillary breakdown, and result in bleeding and deficient healing. Vitamin C has also been known to stimulate cortisone production, participate in epinephrine production, and assist the white blood cell in its pathogenic attack.

Food resources of Vitamin C include: rose hips (the largest percentage of Vitamin C is found in this source), oranges, spinach, watercress, guava, strawberries, green peppers, black currants, broccoli, and Brussels sprouts.

The suggested dosage for vitamin supplements varies, as per patient condition. However, an example of a commonly recommended dose would be 50 mg PO per day and 100 mg-2 g IM, SQ, or IV. For more serious deficiency cases, Vitamin C toxicity could lead to burning with urination and GI upset such as diarrhea, but generally occurrences of severe side effects are rare. Remember, Vitamin C is water-soluble and large amounts are excreted through the urine.

B Complex Vitamins

The B complex vitamins (Vitamins B_1, B_2, B_3 and B_{12}) are also water-soluble and large amounts are excreted through the urine. Side effects reported with B_1 use include tightness in chest, cyanosis, severe itching, flushing, and nausea. Side effects reported with B_{12} use include abdominal pain, nausea/vomiting, severe flushing and itching.

Vitamin B_1 (Thiamin) is a coenzyme involved in carbohydrate and sugar metabolism. Insufficiency of this vitamin may result in a condition called Beriberi and produce symptoms such as muscle weakness, anorexia, cardiac arrhythmias, and lower extremity edema. Alcoholics and diabetics are at high risk for complications especially if they are also deficient in thiamin.

Common food sources include: wheat germ, pork, whole grains, and yeast. Suggested supplemental doses may range from 5-30 mg PO daily, 10-20 mg IM, and 10-30 mg IV daily for more severe cases.

Vitamin B_2 (Riboflavin) is converted into two coenzymes which work in the body to produce energy through cellular respiration. Deficiency of this vitamin results in lesions of the skin, mouth and tongue as well as ocular symptoms such as burning, itching, tearing, and light sensitivity. Usually this deficiency will occur in conjunction with other B complex deficiencies and is therefore treated with a B complex regime.

Food sources of Riboflavin include: milk, dairy products such as eggs and cheese, green leafy vegetables, organ meats, and whole grain cereals. The suggested supplemental dose may be 5-10 mg PO per day.

VITAMINS

VITAMIN	SOURCE / DOSAGE

B Complex Vitamins (cont'd)

Vitamin B$_3$ (**Niacin**) is also known as **nicotinic acid** though it bears only a slight chemical resemblance to nicotine. Niacin plays an important role in cellular oxidation and reduction as well as in the metabolism of fats, proteins, and carbohydrates. Deficiencies of Niacin may result in a disorder called **Pellagra**, which is characterized by insomnia, nervousness, dermatitis, GI distress, and in severe cases: dementia, hallucinations, depression, and reddened swollen tongue could occur.

Food sources of Niacin are lean meats, organ foods such as liver, green vegetables, fish, enriched bread, peanut butter, and potatoes. The suggested supplemental dose may be 10-20 mg daily PO for niacin deficiency and up to 500 mg PO daily for the treatment of Pellagra.

Vitamin B$_{12}$ (**cyanocobalamin**) is essential for cell reproduction, fat metabolism, and myelin and blood cell manufacture. Deficiency of this vitamin could result in two types of anemia (pernicious and megaloblastic) and in severe cases, peripheral nerve and spinal cord damage. People at risk to develop B$_{12}$ deficiency are strict vegetarians and those with GI dysfunction (any condition which leads to a reduction of the **intrinsic factor**, a protein normally secreted by the stomach that aids in the absorption of cyanocobalamin).

Food sources of B$_{12}$ include: dairy products, seafood, and meats. Also this vitamin may be stored in the body and some sources suggest that a deficiency may not occur for 5-6 years of insufficient intake. The suggested supplemental dosage may be 3 mcg PO daily.

Vitamin K

Vitamin K (also known by the trade names, **Synkayvite**, **Mephyton**, **Konakion** and **AquaMephyton**) is essential to prothrombin production and therefore integral to the blood clotting process. Clotting factors II, VII, IX, and X rely on this vitamin to activate their function. This vitamin will also counteract oral anticoagulants (e.g., coumadin) and may be used in cases of anticoagulant overdosing. On the average, a well balanced diet will provide enough Vitamin K for the blood clotting process to function normally. However, infants are at risk for a Vitamin K deficiency as they are born without the intestinal bacteria that synthesizes Vitamin K. To address this, they are given a dose of 500-1000 mcg after birth. This treatment will decrease clotting time and prevent bleeding until such time as intestinal bacteria begins to grow in the infant's intestine. Although Vitamin K deficiency is rare in adults, the symptoms may include nose bleeds, blood in the urine, blood in vomitus, and bruising.

Except in infants (see description at left) Vitamin K is synthesized by the intestinal bacteria and this is the body's greatest overall source. However, food sources of this vitamin include: cheddar cheese (the highest percentage of this vitamin), other cheeses, Brussels sprouts, alfalfa, green leafy vegetables, liver, and egg yolks. Toxicity of this vitamin is rare as it is not stored in the body as long as other fat-soluble vitamins. Newborns, however, may experience severe side effects of this vitamin such as **hyperbilirubinemia** (high levels of serum bilirubin), which is characterized by jaundice and could lead to brain damage or even death. The suggested supplemental dose is 5-10 mg PO per day or 5-15 mg IM, IV, or SQ.

VITAMIN	SOURCE / DOSAGE

Vitamin A

Vitamin A (trade name **Aquasol A**) is stored in the liver and requires bile salts, pancreatic lipase, and fat in order to be adequately absorbed. Therefore, conditions such as biliary or pancreatic disease, colitis, cirrhosis, Chrohn's Disease, and poor dietary intake would contribute to a deficiency of this vitamin. Vitamin A prevents growth retardation, preserves skin integrity, and assists in eye adaptation to night vision. Therefore a deficiency of this vitamin could result in insufficient night vision, fetal malformation, drying of the skin, and possible lowering of resistance to infection.

Food sources of Vitamin A include: yellow and green vegetables, dairy products, organ foods, and shellfish. Liver contains the largest percentage of this vitamin. The suggested supplement dosage is dependent upon patient condition and will vary widely. For example, the range may be from 5,000-500,000 IU (international units) PO per day. Overdosage may result in fatigue, abdominal pain, drying of the skin, hair loss, dizziness, and bone pain.

Vitamin E

Vitamin E, also known by the trade name **Aquasol E**, is used for the prevention and treatment of Vitamin E deficiency. The exact therapeutic function, according to most resources, is undetermined. Some researchers believe Vitamin E helps protect our cells from the oxidation (aging) process and others believe that Vitamin E neutralizes the damaging effects of oxygen on unsaturated fat (the turning of fluid fat to solid fat leading to cell death). Some researchers have even claimed that Vitamin E can be helpful in the treatment of cystic breast disease, scarring, leg cramps and pain, and the healing of wounds.

Food sources of Vitamin E include: wheat germ, cottonseed oil, almond oil, sunflower seeds, and nuts. Vitamin E however, is destroyed when frozen and does not do well in heat. The suggested daily supplement is 12-15 IU, PO per day and any toxic or side effects have been rare.

Vitamin D

Vitamin D helps to regulate calcium metabolism and is often used to treat rickets (bone development disorder exacerbated by lack of sunlight and vitamin D deficiency) in children. Some sources claim Vitamin D is also used to preserve healthy blood clotting and heart function.

Food sources of Vitamin D include: cod liver oil (the greatest source), fish such as salmon, sardines and tuna, milk and egg yolks. Sunlight is also a major source for this vitamin. *Vitamin D can be toxic if taken in large enough doses.* The daily supplemental intake should not exceed 400 IU. Persons at risk for developing toxicity include elderly women with the diagnosis of osteoporosis. Symptoms of toxicity include: nausea, vomiting, weakness, high cholesterol, and diabetic-like symptoms (loss of appetite, excessive thirst, urination, ketones in the urine). Vitamin D preparations are available in many trade names: Calderol, Rocaltrol, Hytakerol, and Calciferol.

VITAMIN CHART

GENERIC NAME	TRADE NAME	ROUTE
VITAMINS		
Ascorbic Acid, Vitamin C	Cevalin	PO
	Various	PO
Beta-Carotene	Solatene	PO
	Various	PO
Cyanocobalamin, Vitamin B_{12}	Various	PO, Injectable
Niacin, Vitamin B_3	Nicobid	PO
	Slow-Niacin	PO
	Nicolar	PO
	Various	PO
Pantothenic Acid, Vitamin B_5	Various	PO
Pyridoxine, Vitamin B_6	Various	PO, Injectable
Ribloflavin, Vitamin B_2	Various	PO
Thiamine, Vitamin B_1	Various	PO, Injectable
Vitamin A	Aquasol A	PO, Injectable
	Unilife-A	PO, Injectable
	Various	PO, Injectable
Ergocalciferol, Vitamin D_2	Various	PO
Calcifediol, Vitamin D_3 (analog)	Calderol	PO
Calcitriol Vitamin D_3 (analog)	Rocaltrol	PO
	Calcijex	Injectable
Dihydrotachysterol, Vitamin D_3 (analog)	DHT	PO
	Hytakerol	PO
	Various	PO
Vitamin E	Aquasol E	PO
	Various	PO
Phytonadione, Vitamin K_1	Mephyton	PO
	Aquamephyton	Injectable
	Konakion	Injectable

KEY CONCEPTS

✔ The function of vitamins is mainly that of a coenzyme that can effect many biochemical reactions in the body. Coenzymes are substances that activate enzymes.

✔ RDA's (recommended daily allowances) of vitamins are calculated to address both males and females and include a breakdown according to age.

✔ Water-soluble vitamins include vitamin C (ascorbic acid) and the B-complex vitamins, e.g., Vitamin B_1 (thiamin), Vitamin B_2 (riboflavin), Vitamin B_3 (niacin), and Vitamin B_{12} (cyanocobalamin).

✔ Fat-soluble vitamins include Vitamins A, D, E, and K. They are stored in fat and used as needed.

✔ Vitamin C is used to prevent and treat Vitamin C deficiencies, including the disorder scurvy.

✔ Vitamin B_1 is a coenzyme involved in carbohydrate and sugar metabolism. Deficiency may result in Beriberi and produce symptoms such as muscle weakness, anorexia, and cardiac arrhythmias.

✔ Vitamin B_2 is converted into two coenzymes that work to produce energy through cellular respiration. Deficiency can result in various lesions and ocular symptoms.

✔ Vitamin B_3 plays an important role in cellular oxidation and reduction as well as in the metabolism of fats, proteins, and carbohydrates. Deficiencies may result in a disorder called Pellagra.

✔ Vitamin B_{12} is essential for cell reproduction, fat metabolism, and myelin and blood cell manufacture. Deficiency could result in two types of anemia (pernicious and megaloblastic).

✔ Vitamin K is essential to prothrombin production and therefore integral to the blood clotting process.

✔ Vitamin A prevents growth retardation, preserves skin integrity, and assists in night vision.

✔ The exact therapeutic function of Vitamin E, according to most resources, is undetermined.

✔ Vitamin D helps to regulate calcium metabolism and is often used to treat rickets in children.

CHOOSE THE BEST ANSWER.

answers are in the back of the book

1. Which of the following vitamins is not fat soluble?
   a. vitamin A
   b. vitamin B_6
   c. vitamin D
   d. vitamin E

2. Which of the following vitamins are measured in International Units?
   a. vitamin A
   b. vitamin D
   c. vitamin E
   d. all of the above

3. Of the following vitamin and medical disorder combinations, which one is not correct?
   a. vitamin B_3 / Pellagra
   b. vitamin C / Beriberi
   c. vitamin D / Rickets
   d. vitamin K / blood clotting disorder(s)

4. Of the following vitamin and source combinations, which one is not correct?
   a. vitamin A / yellow and green vegetables
   b. vitamin E / cod liver oil
   c. vitamin D / sunlight
   d. vitamin K / cheddar cheese

NATURAL AGENTS

Natural medicine has been used successfully for thousands of years and is currently seeing a dramatic resurgence in its popularity. *Herbal* and *botanical* preparations (both oral and topical), natural vitamins and nutrients, and even aromatherapies are hailed by many as therapeutically effective. Stand alone clinics, as well as offices attached to traditional medical facilities, are providing opportunities to offer this form of prevention and treatment to the millions of people who believe this alternative form of medicine works! Some of the most common natural agents include: antioxidants (vitamin E, beta carotene or vitamin A, and vitamin C), aloe, shark cartilage and oil, St. John's Wort, chamomile, garlic, and ginseng.

Though they sometimes produce similar effects, natural medicine products are not regulated as drug products in the United States and many other nations.

In the U.S., they are considered *dietary supplements* and are subject to laws specific to such supplements. These supplements include vitamins, minerals, proteins, herbals and botanicals, and other similar nutritional substances (e.g., ginseng, garlic, fish oils, enzymes, etc.).

A basic knowledge of natural medicines is increasingly valuable to health care professionals because of their wide usage and potential effects and interactions.

Because natural medicines are not as closely regulated, patients often self-medicate and there is a potential for both adverse effects and interactions. At a minimum, understanding what regulations do and don't allow and how people are using these "supplements" is important to health care professionals. Also, as these "medicines" increase in popularity, more scientific attention is being paid to this area, more research is being done, and more information is becoming available. With time, there may also be more standards and regulation.

Lack of Equivalency

It is important to note that there are not the same manufacturing standards for the potency of drug ingredients in dietary supplements as there are for drug products. As a result, similar products from different manufacturers may have very different effects. It is also worth noting that recommended doses for natural agents vary according to the source.

LABEL STATEMENTS

In the United States, the labels of natural products may contain various statements regarding their nutritional value and effect. *However, they are limited in what they can suggest regarding their therapeutic value.* They cannot make claims about the product's ability to:

➡ diagnose.

➡ prevent.

➡ mitigate.

➡ treat.

➡ cure a specific disease.

For example, a product cannot be claimed to cure cancer or treat asthma. They may, however, put accepted health claims on the label such as the claim that calcium may reduce the risk of osteoporosis provided, however, that their product contains calcium.

Any time herbal or natural medicines include statements about health on the label, they must also have this statement:

"This statement has not been evaluated by the Food and Drug Administration. This product is not intended to diagnose, treat, cure, or prevent any disease."

In effect, herbal and natural medicine products are subject to regulations similar to those for foods. They must:

➡ provide ingredient and nutritional information.

➡ not be misleading.

➡ identify the product as a dietary supplement.

Aloe (Aloe Barbadensis)

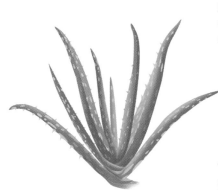

Aloe is a tropical herb that is available in several forms including gel, tablets, capsules, fluid extract, and powder. Due to its analgesic and antihistamine effects, this natural agent has found a wide range of uses, including the treatment of:

- skin irritations.
- insect bites.
- allergies.
- constipation.
- gastritis.

The emollients aloe contains also act as skin moisturizers. Caution is advised if the user is pregnant or diagnosed with a serious gastrointestinal disease. The recommended dosage should not be exceeded as the laxative action of aloe is powerful. Side effects may include abdominal cramping and diarrhea.

St. John's Wort (Hypericum Perforatum)

Derived from a flower, this popular herbal preparation is used as:

- an anti-inflammatory and germicidal agent.
- an antidepressant.

The chemicals, called **flavonoids**, which are contained in St. John's Wort, are thought to positively affect the immune system. However, some of the possible side effects include nausea/vomiting, headache, and high blood pressure. Caution should be taken if the user has hypertension or is especially sensitive to sunlight and sunburn.

botanical generally, a product derived from plants.

dietary supplement nutritional substances, including vitamins, proteins, herbals and botanicals, and other similar products.

flavonoid a compound found in many plants.

herbal a product derived from an herb, as opposed to other plants.

NATURAL AGENTS

Chamomile (Matricaria Recutita)

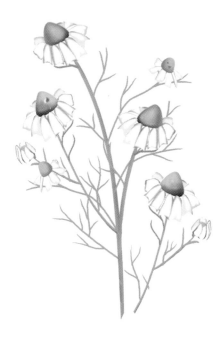

The use of this agent, derived from the chamomile plant, dates back thousands of years. Historically, the oil from this plant has been used in the treatment of:

➡ nervousness,

➡ GI upset,

➡ bladder infection, and

➡ menstrual cramps.

Topically, this product is used to reduce:

➡ skin inflammation,

➡ reduce hemorrhoids, and

➡ decrease joint pain and swelling.

Chamomile is available as a tea, oil or tincture. Although allergies and/or side effects of chamomile are rare, any signs of allergic response should be reported to a physician.

Gingseng (Panax Quinquefolius–American, Panax Ginseng–Asian, Eleutherococcus Senticosus–Siberian)

The use of this root dates back centuries to ancient China where it was believed to be "the essence of earth in the form of a man" and to Native Americans who believed Ginseng would ease childbirth pain and rejuvenate the elderly.

Used to treat medical conditions from depression to fatigue to colds, American ginseng is milder than Asian and more potent than Siberian. Therefore, side effects (such as insomnia, headache, and possible cardiac arrhythmias, asthma or hypertension) would be less serious.

Ginseng is available as a tea, powder, tablet, capsule, and rock candy. Caution should be exercised (especially with Asian ginseng) if the user has a medical history of hypertension, asthma, diabetes and cardiac pathologies.

Garlic (Allium Sativum)

This spice has become increasingly known for the therapeutic effects of it's active ingredient allicin. Garlic is available as tablets or in its natural form as cloves or powder and is used as a remedy for:

➥ colds,

➥ high cholesterol,

➥ high blood pressure,

➥ arthritis,

➥ diarrhea, and

➥ food poisoning.

It may be applied externally in the treatment of skin conditions such as pinworm, ringworm and athlete's foot. It is possible to develop a local skin reaction to the external product or a slight dermatological reaction if it is taken internally. However, side effects are rare. Caution should be exercised if the user is pregnant or has a prolonged blood clotting time as garlic contains an agent that may increase clotting time.

Shark Cartilage and Oil

Shark cartilage has been claimed to be useful as a treatment for certain forms of cancer (i.e., tumor producing, particularly GI). The theory contends that shark cartilage suppresses the development of new blood vessels and in so doing prevents the growth of cancerous tumors. A well known researcher in this field is Dr. Gaston Naessen and the clinical trials that he has worked in are available for inquiry. Few side effects had been noted from the taking of shark cartilage, although allergic reaction was listed as a possibility. Shark liver oil may be classified as a natural antihemorrhoidal preparation. It acts as a skin barrier or protectant and contains large amounts of vitamin A. This product is to be applied topically only. In the case of continued hemorrhoidal condition, a physician should be consulted.

NATURAL AGENTS CHART

Plant Name	Scientific Name	Trade Name	Route
Aloe	Aloe Barbadensis	Various	PO, Topical
Chamomile	Matricaria Recutita	Various	PO
Cone flower	Echinacea	Echinaforce	PO
		Esberitox	PO
		ViraMedx	PO
		Various	PO
Feverfew	Tanacetum parthenium	Various	PO
Garlic	Allium sativum	Kwai	PO
		Kyolic	PO
		GarliPure	PO
		Various	PO
Ginger	Zingiber officinale	Various	PO
Ginko	Ginko biloba	Various	PO
Ginseng	Panax ginseng	Ginsana	PO
		Various	PO
Kava Kava	Piper methysticum	Kavatrol	PO
		Various	PO
Milk Thistle	Silybum marianum	Various	PO
Saw Palmetto	Serenoa repens	Various	PO
St. John's Wart	Hypericum perforatum	Various	PO
Valerian	Valeriana officinalis	Various	PO

KEY CONCEPTS

✔ In the U.S., natural agents are considered dietary supplements and are subject to laws specific to such supplements. Dietary supplements include vitamins, minerals, proteins, herbals and botanicals, and other similar nutritional substances (e.g., ginseng, garlic, fish oils, enzymes, etc.).

✔ There are not the same manufacturing standards for the potency of drug ingredients in dietary supplements as there are for drug products. As a result, similar products from different manufacturers may have very different effects.

✔ In the United States, any time herbal or natural medicines include statements about health on the label, they must also include: "This statement has not been evaluated by the Food and Drug Administration. This product is not intended to diagnose, treat, cure, or prevent any disease."

✔ Due to its analgesic and antihistamine effects, aloe has found a wide range of uses, including the treatment of skin irritations, insect bites, allergies, constipation , and gastritis. The emollients aloe contains also act as skin moisturizers.

✔ St. John's Wort is used as an anti-inflammatory and germicidal agent, and an antidepressant.

✔ The oil from the chamomile plant has been used in the treatment of nervousness, GI upset, bladder infection, and menstrual cramps. It is used topically to reduce skin inflammation, hemorrhoids, and joint pain and swelling.

✔ Ginseng is used to treat medical conditions from depression to fatigue to colds.

✔ Garlic is available as tablets or in its natural form as cloves or powder and is used as a treatment for colds, high cholesterol, high blood pressure, arthritis, diarrhea, and food poisoning.

✔ Shark cartilage has been claimed to be useful as a treatment for certain forms of cancer (i.e., tumor producing, particularly GI).

CHOOSE THE BEST ANSWER.   *answers are in the back of the book*

1. Of the following statements, which one is false?
   a Herbal preparations are derived from herbs.
   b. Herbal preparations are considered dietary supplements.
   c. Herbal preparations are not drugs, therefore they are relatively safe.

2. This product is known for the therapeutic effect of its active ingredient allicin.
   a. chamomile
   b. garlic
   c. ginseng
   d. St. John's Wart

3. Matricaria Recuitita is the same as:
   a. chamomile
   b. garlic
   c. ginseng
   d. St. John's Wart

4. Derived from a flower, this herbal preparation is a popular natural antidepressant.
   a. chamomile
   b. garlic
   c. ginseng
   d. St. John's Wart

ANSWERS TO SELF TESTS

Chapter 1
1. b
2. d
3. a
4. d

Chapter 2
1. d
2. c
3. a
4. a

Chapter 3
1. b
2. b
3. d
4. d

Chapter 4
1. b
2. b
3. c
4. c

Chapter 5
1. e
2. f
3. b
4. h
5. i
6. a
7. g
8. c
9. d
10. q
11. k
12. m
13. l
14. n
15. j
16. p
17. o
18. r
19. u
20. v
21. w
22. t
23. s

Chapter 6
a. 500,000 mg
b. 10,000 g
c. 0.25 L
d. 0.325 g
e. 0.12 mg
f. 224.4 lb

g. 3560 g
h. 0.473 L
i. 65.9 Kg
j. 30,000,000 mg
k. 7.8°
l. 3 ml
m. 2.5 ml
n. 142.85 dext 70% and 357 ml sterile water
o. b
p. c
q. c
r. d
s. d
t. a
u. a
v. b
w. b

Chapter 7
1. d
2. d
3. c
4. b

Chapter 8
1. a
2. d
3. c
4. a

Chapter 9
1. Androgens
2. Enzymes
3. Antianxiety agents
4. Antihypertensives
5. Local anesthetics
6. Cephalosporins
7. Penicillins
8. Anti-fungals
9. Cortisone derivatives
10. Antibiotics
11. Estrogens
12. Progestins
13. Monoclonal antibodies
14. Steroids
15. Antibiotics (quinolone derivatives)
16. Coronary vasodilators

17. Prednisone derivatives
18. Antihypertensives (ACE inhibitors)
19. Antibiotics (sulfonamide derivatives)
20. Calcium channel blockers (diltiazem derivatives)
21. Oxytocin derivatives
22. Antimetabolites (folic acid derivatives)
23. Antidepressants
24. Antihyperlipidemics (HMG-CoA inhibitors)

Chapter 10
match
1. Tylenol
2. Voltaren
3. Advil
4. Indocin
5. Actron
6. Demerol
7. MS Contin
8. Relafen
9. Aleve
10. Daypro
11. Darvon
12. Ultram
best answer
1. b
2. c
3. d
4. c

Chapter 11
1. c
2. d
3. d
4. b

Chapter 12
match
1. Zovirax

2. Amoxil
3. Augmentin
4. Cefzil
5. Ceftin
6. Keflex
7. Biaxin
8. Vibramycin
9. Garamycin
10. Levaquin
11. Macrobid
12. Retrovir
best answer
1. b
2. b
3. a
4. c

Chapter 13
1. b
2. d
3. d
4. a

Chapter 14
match
1. Lotensin
2. Lanoxin
3. Cardizem
4. Cardura
5. Plendil
6. Lasix
7. Prinivil
8. Lopressor
9. Procardia
10. Dilantin
11. Calan
12. Coumadin
best answer
1. c
2. a
3. d
4. d

ANSWERS TO SELF TESTS

Chapter 15
1. a
2. b
3. d
4. a

Chapter 16
1. b
2. d
3. b
4. a

Chapter 17
match
1. Dulcolax
2. Alka-Seltzer
3. Tagamet
4. Propulsid
5. Colace
6. Pepcid
7. Prevacid
8. Maalox
9. Citrucel
10. Prilosec
11. Metamucil
12. Zantac
best answer
1. c
2. a
3. a
4. a

Chapter 18
1. c
2. c
3. c
4. a

Chapter 19
match
1. Miacalcin
2. Clomid
3. Premarin

4. Desogen
5. Glucotrol
6. Glynase
7. Humulin
8. Synthroid
9. Glucophage
10. Tapazole
11. Pitocin
12. Rezulin
best answer
1. c
2. c
3. b
4. d

Chapter 20
1. a
2. a
3. d
4. c

Chapter 21
1. b
2. c
3. d
4. d

Chapter 22
1. b
2. c
3. b
4. b

Chapter 23
1. c
2. c
3. c
4. c

Chapter 24
match
1. Xanax
2. Elavil

3. Tegretol
4. Thorazine
5. Valium
6. Sinequan
7. Prozac
8. Ativan
9. Zyprexa
10. Paxil
11. Nardil
12. Depakene
best answer
1. a
2. c
3. d
4. a

Chapter 25
match
1. Mucomyst
2. Proventil
3. Zyrtec
4. Benadryl
5. Adrenalin
6. Allegra
7. Flonase
8. Robitussin
9. Atrovent
10. Claritin
11. Alupent
12. Neo-Synephrine
best answer
1. a
2. b
3. b
4. d

Chapter 26
1. b
2. d
3. b
4. b

Chapter 27
1. c
2. b
3. a
4. d

GLOSSARY A-D1

ACE inhibitors the "-pril" drugs, they relax the blood vessels. Note: the "-sartan" drugs are considered a subgroup of ACE inhibitors.

active immunity immunity resulting from the production of antibodies in response to contraction of a disease.

active transport the movement of drug molecules across membranes by active means, rather than passive diffusion.

acute viral hepatitis a virus caused systemic infection that causes inflammation of the liver.

additive effects the increase in effect when two drugs with similar pharmacological actions are taken.

admixture the resulting solution when a drug is added to a parenteral solution.

adsorb attachment of one chemical to another.

adverse effect an unintended side affect of a medication that is negative or in some way injurious to a patient's health.

adverse effect an undesired effect of drug therapy.

agonist drugs that activate receptors to accelerate or slow normal cell function.

alopecia hair loss.

Bipolar Disorder also known as Manic-Depression, symptoms are mood, energy, and behavior swings from periods of elation to episodes of depression.

alveolar sacs (alveoli) the small sacs of specialized tissue that transfer oxygen out of inspired air into the blood and carbon dioxide out of the blood and into the air for expiration.

Alzheimer's a progressive dementia often classified as a psychiatric disorder that has been linked to neurotransmitter abnormalities.

aminoglycosides antibiotics that work by interfering with bacteria's ability to synthesize protein.

ampules sealed glass containers with an elongated neck that must be snapped off.

analgesia a state in which pain is not felt even though a painful condition exists.

anaphylactic shock a potentially fatal hypersensitivity reaction producing severe respiratory distress and cardiovascular collapse.

androgens male sex characteristic hormones.

anemia a decrease in hemoglobin or red blood cells.

anions a negatively charged ion.

antacids agents that act to neutralize existing acid, as opposed to inhibiting its production.

antagonist drugs that bind with receptors but do not activate them. They block receptor action by preventing other drugs or substances from activating them.

antianginals agents used to treat cardiac related chest pain (angina) resulting from ischemic heart disease.

antiarrhythmics agents used to treat irregular heart rhythms..

antibiotic (antimicrobial) drug that destroys microorganisms.

antibody (immunoglobulin) a substance in the body that attacks and destroys pathogens.

anticoagulants agents used to prevent clot formation.

antidote a drug that antagonizes or blocks the toxic effect of another drug.

antiemetics agents that treat the urge to vomit by reducing the hyperactivity of stimuli receptors and lower the impulse rate.

antifungal drug that destroys fungi or inhibits its growth.

antihelminthic drug that destroys worms.

antihistamines agents that act to respond to the release of histamine or inflammation producing substance from white blood cells that occurs with an injury or allergic reaction.

antihyperlipidemics agents used to lower high levels of cholesterol.

antihypertensives agents used to reduce a sustained elevation in blood pressure.

anti-infectives agents that treat disease produced by microorganisms such as bacteria, viruses, fungi, protozoa and parasitic worms.

antimicrobial (antibiotic) drug that destroys microorganisms.

antimycobacterial drug that attacks mycobacteria, the organisms that cause tuberculosis and leprosy.

antineoplastic a cancer fighting agent.

antiperistalsis drugs agents used to treat diarrhea by slowing the movement of the intestinal contents to allow for greater water and electrolyte absorption.

antiprotozoal drug that destroys protozoa.

anti-pyretic reduces fever.

antitoxin a substance that acts against a toxin in the body; also, a vaccine containing antitoxins, used to fight disease.

antitussives agents that treat both productive (with phlegm) and non-productive (without phlegm) coughs.

antiviral drug that attacks a virus.

anxiety a condition in which an individual can be abnormally tired or energetic, withdrawn, tremorous, tense, and restless and may suffer from insomnia, phobias, and panic attacks.

apnea absence of breathing.

aqueous water based.

arrhythmia an abnormal heart rhythm.

ascorbic acid vitamin C.

aseptic techniques techniques that maintain sterile condition.

asthma a disorder of chronic airway inflammation related to stimuli hyperresponsiveness, resulting in airflow obstruction with symptoms such as wheezing and potentially acute spasms and breathlessness.

bactericidal bacteria killing.

bacteriostatic bacteria inhibiting.

barbiturates a group of drugs derived from barbituric acid that depress the CNS, respiration, and heart rate, and lower blood pressure and temperature.

B-cells with T-Cells, one of the primary lymphocytes.

benzodiazepines a group of CNS depressing agents with the potential for abuse and/or dependence and that should not be taken by pregnant or breast feeding women or taken along with alcohol consumption.

beta blockers   drugs that reduce the oxygen demands of the heart muscle.

bevel   an angled surface, as with the tip of a needle.

bioavailability   the relative amount of an administered dose that reaches the general circulation and the rate at which this occurs.

biocompatibility   not irritating or infection or abscess causing to body tissue.

bioequivalence   the comparison of bioavailability between two dosage forms.

biopharmaceutics   the study of the factors associated with drug products and physiological processes, and the resulting systemic concentrations of the drugs.

blocker   another term for an antagonist drug, because antagonists block the action of neurotransmitters.

blood concentration-time profile   a graph of the blood concentration of a drug over time.

blood counts   analysis of blood for various factors (red blood cells, white blood cells, platelets, or other indices).

blood–brain barrier   a barrier membrane between the blood and the brain that blocks certain harmful substances from entering the brain.

body surface area   a measurement given in square meters based on a person's height and weight and used in children's doses and chemotherapy.

botanical   generally, a product derived from plants.

bronchodilators   drugs that act to relieve bronchospasm, i.e, an "asthma attack."

bronchospasm   a narrowing of the bronchi, accompanied by wheezing and coughing, i.e., an "asthma attack."

buffer system   ingredients in a formulation designed to control the pH.

calcitonin   a hormone secreted by the parathryroid glands involved with serum calcium and phosphorus level regulation.

calcium channel blockers   rugs that relax the heart by reducing heart conduction.

carcinogenicity   the ability of a substance to cause cancer.

cardiac cycle   the contraction and relaxation of the heart that pumps blood through the cardiovascular system.

cations   a positively charged ion.

cephalosporins   antibiotics that work by inhibiting cell wall synthesis in bacteria.

cerebellum   part of the brain that controls balance and muscle coordination.

cerebrum   part of the brain concerned mostly with learned behavior, thought, memory, sensation and voluntary motion.

cholesterol   an essential lipid in the body that is measured as total cholesterol, LDL (low-density lipoprotein), and HDL (high-density lipoprotein). Excess amounts of LDL can lead to blocked blood vessels and cardiovascular problems.

chyme   the semi-liquid form of food as it enters the intestinal tract.

cirrhosis   a chronic and potentially fatal liver disease causing loss of function and resistance to blood flow through the liver.

clinical trials   the testing of a new drug on people (as opposed to animal or laboratory testing) to determine whether it merits FDA approval.

clotting factors   factors in the blood coagulation process.

coenzyme   a substance that activates enzymes.

colloids   particles up to a hundred times smaller than that those in suspensions that are, however, likewise suspended in a solution.

complex   when molecules of different chemicals attach to each other, as in protein binding.

compliance   doing what is required.

conjunctiva   the eyelid lining.

conjunctivitis   inflammation of the conjunctiva (eyelid lining).

contraceptive   device or formulation designed to prevent pregnancy.

controlled substance mark   the mark (CII-CV) that indicates the control category of a drug with a potential for abuse.

controlled substances   (U.S.) five groups or schedules of drugs that have the potential for abuse and therefore have strict guidelines on their distribution.

COPD (chronic obstructive pulmonary disease)   a disorder of abnormal lung function that generally encompasses both emphysema and chronic bronchitis that is present at least for 3 months a year for 2 consecutive years.

coring   when a needle damages the rubber closure of a parenteral container, causing fragments of the closure to fall into the container and contaminate its contents.

corticosteroids   hormones secreted by the adrenal cortex that regulate the body's ability to handle stress, resist infection, effect glucose, fat, protein and carbohydrate metabolism and maintain salt and water balance.

cyanocobalamin   vitamin B_{12}.

decongestants   agents that cause mucous membrane vasoconstriction, reduction of nasal passage drainage and relief of stuffiness

degradation   the changing of a drug to a less effective or ineffective form.

depression   a condition characterized by mood disturbances that may be mild (e.g., lack of interest or inability to experience joy) or severe (e.g., physical aggression or suicide attempts

depth filter   a filter placed inside a needle hub that can filter solutions being drawn in or expelled, but not both.

dermatological   a product used to treat a skin condition.

dermis   the middle layer of the skin beneath the epidermis.

diabetes mellitus   a condition in which the body does not produce enough insulin or is unable to use it efficiently.

dialysis   movement of particles in a solution through permeable membranes.

diastolic pressure   the minimum blood pressure when the heart relaxes; the second number in a blood pressure reading.

dietary supplement nutritional substances, including vitamins, proteins, herbals and botanicals, and other similar products.

diluent a liquid that dilutes a substance or solution.

displacement when one drug displaces another from a protein binding site, increasing the concentration of the displaced drug in the blood.

disposition a term sometimes used to refer to all of the ADME processes together.

dissociation when a compound breaks down and separates into smaller components.

diuretics drugs that decrease blood pressure by decreasing blood volume. They decrease volume by increasing the elimination of salts and water through urination.

dose response curve a graph of the responses in different patients to a series of doses .

DPT a combination vaccine for diptheria, pertussis, and tetanus.

drug-diet interactions when elements of ingested nutrients interact with a drug and this affects the disposition of the drug.

dyspnea labored breathing.

electrocardiogram (EKG or ECG) a graph of the heart's rhythms.

electrolytes a substance that in solution forms ions that conduct an electrical current.

embolism, embolus a clot that has traveled in the bloodstream to a point where it obstructs flow.

emphysema a disorder of chronic airway obstruction due to lung hyperinflation and diminished oxygen intake, characterized by breathlessness and flushed color.

emulsions mixture of two liquids that do not dissolve into each other in which one liquid is spread through the other by mixing and use of a stabilizer.

endocrine system the system of hormone secreting glands.

enema a solution injected into the rectum that creates the urge to defecate.

enteral the drug route involving the alimentary tract, i.e., the tract from the mouth to the rectum.

enteric coating a coating on tablets to prevent their degradation by stomach acid and ensure that the drug reaches the intestine.

enterohepatic cycling the transfer of drugs and their metabolites from the liver to the bile in the gall bladder and then into the intestine.

enzyme a complex protein that causes chemical reactions in other substances.

enzyme induction the increase in enzyme activity that results in greater metabolism of drugs.

enzyme inhibition the decrease in enzyme activity that results in reduced metabolism of drugs.

enzyme therapy in gastrointestinal therapy, enzymes from the pancreas may be used to break down starches and fats.

epidermis the top or external layer of skin.

epilepsy a neurologic disorder associated with neuron transmission instability and characterized by recurrent seizure activity.

estrogen female sex characteristic hormones involved in calcium and phosphorus conservation.

expectorant an agent that increases the production of respiratory secretions and decreases irritation caused by dryness in the airways. Guaifenesin is the only FDA agent in this class.

extracellular fluids the fluid outside the body's individual cells found in plasma and tissue fluid.

fat-soluble vitamins vitamins stored in body fat for later use (e.g., A, D, E, K).

fibrin the fiber that serves as the structure for clot formation.

fibrinogen clotting factor I.

final filter a filter that filters solution immediately before it enters a patient's vein.

first pass metabolism the substantial degradation of a drug caused by enzyme metabolism in the liver before the drug reaches the systemic circulation.

flavonoid a compound found in many plants.

flexor movement an expansion or outward movement by muscles.

flow rate the rate (in ml/hour or ml/minute) at which the solution is administered to the patient.

formulary a list of drugs that are approved for use, from which individual drugs may be selected.

gastric emptying time the time a drug will stay in the stomach before it is emptied into the small intestine.

gastric reflux a condition in which gastric hyperacidity travels toward the chest and throat area via the esophagus.

gastrointestinal agents agents used to treat disorders of the stomach and/or the intestines.

gauge a measurement– with needles, the higher the gauge, the thinner the lumen.

general anesthesia when the CNS (central nervous system) is depressed to the level of unconsciousness.

glaucoma disorders characterized by abnormally high pressure within the eye that leads to optic nerve damage and loss of vision.

glomerular filtration the blood filtering process of the kidneys.

glucagon a hormone that helps convert amino acids to glucose.

gout a painful inflammatory condition in which excess uric acid accumulates in the joints.

grain a weight measurement: one grain equals 64.8 milligrams.

gram stain (positive/negative) a laboratory method for identifying microorganisms based on staining characteristics.

hematopoietics drugs used to treat anemia.

hemorrhoid painful swollen veins in the anal/rectal area, generally caused by strained bowel movements from hard stools.

hemostatic drugs drugs that prevent excessive bleeding.

HEPA filter a high efficiency particulate air filter.

heparin lock an injection device which uses heparin to keep blood from clotting in the device.

hepatic disease liver disease.

hepato a prefix meaning "of the liver."

herbal a product derived from an herb, as opposed to other plants.

histamine receptor antagonists agents (e.g., cimetidine) that inhibit the secretion of gastric acid by blocking the effects of histamine.

HMG-CoA reductase inhibitor agents that inhibit the coenzyme HMG-CoA reductase to reduce cholesterol biosynthesis.

homeostasis the state of equilibrium of the body.

hormone a chemical secretion that influences or controls an organ or organs in the body.

human genome the complete set of genetic material contained in a human cell.

hydrates absorbs water.

hydrophilic capable of associating with or absorbing water.

hydrophobic water repelling; cannot associate with water.

hypercalemia a condition of high calcium levels often caused by hyperparathyroidism.

hypercholesterolemia excessive amount of cholesterol in the blood.

hyperkalemia is a condition of high potassium levels manifested by muscle weakness, possible paralysis and loss of feeling in the legs, traveling up to the arms.

hypermagnesemia a condition of high magnesium levels with symptoms of muscle weakness and diminished reflexes that in severe cases can result in paralysis, coma, or death.

hypernatremia the condition of having too much sodium.

hypersensitivity an abnormal sensitivity generally resulting in an allergic reaction.

hyperthyroidism a condition in which thyroid hormone secretions are above normal, often referred to as an overactive thyroid.

hypertonic when a solution has a greater osmolarity than another.

hypnotics often referred to as "sleeping pills," these agents are designed to induce and, in some cases, prolong sleep. This group includes barbiturates such as secobarbital and pentobarbital.

hypocalemia low calcium levels that may be related to hypoparathyroidism, vitamin D deficiency, GI diseases, or surgery.

hypokalemia a condition of low potassium levels that is often attributed to dehydration and fluid loss.

hypomagnesemia a condition of low magnesium levels with symptoms of hyperreflexes, muscle twitching, depression, confusion, delirium, and ventricular arrhythmias.

hyponatremia a sodium deficit that causes fluid to move out of the cells in an effort to increase blood volume and make up for the extracellular loss.

hypothalamus a gland attached to the thalamus that controls blood sugar levels, body temperature, emotions, appetite and sleep.

hypothyroidism a condition in which thyroid hormone secretions are below normal, often referred to as an underactive thyroid.

hypotonic when a solution has a lesser osmolarity than another.

idiosyncrasy an unexpected reaction the first time a drug is taken, generally due to genetic causes.

infusion the slow continuous introduction of a solution into the blood stream.

injunction a court order preventing a specific action, such as the distribution of a potentially dangerous drug.

inspiration breathing in.

insulin a hormone that controls the body's use of glucose.

insulin dependent diabetes (IDDM) a diabetic condition that requires insulin injections as treatment.

integumentary system the skin.

interference when one drug interferes with the elimination of another, increasing its concentration in the blood as a result.

international units units used to measure the activity potential of chemicals from natural sources, including vitamins and drugs such as penicillin.

interstitial fluid tissue fluid.

intracellular fluids cell fluid.

intraocular inside the eye.

investigational new drug (IND) what a proposed new drug is called during the clinical trial phase of testing prior to FDA approval.

ions electrically charged particles.

Islands (or Islets) of Langerhans specialized cells of the pancreas that secrete insulin.

isotonic when one solution has an osmolarity equivalent to another.

IUD an intrauterine contraceptive device that is placed in the uterus for a prolonged period of time.

labeling important associated information that is not on the label of a drug product itself, but is provided with the product in the form of an insert, brochure, or other document.

lacrimal canalicula the tear ducts.

lacrimal gland the gland that produces tears for the eye.

laminar flow continuous movement at a stable rate in one direction.

laxatives agents that promote defecation without stress or pain and are often suggested for use prior to certain medical procedures. There are several types: bulk forming, stimulant, saline, and osmotic.

legend drug any drug which requires a prescription and either of these "legends" on the label: "Caution: Federal law prohibits dispensing without a prescription," or "Rx only."

limbic system an interconnecting network of brain cells inside the brain that affects behavior, emotions, sociosexual drives, motivation, learning, and memory storage and retrieval.

lipoidal fat like substance.

local anesthesia when pain conduction from peripheral nerves to the central nervous system is blocked without causing a loss of consciousness.

local effect when drug activity occurs at the site of administration.

lumen the hollow center of a needle.

lymphocyte a type of white blood cell that releases antibodies that destroy disease cells.

lymphocytes a white blood cell that helps the body defend itself against bacteria and diseased cells.

lyophilized freeze-dried.

macrolide antibiotics antibiotic agents used against a wide range of microorganisms that are primarily bacteriostatic.

macronutrients amino acids and dextrose in the base parenteral nutrition solution.

materia medica generally pharmacology, but also refers to the drugs in use (from the Latin materia, matter, and medica, medical).

medulla oblongata (brain stem) part of the brain that controls processes that affect the heart, breathing, temperature control and circulation.

medullary paralysis an overdose of anesthesia that paralyzes the respiratory and heart centers of the medulla, leading to death.

membrane filter a filter that attaches to a syringe and filters solution through a membrane as the solution is expelled from the syringe.

metabolite the substance resulting from the body's transformation of an administered drug.

metastasis when cancer cells spread beyond their original site.

micronutrients electrolytes, vitamins, and trace elements added to a base parenteral nutrition solution.

midbrain part of the brain that works to control blood pressure.

migraines severe headaches that may be linked to arterial vasoconstriction or inflammation of nerve endings in the brain.

mimetic another term for an agonist, because agonists imitate or "mimic" the action of the neurotransmitter.

minimum effective concentration (MEC) the blood concentration needed of a drug to produce a response.

molecular weight the sum of the atomic weights of one molecule of a substance.

moles the molecular weight of a drug in grams.

monoamine oxidase inhibitors MAOIs a group of drugs used to treat depression that can have toxic or fatal interactions with other drugs and with certain foods containing tyramine. Example of MAOIs are: phenelzine, tranylcypromine, and isocarboxazid.

mucolytic drugs agents that act to liquefy thickened bronchial mucous and assist in clearing airways are included in this category by some sources.

mydriatics drugs that dilate the pupil.

myocardium heart muscle.

nasal cavity the cavity behind the nose and above the roof of the mouth that filters air and moves mucous and inhaled contaminants outward and away from the lungs.

nasal inhaler a device which contains a drug that is vaporized by inhalation.

nasal mucosa the cellular lining of the nose.

NDC (National Drug Code) number the number assigned by the manufacturer. The first five digits indicate the manufacturer. The next four indicate the medication, its strength, and dosage form. The last two indicate the package size.

necrosis the death of cells.

negligence failing to do something that should or must be done.

neoplasm abnormal new tissue growth, often used to refer to cancer cells.

nephron the functional unit of the kidneys.

nephrotoxicity the ability of a substance to harm the kidneys.

neurohormones along with neurotransmitters, a chemical that transmits nerve impulses across synapses.

neuroleptic malignant syndrome a potentially fatal reaction to antipsychotic agents with symptoms of rigidity, stupor, high temperature, etc.

neurotransmitters along with neurohormones, a chemical that transmits nerve impulses across nerve synapses.

niacin vitamin B_3.

nomenclature a system of names specific to a particular field.

non-insulin dependent diabetes (NIDDM) a diabetic condition that may be treated through diet, exercise, and various oral agents.

normal saline a solution of 0.9% sodium chloride and distilled water, having an ion concentration similar to blood serum.

NSAIDs – non-steroidal anti-inflammatory drugs that have an analgesic and anti-inflammatory action and are used for mild to moderate pain.

obstructive jaundice an obstruction of the bile excretion process.

onset of action the time MEC is reached and the response occurs.

ophthalmic related to the eye.

opiates narcotic analgesics that are used for severe pain and have a high abuse potential.

osmolarity a characteristic of a solution determined by the number of dissolved particles it has in Osmoles per liter.

osmoles the molecular weight of a drug divided by the number of ions it forms when dissolved in a solution.

osmosis the action in which drug in a higher concentration solution passes through a permeable membrane to a lower concentration solution.

osteoarthritis a disorder characterized by weight-bearing bone deterioration, decreasing range of motion, pain, and deformity.

panacea a cure-all (from the Greek "panakeia," same meaning).

parasympathetic nervous system the part of the nervous system that slows the metabolism.

parasympathomimetic a drug whose actions mimic those of the parasympathetic nervous system.

parenteral any drug route other than the enteral, e.g., intravenous, inhalation, vaginal, etc.

Parkinson's Disease a progressive neuromuscular condition associated with low levels of dopamine in the brain and increased levels of acetylcholine that usually affects patients above 50 years of age.

passive diffusion the movement of drugs from an area of higher concentration to lower concentration.

passive immunity immunity resulting from the introduction of preformed antibodies.

pathogen viruses or microorganisms that cause disease.

pediatric having to do with the treatment of children.

percutaneous the absorption of drugs through the skin, often for a systemic effect.

peristalsis the wave like motion of the intestines that moves food through them.

pH the pH scale measures the acidity or the opposite (alkalinity) of a substance. 7 is the neutral midpoint of the scale, values below which represent increasing acidity, and above which represent increasing alkalinity.

pharmaceutical alternative drug products that contain the same active ingredients, but not necessarily in the same amount or dosage form.

pharmaceutical equivalent drug products that contain identical amounts of the same active ingredients in the same dosage form.

pharmaceutical of or about drugs; also, a drug product.

pharmacology the study of drugs–their properties, uses, application, and effects; from the Greek pharmakon for drug, and logos for word or thought.

pharmacopeia an authoritative listing of drugs and issues related to their use.

piggybacks small volume solution added to an LVP.

pineal gland a gland that secretes the hormone melatonin which effects the body's biological rhythms.

pituitary gland also known as the "master gland" because it regulates the activities of the entire endocrine system.

placebo an inactive substance given in place of a medication.

pneumonia an infectious process of either bacterial or viral origin in which fluid accumulates in the lungs, inhibiting air exchange at the alveolar level.

pons part of the brain that bridges from the medulla oblongata to the cerebellum and also works on muscle coordination.

prodrug an inactive drug that becomes active after biotransformation occurs inside the body.

progesterone a female sex characteristic hormone that is involved in ovulation prevention.

protein binding the attachment of a drug molecule to a plasma or tissue protein, effectively making the drug inactive, but also keeping it within the body.

prothrombin time testing (PTT) tests that assess a patient's clotting time. It measures the plasma's prothrombin or natural clotting factor.

PTH (parathyroid hormone) a hormone secreted by the parathyroid glands involved with serum calcium and phosphorus level regulation.

pyrogens chemicals produced by microorganisms that can cause pyretic (fever) reactions in patients.

quinolones antibiotics that inhibit DNA replication in bacteria.

RDA's recommended daily allowances for intake of vitamins and other nutrients.

recall the action taken to remove a drug from the market and have it returned to the manufacturer.

receptor the cellular material at the site of action that interacts with the drug.

remission a state in which cancer cells are inactive.

Reye's Syndrome a potentially fatal reaction to aspirin in children having Chicken Pox.

rheumatoid arthritis a chronic and often progressive inflammatory condition with symptoms that include swelling, feelings of warmth, and joint pain.

riboflavin vitamin B_2.

schizophrenia a condition characterized by extreme and inappropriate behavior and dysfunctional daily routine. Hearing "voices," experiencing delusions, becoming agitated or hostile and perhaps a lack of response at all are examples of schizophrenic behavior.

sedatives drugs that are intended to relax and calm. Antianxiety medications that include benzodiazepines (e.g., diazepam and chlordiazepoxide) are included in this group.

selective action the characteristic of a drug that makes its action specific to certain receptors and the tissues they affect.

selective serotonin reuptake inhibitor (SSRI) antidepressant agents that inhibit the reuptake of serotonin and are generally better tolerated than tricyclic agents.

serum glucose blood sugar.

sharps needles, jagged glass or metal objects, or any items that might puncture or cut the skin.

site of action the location where an administered drug produces an effect.

solvent a liquid that dissolves another substance in it.

Status Epilepticus a very serious condition in which the patient is in a constant state of grand mal seizure activity.

sterile a sterile condition is one which is free of all microorganisms, both harmful and harmless.

stool softeners agents that promote the mixing of fatty and watery intestinal substances to soften the stool's contents and ease the evacuation of feces.

subcutaneous tissue the tissue beneath the dermis.

sublingual under the tongue.

sulfonamides antibiotics that work by interfering with folic acid synthesis in bacteria.

surgical anesthesia the stage of anesthesia in which surgery can be safely conducted.

sympathetic nervous system the part of the nervous system that increases metabolism in a fight or flight situation.

synapses the spaces between nerve cells.

synergism (potentiation) when two drugs with different sites or mechanisms of action produce greater effects when taken together than when taken alone.

synthetic man-made; with chemicals, combining simpler chemicals into more complex compounds, to create a new chemical not found in nature.

systemic effect the effect caused when a drug is introduced into the circulatory system and carried throughout the body.

systolic pressure the maximum blood pressure when the heart contracts; the first number in a blood pressure reading.

T-cells with B-Cells, one of the primary lymphocytes.

teratogenicity the ability of a substance to cause abnormal fetal development when given to pregnant women.

testosterone the primary androgen.

thalamus a gland attached to the brain that receives sensations such as heat, cold, pressure and pain.

therapeutic equivalent pharmaceutical equivalents that produce the same effects in patients.

therapeutic window a drug's blood concentration range between its minimum effective concentration and minimum toxic concentration.

therapeutic serving to cure or heal.

thiamin vitamin B_1.

third party insurance a party other than the dispenser or the patient that pays for all or part of the cost of a prescription.

thrombolytics agents used to dissolve blood clots.

thrombus a blood clot.

thyroid gland the gland that secretes the hormones Thyroxine (T_4) and triiodothyronine (T_3) that affect metabolism, growth, and central nervous system development.

tissue plasminogen activator a drug used to dissolve blood clots.

topical hemostatics drugs used for minor bleeding when sutures are not appropriate.

topical applied for local effect, usually to the skin.

toxoid a toxin that has had its toxicity destroyed but that will stimulate the production of antibodies.

transcorneal transport drug transfer into the eye.

trauma an injury.

tricyclic antidepressants common antidepressant agents with side effects that include dry mouth, blurred vision, constipation, sedation, and sexual dysfunction.

TSH (thyroid stimulating hormone) a hormone in the circulating blood that stimulates the thyroid to produce thyroxine and triiodothyronine, the primary thyroid hormones.

uricosuric drugs drugs used to treat gout that increase the elmination of uric acid.

vaccine a suspension containing infectious agents used to boost the immune response.

vasodilators drugs that relax and expand the blood vessels.

vasopressors agents that act to increase blood pressure.

vial a small glass or plastic container with a rubber closure sealing the contents in the container.

virustatic drug that inhibits the growth of viruses.

viscosity the thickness of a liquid.

vitamin A also known by the trade name Aquasol A, a vitamin stored in the liver.

vitamin B_1 also known as thiamin, a coenzyme involved in carbohydrate and sugar metabolism.

vitamin B_{12} also known as cyanocobalamin, essential for cell reproduction, fat metabolism, and myelin and blood cell manufacture.

vitamin B_2 also known as riboflavin, converts in the body into two coenzymes that work to produce energy through cellular respiration.

vitamin B_3 also known as niacin and nicotinic acid, plays an important role in cellular oxidation and reduction as well as in the metabolism of fats, proteins, and carbohydrates.

vitamin C also known as ascorbic acid and trade name Cevalin and used to prevent and treat Vitamin C deficiencies.

vitamin D a vitamin that helps regulate calcium metabolism and is often used to treat rickets in children.

vitamin E also known by the trade name Aquasol E, a vitamin for which the function is not yet determined.

vitamin K also known by the trade names, Synkayvite, Mephyton, Konakion and AquaMephyton, an essential vitamin for prothrombin production and therefore integral to the blood clotting process.

water soluble the property of a substance being able to dissolve in water.

water-soluble vitamins vitamins stored in water for quick usage by the body (e.g., C and B-Complex).

wheal a raised blister-like area on the skin, as caused by an intradermal injection.